At Risk?

To Gloria
2nd prize Draw
with best
wishes

Christmas
Nov. 15/09

Other Books by Rivkah Roth DO DNM®

At Risk? Expanded Workbook

Diabetes Prevention, Not Like the Last Thirty Years

DIABETES-Series Little Books:

Risk of Diabetes

Low-Carb for Diabetes

Gluten-Free & Diabetes

Minerals for Diabetes

Spices for Diabetes

Teas for Diabetes

Visible Risks of Diabetes

Das Kochbuch aus Zuerich

Das Kochbuch aus dem Bernbiet

At Risk?

Avoid DIABETES by Recognizing Early Risk
A Natural Medicine View

Rivkah Roth DO DNM®

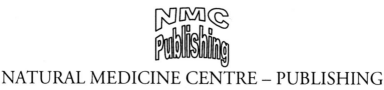

NATURAL MEDICINE CENTRE – PUBLISHING
Toronto

Disclaimer

This book and its recommendations are not designed to replace a professional medical diagnosis and treatment.

It is the sole intent of the author to offer knowledge of a general nature and to create an understanding for the complex natural processes involved in metabolic diseases that may lead to pre-diabetes and diabetes. None of the information contained in this book is intended for diagnostic or treatment related purposes. The author and publisher disavow any responsibility for any decisions or actions with regards to and not limited to self-care, self-diagnosis, and self-prescription that you may want to undertake based on this book. The author and publisher strongly recommend that you seek medical help from your own licensed healthcare provider.

The statements and information in this book have not been evaluated by the American Food and Drug Administration (FDA) or by other National Health commissions.

Library and Archives Canada Cataloguing in Publication

Roth, Rivkah, 1950-
    At risk? : avoid diabetes by recognizing early risk : a natural medicine
view / Rivkah Roth. -- 2nd ed.

Includes bibliographical references and index.
ISBN 978-0-9812297-0-6

    1. Diabetes--Risk factors. 2. Diabetes--Prevention. 3. Diabetes--Popular
works. I. Title.

RC660.4.R68 2009   616.4'62   C2009-902637-6

To order additional copies or volume orders of this book, contact:

 Natural Medicine Centre–Publishing
"AvoidDiabetes"
www.avoidiabetes.com
nmcpublishing@ymail.com   ISBN Paperback 978-0-9812297-0-6.

Contents

Table of Illustrations

TO DATE THERE IS NO CURE
FOR DIABETES BUT THE CURE YOU
TAKE INTO YOUR OWN HANDS

To my patients who have opened my eyes
To my patients who make me search for solutions
To my patients for their feedback
To my patients who have turned their lives around
And to those patients who still struggle

Acknowledgements

I am blessed with friends and several proactive patients who successfully manage their late-diagnosed diabetes naturally and with lifestyle changes. Their attitude helps to keep the burden off our heavily overextended healthcare systems. They act as role models and encourage others at risk of diabetes to proactively take their health and wellbeing into their own hands. These individuals truly exemplify why we say, "The best doctor is the patient."

I also must acknowledge my eighty-some year-old mother who lives in Europe. Following "doctor's orders" she pumps herself full of medications for her diabetes; all under the guise of continuing to enjoy what she considers necessary carbohydrate and sweet food treats. To make matters worse, none of her physicians pointed out that grains may not work for her. Considering that I, her daughter, am affected by full-blown celiac disease it is more than likely that she too suffers from an underlying gluten-sensitivity.—But, more later about such a possible link between diabetes and gluten-sensitivity!

To add another facet to my mother's diabetes story: The medications her doctors prescribe have long been banned on the North-American continent and have just recently brought her to the brink of acute lactic acidosis and several emergency stays at the hospital. Needless to say, she now is on additional medications, suffers from added side-effects, and pays the price for insisting on blindly following her doctor's orders. How much easier it could have been to look after her body by eating reasonably! Many lessons for me to learn from… some painful ones! Yet, without having to witness such self-destructive behaviors this book might not have happened.

Over the years many of my friends have supported me in more ways than simply by acts of their friendship. Without them I would not be in a position today to focus on writing and disease avoidance campaigns. These individuals all follow their inner calling and greatly support others on that same path. The world is a richer place for them.

Without a doubt, I am most grateful to my teachers and colleagues. They stirred in me a never-ending curiosity. They awakened in me an inquisitive mind that is not satisfied with simple answers but has learned to look at the complexities of the issues from many angles. Most importantly, they helped me understand that, sometimes, it is just fine not to come up with a definite answer. They helped me acknowledge that there never is an end to knowledge and understanding. I learned that new questions must be asked and old answers questioned.

I am priviledged to acknowledge several special friends and colleagues who have read the initial draft pages of this book and have helped me come up with its present concept. Two of them I would like to single out: Dr. Sir Paul Guppy MD who much contributed with his clear and concise comments during the initial phases of *At Risk?*, and Dr. George Milne DC ND who, in his chiropractic and naturopathic practice, for decades has fought for a healthier lifestyle and has kept me going when the going got tough. No acknowledgement would be complete without mentioning the tireless and patient input of my friends Chaim and Al. Many of their ideas find themselves reflected in the cover design of *At Risk?* and in the entire planning of our *Early Diabetes Risk Recognition and Avoidance Campaign.*

Last, but not least, I want to thank my co-op students for the many hours they spent faithfully researching, printing, and filing research reports in preparation of this book.

A big thank you to all of you! Your individual and cooperative contributions have made this book possible. May there be a time when we learn to deal with illnesses in ways other than by suppressing them! And may there soon be a time when illnesses like diabetes once again disappear from our screens; when we concede (every single one of us) that we are in charge of our own state of health or disease, and when we will have the courage and strength to acknowledge that diabetes and other health challenges respond to lifestyle changes and truly are largely avoidable.

King City, Ontario, Canada – 2008

Rivkah Roth DO DNM® DAc DTCM

Preface

When ailments affect our daily ability to function it is easy to remember their signs and symptoms. However, as soon as we feel better we seem to forget the sometimes painful ways our body uses to communicate its needs to us. For this reason I have written *At Risk?* not only as an informational book but also as a working manual. Call it your "health diary." I have designed *At Risk?* in a way that allows you to recognize a possible risk of pre-diabetes and diabetes by your personal state of health and your minor or major signs and symptoms of illness and disease. Because I want you to be able to read this book not only cover to cover but also pick out individual sections you may find the odd duplication. Not to worry, these repetitions concern information that you simply must not forget.

Most books dealing with diabetes talk about diabetes proper or, at best, the stage of pre-diabetes. Both stages (pre-diabetes and diabetes), according to our natural medicine view, are late-stage occurrences of metabolic disease. There is no doubt that prevention is the name of the game. However, prevention must start at a much earlier point than promoted by our present healthcare systems. Those systems promote prevention once a patient has been diagnosed with pre-diabetes; that is not early enough.

Just as diabetes is not the beginning of the disease, neither is pre-diabetes. A risk of pre-diabetes and diabetes is detectable earlier—much earlier. When I started to tally up the numbers I found that independent research has shown well over fifty conditions that may indicate a link or correlation with the future development of diabetes. In some cases the connection is clear, and diabetes is considered the logical progression. In many other cases, a single occurrence of one of these conditions may be of no significance for a possible future risk assessment of pre-diabetes or diabetes. However, any repeat occurrence "for no particular reason" of such a condition—or the simultaneous presence of three or four of these over fifty conditions—may present clear indications of a potential future risk. The writing is on the wall. It is up to the reader to become proactive.

It is with this understanding that I have written *At Risk?* in such a way that, following the description of each individual condition, you find a short FACT Summary ("Favor," "Avoid," "Consult," "Test"), a simplified "blanket recommendation" for your lifestyle choices, and also a space for "Your Personal Notes." Latter is designed for you to fill in anytime you notice one of the respective signs or symptoms. We all know how quickly and easily we forget any physical changes once we feel better again. *At Risk?* will serve you as a central place of record keeping: this book will become a testimony to your personal health inventory.

Have your copy of *At Risk?* accompany you to your medical appointment: With your notes complete—date, type of problem, description of symptoms, and more—you no longer will forget to pass on important information to your healthcare giver. Potentially, this represents a big step in your effort to assess your personal risk of pre-diabetes and diabetes early. Most of all, it might help you avoid future, more severe problems by allowing you to properly interpret your early signs and attend to them in good time.

Prevention and avoidance start with your awareness, your knowledge and your willingness to listen to what your body tries to tell you. So, open your mind, your heart, your eyes, and your ears; read and start listening to your body today!

PART ONE - The Basics

Your pain is the breaking of the shell
that encloses your understanding.

Kahlil Gibran

Diabetes Avoidance is Key

You might be the one in two people worldwide who is at risk of developing pre-diabetes and diabetes. Mostly a lifestyle disease, diabetes is largely avoidable. To date, research has linked well over fifty health conditions to an increased risk of metabolic syndrome or diabetes. Eight to fourteen years of a variety of more or less serious health problems predate the diagnosis of diabetes by a mainstream medicine system that bases its findings mostly on your elevated blood sugar levels. Recognizing your full risk early, therefore, is paramount if you want to live a life free of diabetes and its dreaded complications.

Why is it that few healthcare professionals and even fewer private individuals are aware of the presence of this decade spanning at-risk window? Even more pressingly: Why is the public not being informed on how to recognize their very earliest risk factors that may lead them to avoid—or at least postpone—pre-diabetes and diabetes during those eight to fourteen years?

It is simply not sufficient to point towards the infamous three factors: increased thirst, frequent urination, and hunger pangs. The list of possible imbalances or health conditions that have the potential of alerting you to an existing risk of pre-diabetes or diabetes is far longer and considerably more elaborate than what you are commonly led to believe. Many lifestyle factors and food choices lead to inflammations. Inflammations result in absorption problems and malfunctions. Absorption problems are the beginning of mineral deficiencies. Deficiencies open the door to disease. It is easy to imagine how this may turn into a vicious cycle.

Over the course of these pages, I will introduce you not just to the most common three or four complaints, but to over fifty conditions that have been linked to an increased risk of the metabolic syndrome and diabetes, and whose presence might serve you as an early warning of on impending risk of pre-diabetes and diabetes. A one-time occurrence of many of the signs and symptoms that I will mention here should not disquiet you. However, any repeat occurrence or a chronic state present for longer than ten days to one month should ring a definite warning bell. If that happens—and if you experience three or more of these conditions at the same time—you might well want to look deeper into the presence of a possible risk of pre-diabetes and diabetes.

Diabetes is not a simple illness; it is a disease complex. Diabetes does not hit you out of the blue. It is not the beginning of an illness but the culmination of a long line of biochemical misfirings that, over time, succeed in breaking down your body's self-regulating system. Anytime your blood sugar level exceeds a reading of 7.0 mmol/L (USA: 126 mg/dl) for any length of time some of your cells stand to suffer damage; sometimes irreversible damage. Your body's functional or organic weakest link determines where such damage will occur first.

No matter what, your blood sugar high is not the problem; what has allowed your blood sugar to go out of control is! If you read this book pencil in hand I want you to double-underline this preceding sentence. I strongly believe that—in order to be able to stem the diabetes epidemic—we must move away from the mainstream medicine model that mostly looks at controlling blood sugar levels. Instead, we must develop a more inclusive, yet individualized approach that identifies a person's underlying conditions, some of which may end up in loss of blood sugar control. If you don't want to go down the road towards a possible future with diabetes you need to be able to identify your own personal weak link or links. Once you find out where and what these are you can start your mending process.

When you consider the widespread doctor shortage and the fact that most of our healthcare systems are designed to deal with the ill only, not those individuals who still function marginally, it becomes blatantly obvious that the person with the greatest possible impact on your health and wellbeing is you. The better you learn to understand the natural functions and needs of your body, the easier it will be for you to avoid and—in some cases—reverse serious cell damage and illness.

Your human body works according to a simple, unwritten contract: You provide your body with the essentials from which it can extrude, manufacture, and make available the substances and processes to run itself. In return you get to enjoy a life full of vigor and health. If you don't uphold your end of the deal your body may be forced to cut corners. Sooner or later you will experience lack of vitality and minor or major ailments.

How wonderful that this body of yours has a built-in safety system! Your body replaces its cells, few at a time, roughly every three months. What this means for you is that it is hardly ever too late to start upholding your end of the contract. As soon as you provide your body with the necessary building blocks and eliminate any destructive habits, new (and healthier) cells will be able to replace the ones previously damaged. This is what is meant by disease reversal or by healing.

If you are prepared to introduce the necessary changes to your lifestyle you do stand a fair chance of avoiding full-fledged diabetes and its ugly complications. No one brings diabetes on you; in most cases you are bringing it on yourself by unwise nutritional and lifestyle choices. While you cannot change your inherited genetic weaknesses and strengths you can learn to recognize your modifiable weak points and work with them. Prevention, mostly by avoidance, can be surprisingly simple and, best of all, it works!

Before getting into greater details on how to recognize your issues and to work on remedial approaches let us take a brief look at how disease progresses and how your body loses its physical and functional balance:

At the beginning of the twentieth century a German medical doctor and homeopath, Dr. Hans-Heinrich Reckeweg (1877-1944), formulated the concept of disease and reversal of disease (healing). In his "Six-Phase Table" he postulated that whenever a pathogen enters your body, your body will attempt to emit it (the diarrhea or cold sweat in the nape many pre-diabetics experience). He called this the "Excretion Phase."

If your body is unsuccessful in this attempt of ridding itself of the offender it responds to an acute infection with an equally acute inflammation (conditions ending in –itis, such as colitis, pancreatitis). Such an inflammation may not necessarily occur in the area the pathogen first invaded. Dr. Reckeweg called this the "Inflammation Phase," the second stage of disease progression.

As you see, disease progresses and moves deeper unless it can be reversed methodically stage by stage. An unresolved or suppressed inflammation may lead to a deeper-seated and chronic problem when it affects the fluid surrounding your cells in what Dr. Reckeweg called the "Deposition Phase." This third stage taxes your antibodies to their maximum (water retention, changes in body acidity, suppressed chronic inflammations). Consequently, your energy levels drop, brain fog sets in, and sleep issues are sure to follow.

If at this third stage your lymph system fails to bind a pathogen and flush it out of your system, the disease may progress to the "Impregnation Phase." This he called the fourth stage in which an offender finds its way into some of your actual tissue cells. It is at this stage where glucose intolerance, malabsorption issues, autoimmune deficiencies, irritable bowel disease, ulcerative colitis, Crohn's disease, fibromyalgia, and a long list of other conditions show up.

Unfortunately, as we shall see later, mainstream laboratory tests rarely do indicate changes before stage five. In mainstream medicine the definitive diagnosis of any of the above mentioned stage-four or earlier diseases, therefore,

Rivkah Roth DO DNM®

is rare unless infection levels are acutely high. If you are being sent from inconclusive test to inconclusive test it is quite likely that you are finding yourself in one of the stage-four patterns.

If the healing attempts continue to remain unsuccessful, and the condition lingers in this stage for any length of time, phase five will start to develop, the "Degeneration Phase." At this stage your cell functions and processes are undergoing changes. In most cases it is not until this fifth stage where, finally, initial problems start showing up in your laboratory test results. The diagnosis of diabetes falls into this fifth phase.

If diagnosis at this level is missed yet again, or delayed, the outcome may be the impairment or shut down of cell or even organ functions. A disease may shift and spread to other organs—diabetic complications. In its extreme form this stage may lead to the excessive replication of altered cells such as in cancer. Alternatively, cell death may occur. Dr. Reckeweg called this sixth stage the neoplastic or "Dedifferentiation Phase."

At any stage illness can be reversed; easier from the first three or four phases, more difficult from the last two phases due to the presence of cell damage. In what natural medicine has termed a "healing crisis" any reversal (healing) process must be expected to proceed in reverse order if it wants to be successful. Stage five diseases heal into stage four conditions. Illnesses belonging to stage three may follow and a sudden surfacing of an acute inflammation may indicate reversal to stage two. This retracing pattern is what frequently leads to seemingly odd sequences of illnesses. Once the third stage has passed where the interstitial fluid becomes exposed to the pathogen it is anyone's guess what organ or processes will be involved next. In this way a kidney issue may be cleared via lung and breathing problems or a liver problem may follow a gastrointestinal challenge.

Dr. Reckeweg's linear and progressive disease model explains a majority of the issues we are facing also with today's healthcare system. The inability of our mainstream healthcare system to recognize potential problems early makes it impossible to effectively prevent disease. If, after the initial suppression of an infection or inflammation, a patient has to reach phase five before the warning light in our mainstream medical offices goes on, no wonder that the numbers of the sick are taking on epidemic proportions and the cost of healthcare is exorbitant and ever rising.

Another disease model, frequently cited by natural medicine professionals, is that of inflammations leading to mineral deficiencies. Only a few decades ago, two-times Nobel Prize winner Linus Carl Pauling (1901 to 1994) stipulated that every disease could be traced back to a mineral deficiency. Although this view still has not been adopted by mainstream medicine, Pauling recognized the importance of the biochemical processes for the workings of our human body. Like the European "father of medicine" Paracelsus, who lived four hundred and some years earlier, Pauling stipulated that macro- and micro-mineral deficiencies lead to imbalances and disease. While Pauling largely stressed the action of certain vitamins (in particular vitamin C) Paracelsus, who did not yet know about vitamins, emphasized the minerals and their role in the development of disease and its healing.

Today, we know that minerals act as keys. They enable or block the absorption of most of the vitamins. Minerals are instrumental in the formation of enzymes, hormones, proteins, and many other drivers required for the body to function properly. This role of the minerals is fully acknowledged and, in fact, is being taught in biochemistry, anatomy and physiology classes at medical schools worldwide (see figure 16, p. 273). Why this basic understanding of the workings and interactions of the human body is largely disregarded by mainstream medicine when it comes to treating the body or, even more so, when it comes to preventing illness is beyond my understanding.

The bottom line is: Disease is your body's way of letting you know that something with your internal balance is seriously amiss. Why are we not listening to the initial warning signs? To ignore your individual body makeup spells disaster. To cater to it, on the other hand, may avert pain and long-term illness. It is time for mankind to stop disregarding long-recognized wisdoms and truths; time to drop self-destructive habits.

Before I introduce to you in greater detail the factors that indicate a possible risk of diabetes let me give you an overview of the situation as it presents itself today. With this background knowledge in place it will be easier for you to find and identify your own risk and to counteract the progression of your pre-diabetes and diabetes with its complicating diseases (see figure 1, p. 24).

Rivkah Roth DO DNM®

Type 2 Diabetes
A Progressive Disease

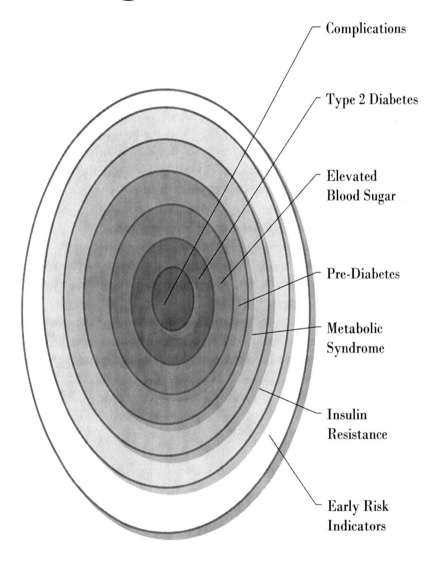

Complications

Type 2 Diabetes

Elevated
Blood Sugar

Pre-Diabetes

Metabolic
Syndrome

Insulin
Resistance

Early Risk
Indicators

Figure 1 Diabetes—A Progressive Disease

Society is its Own Worst Enemy

Diabetes has been known since ancient times. Already the ancient Chinese knew about it and probably were some of the first to systematically look at ways of treating and avoiding it. Individual cases of diabetes or diabetes-like symptoms were reported along with their specific treatments and outcomes. Over the course of many centuries, a large number of traditional Chinese medicine treatises were written and handed down on how to treat *Xiao Ke*, the Chinese name for diabetes.

Traditional Chinese medicine always considers the body as the one indivisible sum-total of a great big number of bodily interactions and functions. Accordingly, no disease occurs in isolation. It, therefore, comes as no surprise that thousands of years ago already connections were recognized between diabetes, kidney disease, and heart problems. Powerful herbs were custom-blended for individual patients. In addition, food-cures were devised and recommended that entailed detailed directions on what foods to eat, what to avoid, and when to eat the meals. The proof was in the pudding, so to speak: if the patient followed the recommendations the disease came under control.

However, throughout the course of history it appears that wide-spread diabetes surfaced and disappeared in waves. So did the plague, you say, and today's flu epidemics. Yet, unlike the uncontrollable dangers of contracting these acute epidemics, you do not contract diabetes. In fact, diabetes is a progressive, chronic condition; you do have a direct stake in triggering or avoiding your diabetes by how you live your life. This is why we call diabetes a metabolic disorder; it directly reflects the way your body handles—or does not handle—food and drink.

It is said that the vast Roman Empire fell because of the ever-increasing indulgence of its citizens. The Roman bucolic feasts are proverbial. Have you ever wondered if some of the ensuing laziness and obesity that impacted the fitness of the Roman centurions might have been diabetes-related and if this contributed to Rome's decline? Rome fell and Europe for centuries plunged into the dark of the Medieval Ages. Much earlier, the ancient Chinese Empire had gone a similar route, so did ancient Egypt, to name but some of the cultures that became extinct after having enjoyed great social wealth.

What these cultures all had in common—just prior to their demise—was not only their great societal wealth leading to an increased and non-discriminatory availability of food, but also their citizens' individual prosperity that allowed for increased availability and consumption of food. Food nourishes; but food also destroys. That is the fine line between health and disease. We experience similar problems today. Food is widely available and we tend to eat more than we need.

It is not too late. We still can learn from history. It is said that, in order to change history, we need to change our present; and that by changing the present we change our future. This is exactly what prevention—in our case the prevention of the threatening metabolic disorder called diabetes—is all about. If you want to avoid ending up on the casualty list of diabetes-related complications there are several things you might want to keep in mind.

Our present-day lifestyle is probably the single greatest contributor to the step-by-step decline of our health into disease. Show me a family among your circle of friends and acquaintances that does not to some degree follow the rush-to-work, eat-on-the-go routine! Stress and fast food are major culprits in the development of conditions such as diabetes and of several of its complications, heart disease, kidney failure, and central nervous system disorders. Avoidable? Yes, absolutely!

Oh no, I cannot help you wriggle out of that job of yours and your obligations, nor can I take off your shoulders these never-ending daily chores that relate to making ends meet. But, there are alternative approaches to dealing with your quagmire of immeasurable stress. Some ways are as simple as learning to prepare easy and quick on-the-go meals that you can pack. Forget the "sand-," stick to the "wi(t)ch!" Traditional sandwiches are out for the person at risk of metabolic disorders. Learn more about how to eat yourself healthy in the *DIABETES-Series Little Books*.

You see, it is your attitude that counts. Often you are your own worst enemy. Maybe you might be more willing to put the *you* first once you recognize that—without you looking after yourself—your world no longer waits at your feet. Without taking care of yourself you will ultimately lack the means of taking care of your family and friends. Your personal disease does not remain yours alone; it impacts your family and your entire social network. Remember this, and it will help motivate you in your desire to improve your lifestyle and health.

Publicly we blame our on-the-go lifestyle and the fast-food industry that caters to it for the growing rates of obesity and diabetes. Yet, despite of this, we promote our societal values as the best path to follow worldwide. We send wheat to peoples who—for centuries—have lived happily in a different manner on locally grown, seasonal, and unadulterated fresh foods. We come up with newly engineered grain, rice and soy seeds that yield yet greater harvests. We establish fast-food chains in every corner of the world and then we are surprised at how much faster obesity and diabetes rates grow in developing countries.

Peoples' genes do not change quickly. Maybe it is time to acknowledge how the change in source-food production has played a huge role in the worldwide spread of metabolic diseases. Our eating habits have been hugely impacted by craving-inducing foods. As time goes by we may have to stop blaming all on the genes and, instead, take a harder look at these food sources of ours as a possible and direct cause of diabetes—in our corner of the world, in the so-called developed countries, and in those regions we so benevolently "support" with our disease-causing lifestyle.

We have mentioned the ebb and rise of ancient civilizations; in this twenty-first century, once again, mankind appears to reach a point of self-indulgence from which there seems to be no return except for radical lifestyle changes. Availability of high-calorie and craving-inducing foods does corrupt our ability to make wise choices; yet, let us not forget that all these choices still are ours to make. So why do we not make use of our freedom to choose our foods and lifestyle in a proper and productive manner?

Education—or the lack thereof—seems to play a great part in this teeter-totter between health and illness. Today, the numbers of kids and young teenagers diagnosed with obesity, hypertension, and even diabetes are shocking. The way it looks we are raising a generation of unhealthy human beings preprogrammed for a future with illness. Nobody wants this. It is time for schools, the public, parents, you, to serve as role models and to initiate effective lifestyle changes now.

Prevention and, specifically, diabetes avoidance must become a personal and public focus for two major reasons: One, if we want to raise a generation of kids who will be able to live a healthy and productive life. Two, if we want to make sure that—in our old age—we will not end up becoming a burden and liability to a younger generation already dealing with even greater disease rates than our own age group tallies up. We must stop thinking in terms of only treating illness and, instead, must work on truly preventing disease. Therefore, instead of treating the sick and except for the much needed emergency services, this is precisely what healthcare should be all about, namely, to promote health early!

Rivkah Roth DO DNM®

Here is what you can do: The four most important steps towards effective avoidance of type 2 diabetes and many of its complications are to:

1. Familiarize yourself with the implications of diabetes.

2. Recognize your personal individual risk factors early.

3. Act upon these insights in a resolute and timely manner by making responsible lifestyle, food, and drink choices.

4. Help others on their path of diabetes avoidance and greater health.

Present Day Statistics

The latest statistics for Canada mention over two million diagnosed diabetics and project three million people to be diagnosed with type 2 diabetes by 2010. At a 2006 healthcare cost of 13 billion Canadian dollars annually a startling eighty percent of all type 2 diabetes patients are classified as obese. Keep this number in mind when we will look in greater detail at an interesting correlation in the chapter about Obesity (p. 98).

For the USA the number of diagnosed diabetics presently stands at 24 million at an annual healthcare cost of 174 billion dollars for 2007—up from 132 billion dollars for 2006. These numbers quite likely represent no more than the proverbial tip of an iceberg. As recent as March 2007, the American Diabetes Association estimated the number of pre-diabetic Americans at 60 million. This figure is significantly higher than its 54 million posted only a few months earlier at the end of 2006. Shockingly enough, this represents more than 40% of the population ages 40 to 74. The question no longer is "if" we are heading for the dreaded one individual out of every two ratio to be pre-diabetic, but "how soon" we will reach and surpass this benchmark. In North-America every 21 seconds around the clock a person is diagnosed with diabetes. Worldwide, every ten seconds two individuals are newly diagnosed.

According to recent numbers compiled by the World Health Organization (WHO) more than 180 million people worldwide are known to suffer from diabetes. By the year 2030 the WHO expects this number to exceed 360 million. But, by the end of 2007, these forecast numbers already have been surpassed significantly according to the International Diabetes Federation (IDF). They put the present number of diabetics worldwide at 246 million and forecast more than 380 million diagnosed diabetics five years earlier than the WHO, namely by the year 2025. In addition, the total known number of those with impaired glucose tolerance, insulin resistance, or pre-diabetes has reached triple the number of those already diagnosed with diabetes. Adding up the numbers of those affected by pre-diabetes and diabetes we are quickly approaching the one billion mark.

As of the writing of this book, complications from diabetes (mostly from cardiovascular disease) lead to one death every ten seconds worldwide. In short, roughly 3.2 million people every year die from diabetes-related causes alone; all of them in addition to those 1.2 millions whose cause of death is given as diabetes itself. Without major changes in our lifestyle WHO predicts a global increase of 50% of diabetes deaths by 2015—eighty percent of which in upper-middle income countries.

A quite recent health comparison published in JAMA of 55 to 64 year old people (the baby-boomer generation) postulates known numbers of 12.5% diabetics in the USA versus 6.1% in Great Britain. It also points to heart disease numbers at 15.1% for the USA versus 9.6% for England and—most frighteningly—sets the numbers for hypertension (one of the predictors of diabetes and heart disease) at 42.4% for the USA and 33.8% for Great Britain. Imagine, nearly half the people of the 55 to 64 year-old age group already are known to experience signs of hypertension! Such high hypertension numbers are most disturbing and should sound alarm bells with regards to their significance as a predictor of diabetes. No question, we are heading for a crisis of epidemic proportions!

According to the type 2 Diabetes symposium held in March 2006 at the Joslin Diabetes Center in the USA, 50% of all newly diagnosed type 2 diabetes patients already suffer from coronary heart disease by the time of their initial diabetes diagnosis. Those are frightening perspectives. Mainstream medicine still considers elevated glucose levels as the indicators for a diagnosis of diabetes and the last step in the development of type 2 diabetes. Participating doctors at the time of the aforementioned symposium were reminded that ten to twelve years of exposure to metabolic imbalances predate their diagnosis of diabetes and that, therefore, their treatment is falling years behind. Pretty scary admission, wouldn't you say? Other sources set the same time period from initial symptoms to a diagnosis of diabetes at eight to fourteen years.

However you look at it, in addition to the above North American numbers, we must assume large numbers of undiagnosed cases of diabetes, particularly in the non-Caucasian population. In fact, India and China presently experience the highest growth in newly diagnosed diabetes cases. Disparities exist for many reasons, not the least due to a shortage of specialized medical professionals from these very population segments. While many of the individuals who elude diagnosis may come from lower income groups, I personally know several well-off and high-profile African Americans who, by all means, could afford the best of healthcare, but who somehow have fallen through the cracks of the medical screening system.

As much as we like to all be alike, when it comes to our bodies we are not. Genetic pools differ; a fact that still needs to be acknowledged by our brilliant twenty-first century medical screening methods. Don't misunderstand me. The medical research community is well aware that different testing ranges and sometimes also methods should be applied to the diverse population segments. In reality this does not happen in your doctor's office, and we are a long way from understanding and properly documenting the respective variances.

Up until recently, most research has been done on Caucasian people or, at best, on mixed racial groups. At the same time, we already know from practical experience and countless research data that the risk for metabolic diseases is disproportionately higher for non-Caucasian groups, such as Native American, African American, Hispanic, and Asian populations. The big question is why does metabolic disease seem to affect these groups more? If diabetes is simply the result of a more sedentary lifestyle and of limited exercise there should not be such a discrepancy in these statistical findings. Read on, I may have some ideas worth investigating.

These days, threats to mankind of a life lived in disease are far greater than those posed by war and terrorism. Only global warming and its set of threats may be comparable to the menacing increase in life-altering illnesses and diseases. While you may attempt to somehow write off the environmental changes you cannot do the same with an illness such as diabetes. Yet, unlike our perception of global events, the widespread understanding of diabetes and related diseases as unavoidable events in a person's life tends to paralyze our very ability to react and defend ourselves against the impending threats. We wait until the inevitable happens, until the diagnosis pronounces, "You are now diabetic." For some odd reason disease prevention still appears to be a dirty word in mainstream medicine circles.

Lucky that you do have choices! Choices that—if made early enough and wisely—allow you to avoid the seemingly inevitable consequences (such as heart disease and diabetes). All the tools are available to you already. How come then, you will explore the inner workings of your bike or your car but show little or no interest in finding out about the wondrous interactions of that body of yours? How come, you spend time and money on all sorts of endeavors and don't realize that without a working brain and a fit body you will not be the one enjoying the fruit of that labor of yours?

History teaches us that we are not the first ones having messed with the gifts we are given. Ancient cultures may not be the last ones wiped off this planet; unless we wake up—quickly!

Diabetes—An Overview and an Outlook

Diabetes is the most common metabolic disease complex of our century. Worldwide it has become the most widespread endocrine disorder. Its onset appears to be triggered by lifestyle. Today, we know that by the time a patient is diagnosed with type 2 diabetes at least a decade of metabolic imbalances must have been present. Why does it take so long then until patients or doctors recognize that there is an impending problem?

Very obviously, preventive measures have a good chance to make a huge difference by avoiding or delaying more acute problems, and possibly even an otherwise almost certain diagnosis of diabetes. However, instead of starting prevention at the diagnosed pre-diabetes level, we must start thinking of avoidance long before we are confronted with glucose absorption or insulin resistance—the defining factors for diabetes. As we have seen in the previous chapter, half of the newly diagnosed diabetics experience severe complications already by the time of their initial diagnosis of type 2 diabetes. It is my goal to provide you with the necessary tools to become proactive; even more importantly, to help you realize at an earlier point in time where and what the weak links in your bodily systems are, and when and how you need to act.

In most cases, diabetes leads to a slew of complicating chronic illnesses. We have seen the high numbers of cardiovascular disease incidences related to diabetes with their two- to four-fold risk when compared to the non-diabetic population. There are other complications: Diabetes is a major cause of kidney failure. 42 percent of all kidney dialysis patients are known to suffer from diabetes. Apart from painful neuropathies foot problems and leg ulcers—due to reduced sensitivity and late detected injuries—often lead to amputations; a menacing threat for many diabetics. Another often overlooked complication of diabetes, retinopathy, is the leading cause of blindness in North America.

Frequently forgotten are the side effects of the supposedly life-saving medications you are prescribed by your caregiver to control the various forms of diabetes and its many complications. Remember, to date there is no definite medical cure for diabetes. Every package insert of diabetes medications still states this fact. Medications control some of your excesses and help achieve more acceptable laboratory results. Most medications do not reverse the disease—even if your lab results appear improved. Proof of this is that, over time, stronger or additional medications are needed to achieve a consistent level of control or to placate the medication-induced side effects of the initially prescribed drugs.

A grim picture for sure, but not without hope for those who are vigilant and willing to learn to look after themselves in good time. Determining that very point of time is key; it comes up long before serious predictors of diabetes start surfacing. Nothing should hold you back from making the necessary changes once you know that diabetes may be looming on the horizon for you. It may yet be avoidable and the specific knowledge about how to achieve this is available to you here!

High Blood Sugar Damage

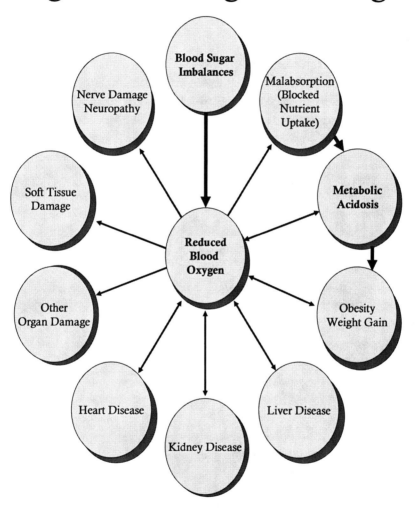

Figure 2 High Blood Sugar Damage

Classifications of Diabetes

It wasn't until I started working with diabetes patients in my daily natural medicine practice that I realized that even within each category of diabetes one patient's diabetes is not equal to the diabetes of another patient. In an effective natural medicine approach there are many ways to support someone diagnosed with diabetes. One basic approach for all will simply not do. Every type 2 diabetes patient displays a different disease complex and experiences slightly different issues and triggers. We, as caregivers, must learn to individualize our preventive and remedial approaches. After all, we treat each individual patient, not the overall disease called diabetes. Precisely in this patient-centered outlook rests the big difference between the individualized natural medicine approach and the disease-focused approach offered by the mainstream, pharmaceutical medical view.

The medical research community is actively looking into the factors leading to diabetes; and many good results will help change the face of this disease. But for now, lifestyle considerations still top the list of possible approaches. According to recently released reports, an uncanny number of young diabetes patients are starting to display type 1 and type 2 diabetes simultaneously, leading to a new terminology of "double diabetes" or "hybrid diabetes." It remains to be seen if this phenomenon is an overlap or a parallel development of problems.

Traditionally, your doctor diagnoses you with type 2 diabetes based on the presence of increased thirst, increased urination, and fatigue, combined with elevated blood glucose levels. Exercise and diet are recommended as the primary treatment approach. However, most doctors will want to put you on medication immediately. The reason for this is that experience has shown them how few people are willing to adjust their eating habits. Mainstream medicine, therefore, focuses on teaching you how to check your blood sugar levels, how and when to take your prescription medication and—if necessary—also how to give yourself insulin shots, and where to buy and store your supplies. In addition and despite the medication, once diagnosed, your health is expected to progressively deteriorate long-term.

As natural medicine professionals, on the other hand, we tend to look further towards your future. We want our patients healthy twenty years from now not just have them get through the next couple of years doing what has gotten them to where they are—in a state of dys-ease.

You successfully can learn to control diabetes naturally, and (hopefully) largely without suppressive medication. However, the predisposition to the condition will remain with you in the background even if you seemingly should have managed to reverse your diabetic issues. Any slip in your regimen may trigger diabetes to raise its ugly head all over again. The weak link in your body's system may crack anytime unless properly supported and catered to— daily and permanently. The bottom line is that you learn to care for yourself. We know that this is not so easy; otherwise, everyone would be doing it. Let me ask you: You care for your aging car; when will you resolve to care for your body? It all starts with consistency in your day-to-day habits and with a clear understanding of what is going on in your system. Changes for the better and healing will soon follow suit.

Although much of the focus of At Risk? is on type 2 diabetes, type 1 diabetics too may draw great benefit from the explanations and suggestions found in this book. For now—and before we dive into the particulars of how to assess the early risk of pre-diabetes and diabetes in greater detail—let us very briefly review the most commonly acknowledged particulars about the various forms of diabetes, type 1 and type 2 diabetes, gestational diabetes, and pre-diabetes as mainstream medicine views them.

Type 1 Diabetes

Type 1 diabetes, or insulin-dependent diabetes, is also called juvenile-onset diabetes or diabetes insipidus. For some time now, type 1 diabetes has been considered to be an autoimmune disorder in which the patient develops antibodies against his or her own pancreatic tissue. Subsequently, the body's insulin production is compromised, and most patients need to be put on additional insulin life-long.

When you read At Risk? you will find out more about the action of your body's natural insulin and its complex interactions with many of the biochemical processes within your body. For now, it is important to understand that insulin (a hormone produced in your pancreas) is instrumental in moving sugar from your blood into your cells where it can be burnt up into energy. Without the presence of insulin this energy-producing process fails with dire consequences.

Most type 1 diabetics need to artificially replace their insulin. Typically, these individuals are on daily insulin injections or puffers. Frequently, they do not realize the extent to which sugar imbalances still continue to wreak havoc with their system—unless they check their blood glucose levels several times during the day, that is. The insulin injections mask the presence of sugar in your blood but cannot totally prevent the damaging effect of excess sugar or sugar fluctuations on your various organs and processes. Cell damage may occur anytime a blood sugar reading of 7.0 mmol/L (European/Canadian system) or 126 mg/dl (US system) is exceeded.

While the present understanding of type 1 diabetes still looks for that genetic link, not all of the type 1 diabetes cases are attributed to your genetic background. Type 1 diabetes appears more frequently in patients suffering from autoimmune diseases such as Addison's disease, Graves' disease, and Hashimoto's thyroiditis. These are all adrenal and thyroid related disorders. Is it a mere coincidence that these latter disorders also are on the rise worldwide?

Viral diseases too are linked to the development of type 1 diabetes. Mumps, rubella (measles), and coxsackie B virus are believed to destroy autoimmune system beta cells—the very cells needed to secrete insulin—and, through this action, these viruses potentially trigger type 1 diabetes. An interesting recent research project is studying if inflamed nerves may play a role in the destruction process of these very same pancreatic beta cells. This research, thus, is looking at a link between inflammation and type 1 diabetes. This connection seems to make sense since we know that, for instance, in your brain your insulin no longer has the function of regulating your blood glucose level. Instead, certain centers of your central nervous system take over this role in cooperation with several of your adrenal hormones; a clear link, thus.

While it does not implicitly talk about diabetes and inflammation, a similar association already is known in the field of homeopathy, one of the natural medicine modalities. Several homeopathic remedies (most of which are made from plants and minerals) in their drug picture suggest their use for viral infections at the same time as a use for inflamed nerves is indicated. Could nature have prepared the cures for us?

It is commonly accepted that individuals with type 2 diabetes best control their disease by lifestyle modifications. Type 1 diabetics too would be well advised to keep in check their blood sugar fluctuations by dietary measures and not simply by adjusting the amount of insulin they inject. In many instances, insulin requirements can be kept to a bare minimum when you no longer aggravate your system with destructive food and lifestyle habits. In this manner, it is possible even for type 1 diabetics to avoid, or at least delay, the common disease complications of diabetes by restricting their glucose rollercoaster.

On another interesting note, gluten-sensitive enteropathy (GSE) and its full-blown form, celiac disease (CD), seem to have an affinity for patients with type 1 diabetes. Or, as I have long suspected, could it be the other way around? Does an underlying gluten-sensitivity, due to its malabsorption syndrome, depress the insulin function sufficiently for patients to be diagnosed as insulin-dependent diabetics? Mineral deficiencies appear to be common to both, diabetics and celiac patients. Minerals play a paramount role in the production and control of many hormones and enzymes. Signs of malabsorption involve chronic deficiencies of essential minerals the likes of chromium, zinc, vanadium, molybdenum and, occasionally, copper, along with several vitamins, which latter need enzymes or co-enzymes in order to be properly absorbed. Every function in our body is interrelated. While I have my own ideas and projections about this correlation, to date, there is little definitive research available about the existence of such links, and definitive answers remain yet to be researched and confirmed.

Type 2 Diabetes

As we shall see, type 2 diabetes shows the greatest variance in appearance and, therefore, is the most widespread form of the disease today. Its diversity makes it the major focus of this book. Frequently, type 2 diabetes is called diabetes mellitus, which translates into age or adult-onset diabetes. Other names you may have heard are non-insulin-dependent diabetes (NIDD) or non-ketotic diabetes. In short, type 2 diabetes is the name for a group of metabolic problems that result in increased glucose levels in your blood.

There are two major causes to be considered: For one, a decrease in the secretion or action of pancreatic insulin may cause your blood sugar highs. Alternatively, your body may experience an insulin resistance on the cellular level, for instance in the muscular tissue. For some reason, your cell walls resist the insulin's function of moving the sugar molecules from your blood into your cells where they should produce energy (ATP). Soon, some of these processes will become easier for you to grasp. Be patient with me and you will see why natural medicine holds that everything in your body is connected.

Other circumstances may temporarily cause and present a picture of diabetes too. Such conditions include chronic pancreatitis or severe malnutrition, especially if you also turn out to be protein-deficient. Type 2 diabetes also may develop secondary to several endocrine system disorders.

Cushing's disease, aldosteronism, and several other conditions are known for their ability to induce insulin resistance. Usually, once these illnesses are resolved so is—with proper management—your diabetes.

What does this tell us? If these other conditions—many of which are the result of biochemical imbalances—are properly addressed and even corrected, diabetes may become a non-issue for you. Was there a misdiagnosis? Was your diabetes cured? Neither one; your predisposition to diabetes will not go away. However, as long as you are able to keep these other factors under control, you should be able to avoid any future encounters with diabetes. It does pay for you to remain vigilant. You may be at greater risk for the rest of your life and will not be able to take risks with your lifestyle choices. Yet, when you know about your weak spot you can deal with it more effectively and, yes, you may successfully avoid diabetes.

Drug-Induced Diabetes

It is known that several of the commonly prescribed diabetes drugs, especially those approved to lower your cholesterol, may cause liver disease. Others, like the diabetes drug Avandia (rosiglitazone), may negatively affect your heart health. This book is not the forum to get into the rather long and frightening list of moderate to severe side effects that are part of your diabetes medications. It is a good idea, however, to discuss with your primary healthcare practitioner in great detail all the possible side effects and complications you might have to expect before you start down the path of prescription medication for diabetes or any of its known complications.

Why does mainstream medicine recognize that prescription medications produce side effects, yet it sees nothing wrong with not informing the patient of these unpleasant facts? To a natural medicine professional, and maybe to you too, wanting to avoid side effects at all cost should be reason enough for choosing to live more healthily and, if at all possible, free of prescription medication.

Less known, or often forgotten, is the fact that many of the common medications prescribed for a variety of other moderate to serious diseases may cause you to become diabetic. Did you know that patients who for longer than one year are on total parenteral nutrition (TPN) stand a fifty percent greater chance of developing type 2 diabetes?

If you are at risk, are already pre-diabetic, or have strong family indicators of a risk for diabetes you should check with your doctor and carefully weigh benefits versus hazards before agreeing to any of the following medications. This list of potentially diabetes-causing drugs does not make any claims of being complete. Still, its extent may rather surprise you:

⇨ Steroids top the list of possible inducers of diabetes and are known to increase your blood sugar levels by depressing the function of your pancreatic beta cells. You are at even greater risk of developing diabetes following the use of steroids if you happen to be obese or have a family history of diabetes.

⇨ Glucocorticoids (hydrocortisone) are a special class of steroid hormones. They may cause hyperglycemia (high blood sugar) by promoting liver glycogen and inducing insulin resistance.

⇨ Several of the commonly prescribed psychiatric drugs, *Clozaril* (clozapine) in particular, but also *Zyprexa* (olanzapine) and, with some contradictory results, *Risperdal* (risperidone) and *Seroquel* (quetiapine) have been earmarked as increasing your risk for diabetes. These drugs, furthermore, induce significant weight gain, increase your cholesterol levels, and are associated with diabetic ketoacidosis, opening the path for severe kidney disease. All of these side effects are putting your heart at risk as well.

⇨ Niacin too may contribute to hyperglycemia and so may other niacinamides. Those at risk for diabetes should avoid this group of drugs or supplements. Even the natural supplements containing niacin should only be administered under the close supervision of a knowledgeable healthcare professional.

⇨ Thiazides are a group of diuretics that affect your electrolyte and calcium balances and are commonly prescribed to treat hypertension. However, they may raise your cholesterol levels or trigger kidney problems (hypokalemia) in addition to causing an imbalance between your sodium and potassium levels.

⇨ *Epivir* (lamivudine) is a common infection-fighting HIV drug. Its drug pamphlet includes hyperglycemia, pancreatitis, liver, and kidney problems, as well as its tendency to produce the proverbial beer-belly (a sure-tell sign of insulin resistance), and to induce lactic acidosis. Once again, all these are signs and symptoms closely connected with an increased risk of diabetes.

⇨ Insulin resistance and diabetes are expected side effects of *Crixivan* (indinavir) and *Norvir* (ritonavir), drugs used to inhibit the protease mechanism in the treatment of HIV.

Other drugs may induce mostly hypoglycemic states and, therefore, add another worrisome component to your diabetes:

⇨ These drugs include sulfonylurea drugs, which are a group of your rather common anti-diabetic drugs.

⇨ Obviously, your dispensing doctor should have made you aware that an overdose of insulin can trigger hypoglycemia. If you are on insulin any changes in food and exercise habits must be very carefully coordinated with how much insulin you will need.

⇨ Among the most common drugs with a side effect of causing hypoglycemia are salicylates (used also as a food preservative and an antiseptic in toothpaste), propranolols (beta-blockers used to control hypertension), and pentamidines (an antimicrobial medication).

⇨ Alcohol intake too may prompt blood sugar imbalances and, in addition, can induce an acute metabolic acidosis.

In summary, taking prescription drugs for any condition, including diabetes, rarely offers a straightforward solution. Provided there is no excessive tissue damage, even western medicine acknowledges that lifestyle modifications have a positive impact on the avoidance, stabilization, or even reversal of your diabetes. Why not try anything humanly possible to develop and stick to a beneficial lifestyle and—hopefully—avoid any of these multifaceted drugs?

Therefore let me repeat it once again, particularly if you recognize your specific risk factors early: Diabetes may be avoidable—it is up to you!

Gestational Diabetes

Gestational or pregnancy-related diabetes often is a transitory form of diabetes. Still, the fact that it surfaces--even temporarily—should serve as a strong warning for the potential and future development of type 2 diabetes in the mother or her baby. You could call gestational diabetes your "diabetes litmus test." Gestational diabetes is considered a form of carbohydrate intolerance and can be more or less severe. Presently available statistics point to a fairly small number (in the single digits) of pregnancies of non-diabetic mothers to be affected by it. However, just as with non-pregnancy related diabetes, the risk for mothers of non-Caucasian origin may be considerably greater.

If you plan on having children, and if you or your partner already are diabetic, it is ultimately important that you get your physician's advice and support before conception; even more so if you are aware that you might be at risk of developing diabetes. The better your blood sugar control at the time of conception—and, obviously also during your entire pregnancy—the better the chances are for your fetus to get a good start on life. For the mother too this can make the difference between getting through pregnancy without major complications and having to face all sorts of undesirable problems along the way. For the mother it does not stop with the delivery of the baby either. An individual who develops gestational diabetes always runs a higher risk of developing type 2 diabetes later in life.

Fathers matter equally! Is it not interesting how—when it comes to pregnancy—the entire focus shifts to the woman? Let us not forget that at conception half of the life-giving input comes from the man's side. The overall quality and motility of male sperm directly reflects the health status of the father. Consider the quality of your sperm "your daily health report!" Does the prospect of a healthy offspring not sound like the biggest incentive for you to attain your own best possible health before planning and starting that family of yours?

For newly pregnant women the general recommendations when dealing with gestational diabetes are straightforward: Monitor your blood sugar daily and get regular check-ups at least on a monthly basis. High HbA1c values around the time of conception and during the first couple of months of the embryo's development have been associated with congenital organ malformations in the fetus. This is an ugly prospect and is entirely avoidable if and when we take serious our responsibility as co-creators in the start of a new life!

It is worth mentioning that orally used hypoglycemic drugs have been shown to cause ear defects, heart, kidney, and spinal defects in the fetus. Therefore, the better you monitor your diet and contributing lifestyle factors, the less medication you may need, and the more predictable and controllable your blood sugar values will be. A healthy mother will be more likely to give birth to a healthy child.

Pre-Diabetes from a Different Angle

While not obvious at first sight, all the signs of oncoming diabetes are already in place years before most doctors or patients pick up on the full-blown disease. Many years ago terms such as Syndrome X and Metabolic Syndrome have been coined. Today we simply call it "pre-diabetes." It has been only quite recent that authorities such as the American Diabetes Association have started calling pre-diabetes a "serious medical condition." This is worth repeating: pre-diabetes already is a serious medical condition!

According to a position statement published by the American Diabetes Association in conjunction with the National Institute of Diabetes and Digestive and Kidney Diseases recent studies show conclusively that diet and lifestyle modification can prevent and even stop type 2 diabetes. This is why we need to look in greater detail at the stages of pre-diabetes. According to our natural medicine understanding, there are signs and symptoms that show even before pre-diabetes. But the at-risk stage prior to diagnosis is still widely ignored by our present mainstream medical systems.

As we have seen earlier, most of the time diabetes shows up long before it is being diagnosed. We know this from the difficulties with establishing reliable statistical predictions. Unpredictable dark figures only all too often are proven wrong just a few years or even months after they have been published. Again and again, it turns out that the initial assumptions in the case of diabetes are largely being underestimated and underreported. Just look at the increase from supposed 41 million pre-diabetic Americans in 2004 to 54 million by the end of 2006 and 60 million by the beginning of 2007. All of these individuals are considered pre-diabetic on the grounds of slightly elevated blood sugar levels; a rather narrow definition of pre-diabetes.

Why wait for pre-diabetes to be diagnosed according to this mainstream definition when, even earlier in what in my clinic is called the at-risk stage, we can recognize the infallible precursors to pre-diabetes and to type 2 diabetes? According to some sources, ten to twelve years—according to others eight to fourteen years—prior to glucose level increases your body already shows signs and symptoms of impending diabetes. Therefore, do not believe your local pre-diabetes programs when they broadcast that you need to be pre-diabetic before you can be considered at risk of diabetes.

However, there is an explanation for such a mainstream approach: Did you realize that many of the early signs are either missed or outright dismissed because lab results at that time still are largely inconclusive or negative? It goes something like this: blood tests mostly reflect levels of substances that run through your body, not of those lodged in your tissues. In order to make up for any shortcomings your blood simply draws the required particles from any of your body tissues and mostly from your skeletal system. Blood, therefore, is the last component of your body to show imbalances. This means that blood tests rarely are predictive indicators—although, to date, they are just about the only tests relied upon in the mainstream medicine environment. Urine tests too present a one-sided picture. Urine tests show you what your body excretes; not what it should get rid of. Neither test shows you what has been deposited in your body's tissues or what essential building blocks your body is deficient in. For this reason, in many cases, underlying diabetes does not become apparent until when—during a medical emergency—you receive treatment for diabetes-related complications such as for a cardiovascular event.

Natural medicine practice takes a different approach. Threatening trends become obvious a long time before blood and urine test results conclusively indicate the presence of diabetes. The reasoning for this is simple and straightforward. It has long been acknowledged that mineral deficiencies predate disease development. In fact, we believe that deficiencies of essential minerals precondition a patient for diabetes and other diseases because such imbalances may open the door to inflammations. Assessing nutritional deficiencies, therefore, may serve as an important warning beacon. The at-risk stage and, to some degree, that of pre-diabetes are when prevention works best because the body's tissues have not yet begun to degenerate.

Unfortunately, mainstream medicine rarely acknowledges other signs and symptoms before the disease becomes irreversible. Most mainstream physicians are too busy caring for those already sick. This leaves the general population with a twofold predicament. Short of creating some kind of a public health police (not something we could or would want to implement in a democratic society) we must empower every private individual to recognize his or her own issues and risk factors early. Once signs of an at-risk stage or of pre-diabetes are recognized or suspected, simple and easy to follow guidelines must be made available to help these patients revamp their lifestyles. You find many cancer treatment retreat centers all over the North American continent but, there are few similar opportunities for those facing metabolic diseases and diabetes.

It is time to give similar support to the large and growing population of those of you who need to cope with new requirements and lifestyle changes following a risk assessment or a diagnosis of diabetes. Educational programs, such as those offered through our natural medicine diabetes avoidance coaching and counseling programs or the natural medicine diabetes prevention retreat model, are designed to fill some of this void on a global scale along with individual consultation sessions and online support programs.

Summary

⇨ Diabetes is not the start of the illness. Years of signs and symptoms and pre-diabetes precede the diagnosis of the disease. Pre-diabetic signs and symptoms, much as diabetes itself, may affect people in different ways and through different stages of health or illness.

⇨ Diabetes is a disease complex and is mostly self-caused by inappropriate lifestyle choices or environment. In other words, it is a combination of what you do to yourself, what others do to you, and what your doctor gives you to "control" some of your health complaints.

⇨ Diabetes can be controlled, occasionally reversed, and certainly avoided or delayed by making appropriate lifestyle modifications. You can remedy much of your problems by learning how to make better choices. This starts with an uncompromising commitment to taking care of your own body and that of all the members of your family; including your newborn babies, toddlers, and teenage kids.

Manmade cars are unforgiving when it comes to proper care. The human body is no less tolerant of insults and omissions. Once you understand the way in which your body converts input (food and exercise) to output (state of health and wellbeing) you will find that it becomes straight forward and rather easy to play along with your body's natural requirements. This opens the door to greater health.

Let us take a step back. How did you find out that you, or someone in your family or among your friends has or may have diabetes? How can you find out if you too may be at risk of developing diabetes?

PART TWO - Figuring Out Your Risk

I can give you nothing
that has not already
its origin within yourself

I can throw open no
picture gallery
but your own

I can help make
your own world visible
that is all.

Hermann Hesse

To Prevent is to Know Your Risk

Your doctor does not live with you at home or at work. It is not your doctor's responsibility to keep you healthy. It is your very own responsibility and liability to lead a healthy life. The bottom line is that we people do not come with a warranty. Unless you develop a heightened level of body awareness you may not find out about impending changes that can lead to early diabetes until its secondary and most dreaded effects start showing up. As we have seen earlier, this may turn out to be at least eight to twelve or fourteen years too late!

What about your kids and those new babies who are born daily into this world of increased carbohydrate, sugar, and toxin consumption? Kids are fathered by men who smoke, drink beer, eat processed foods, and play spectator sports. After conception these babies are nurtured by mothers whose bodies find themselves in a chronic inflammatory stage due to those same unhealthy foods and the same destructive lifestyles.

The vicious cycle of looming illnesses does not begin with birth, however. It starts already pre-birth with less than potent semen and with a deficient nutrient transfer from the mother's placenta to the unborn fetus. Today's youth carries a considerably greater risk of metabolic diseases than did their parent and grandparent generations who grew up in quite a different environment. Let us have a look at some of those differences:

The twentieth century with its great wars and recessions presented its challenges. Foods were scarce during several of those decades; substantial nutritional deficiencies were present in the generations growing up during and after the great wars. Yet, most importantly, the numbers of people suffering from metabolic diseases such as obesity, diabetes, and heart disease were considerably lower than they are today and starting with the baby-boomer generation. Fewer grain-based products and no fast foods were available in those times of post-WWII scarcity.

Today's health issues are blamed on lack of exercise and a predominantly sedentary lifestyle. I believe that there is another, more powerful explanation to the difference between then and now. Today, commercial and processed foods are widely accessible and touted as both convenient and affordable. Most fast foods are made from grain-based products: buns, muffins, pasta, pizza dough, and breading. Grain starch is added to everything from salad dressing to cosmetics and unlikely daily items such as the glue that seals your envelopes. As we shall see, most of these grain-based foods listed above are addictive and habit forming. Not having had this choice, our parent and grandparent generations relied on produce that was seasonal and locally grown under conditions that required less fertilizer and fewer pesticides. On the other hand, the number and amounts of additional nutrients that our generation needs to consume today is mind-blowing; all just to make up for the negative impact of the toxins we take in unknowingly.

Convenience, economics, and savvy marketing are the most likely answers for the considerable amounts of grain-based foods consumed today. Never throughout the course of history has there been available such a variety and amount of processed foods. Even our animals are fed more grains these days. You just need to check the label on your commercial dog food bag to see that the grain content is ever growing. Strange for this traditional meat eater, isn't it! You would be surprised to find out about the growing number of pets that your veterinarian is diagnosing with diabetes and diabetes-related complications. This trend also affects our food source animals. The common feed for our dairy and beef cattle used to be grass and hay (dried grasses). Today, they too are fed mostly grains or sugar-rich corn and are kept in unnaturally restricted spaces.

But, maybe, we cannot blame all our health problems on the availability of grain-based products and fast foods. What if you decide to avoid fast food and stick to fresh greens instead? Why are we still far less healthy today despite of having available a greater variety of fresh produce reaching us from all corners of the world any time of the year? Did you know that the nutritional content from greens produced today is at least five times lower than that of the same produce grown twenty-some years ago in the nineteen-eighties? Let us not forget to mention considerably higher levels of toxins from soil, air, and packaging materials. In your body these toxins either stand in for some of the nutrients that your body is missing, or they completely block the essential nutritional components from being able to function properly. The bottom line is that even from our supposedly healthy vegetables we consume far fewer nutrients and ingest more inflammation producing toxins.

There is no magic wand, no wonder-pill that will make diabetes and its complications go away. Despite the billions of dollars and hours of dedicated medical research the most effective measure against diabetes still is to live a healthy life—even long before a possible diagnosis. Easier said than done! But, in most instances, it is a matter of knowing the facts and understanding the implications. Several thousands of books already talk about diabetes and how to deal with it once you are diagnosed with the disease. In our natural medicine practice we believe that the best way to deal with diabetes is by not having to deal with it! Once again allow me to reiterate: diabetes is largely avoidable!

Such an approach of avoidance puts you in the limelight. You are responsible for yourself, for your kids, your family, and maybe for your friends. The more you know about the very early risk stages the easier it will be for you to hear that wake-up call and to turn the clock around. Isn't it a wonderful thought that, by living a healthy lifestyle, you may not have to deal with a large number of dreaded diseases such as diabetes, heart disease, or kidney disease? And, don't believe anyone who says that it is a "piece of cake," that you "just pop a pill or poke a needle and that life goes on as before." Denial is one way to deal with diabetes; diabetes and, even more so, its ugly complications are not going away by you continuing your destructive habits—never mind the myriad of pills and injections your mainstream doctor prescribes.

This is why prevention by living a healthy lifestyle is key! The big question is how to define such a healthy lifestyle. This is precisely what we will be looking at in *Part Three, Diabetes can be Controlled* (p. 243). In the meantime, let us learn about the many early warning signs that your body gives you in order to indicate your risk.

Signs and Symptoms – Your "Before" Facts

You hear these terms all the time in connection with your medical condition: sign, symptom, syndrome. Many readers—and even some health professionals—find it difficult to distinguish between the definitions of these three terms. Let me try to clear up the confusion before we delve in greater detail into our discussion of risk factors of pre-diabetes and diabetes.

⇨ A "sign" describes a change from the normal physical function. A sign can be observed by you and also by others such as your family, friends, or your doctor.

⇨ A "symptom" also describes a change from the normal physical function. However, unlike a sign, a symptom is what you, the patient, experiences and describes. A symptom is not obvious to others.

⇨ A "syndrome" describes a group of signs and symptoms that generally occur together and make up the picture of a particular illness or condition.

Know how to Evaluate Your Early Signs and Symptoms

You thought that it is normal for a young adult to look for a bathroom every couple of hours! You thought that it is normal for you to feel tired after lunch or too exhausted to get up in the morning! You thought that it is acceptable for you to crave sweets after a breakfast of orange juice, cornflakes and milk! All these signs and symptoms are initial indicators that your body is no longer in homeostasis. Homeostasis is your body's ability to self-regulate and work optimally. When you experience any of the above named symptoms this is your body's way of telling you that it lacks something. Your body directly warns you of greater problems to follow. You better find out quickly what is and what is not spelling trouble for your future state of health.

Your body's health depends on the interaction of many biochemical reactions. Your body turns food into energy and lastly into health. When something along this supply-line of nutrients goes wrong—either by lack of supply, by oversupply, or by the wrong supply—it turns it into disease. Your body's ability to convert food into nourishment and, after sifting out the useful components, to clear out the waste is what we call your metabolic rate. Metabolic imbalances and diseases all are progressive conditions that can only be resolved by radical changes to your input, in other words by how much and what you eat and drink.

Type 2 diabetes is no exception; diabetes is a progressive disease. Ask all those individuals who already are on medication for diabetes, heart disease, or any other serious condition. One problem leads to another. It is no fun; and, it is so avoidable. Take a good look around you. Have you ever wondered how come that all the many people on medication do not heal? After starting on medication you may feel somewhat better. But, strangely enough, very soon after the first prescription medication you will need a second, then a third, and a fourth prescription. In time, you will need additional prescription drugs to counteract the side effects of the first ones. Many of the patients coming to me for natural medicine advice initially are already on eight or more prescription drugs. Talking about a drug cocktail! But, has their health improved?

How can your general practitioner know everything he or she should know about you and your health in a five to fifteen minute consultation? Your mainstream medical doctor mostly relies on lab results. But, as we have seen earlier, in most cases your doctor's diagnosis comes years too late since these lab results rarely indicate changes until your body has reached the level of cell damage. A natural medicine professional has more time available for consultations and may pick up on changes earlier. Yet, even in our customary one to two-hour interviews it is not always that easy to get the proper information from you, the patient. How often do our patients answer in the negative a specific question of ours only to describe five minutes later a symptom that would have made the earlier question a yes-answer in the first place! Your practitioner's skill and experience, therefore, is a huge determinant in how quickly your risk is being assessed—and controlled.

You can help both your medical doctor and your natural medicine professional by developing your own awareness and understanding of your body functions and state of balance. Gather and bring up the facts, but leave the interpretation to your healthcare professional! When you catch a cold you know that it is over when you feel better again. The trouble is, when you catch another cold, it may not be that you simply caught another cold. Only your healthcare professional can determine if perhaps your first cold, or whatever led to it, never fully healed. How many times do I hear from new patients: oh, it's nothing, I always am running a cold! That is wrong! The word "always" here is the operative word. By presenting you with repeat illnesses your body is telling you that it is running on its spare tire and that it is time for you to listen up and improve its condition.

As you see, recognizing the early warning signs and symptoms is not that easy. When you live a certain way that way becomes normal to you. For this very reason I like to get a patient's family involved in the entire trouble shooting and healing process. Your family members may notice subtle changes long before you become aware of these changes. Teamwork and networking, therefore, are great assets when it comes to early risk recognition. Not seeing the forest for the trees is an issue that makes it easy for specific risk factors to be missed. There are so many smaller signs or symptoms that, if taken by themselves, are of no great concern. Their simultaneous appearance, however, should raise a warning flag that you must not miss. Again, your knowledgeable natural healthcare professional should be able to help you sort out the seriousness of these issues.

Keep in mind that a large number of the conditions and problems described in the following chapters might be part of other illness complexes if they occur as isolated instances. Yet, remember that in certain combinations they quickly may indicate an underlying risk, a pre-disposition of pre-diabetes or diabetes. This is precisely why I so adamantly insist that you need to work together closely with your trained healthcare professional. Even more so, it requires from your healthcare professional that he or she be able and willing to effectively communicate with all other healthcare professionals on your "team." Without willingness to network your best interest is at stake and results may be questionable.

A good measure is for you to contact your doctor or other primary healthcare provider as soon as you identify three or four of the telltale signs and possible risk factors described in this book. To help you further, at the end of this book, I have added a link to our *Natural Medicine Diabetes Risk Questionnaire,* which you can use to pre-calculate your level of risk. The signs described speak for themselves. Your body does not lie. In fact, it cries out to you: listen to me and take care of me!

Summary and Outlook

⇨ Diabetes is avoidable if you recognize your causative factors early and adopt habits that lead you to better health.

⇨ The risk of pre-diabetes is high in close to half of the North American population but is even higher in Non-Caucasian populations.

⇨ The age groups at risk are turning increasingly younger.

⇨ Prevention is key and is possible.

⇨ Early risk recognition means learning to recognize your very own and specific early warning signs.

⇨ Don't wait until your body starts losing its coping mechanisms (losing homeostasis and falling into dys-regulation).

⇨ When you experience three or four of the following fifty or so telltale signs you almost certainly need to reassess your level of health, no matter what.

⇨ Identify your individual lifestyle changes that might be called for.

⇨ Get help and adjust your direction today!

Your Family Disease Tree

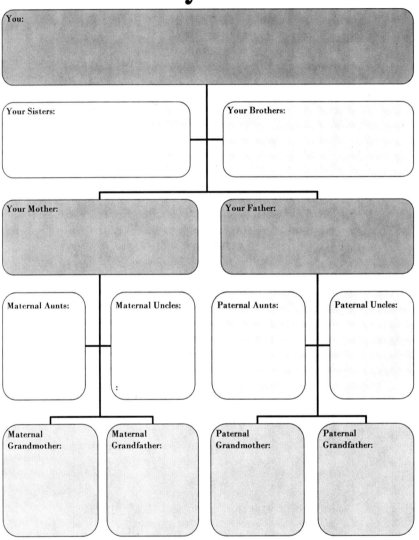

Figure 3 Your Family Disease Tree

Genes are not Everything

You can no longer blame your genes for all your problems. Genes determine a pre-disposition for certain conditions and illnesses; they are not everything. Research has found that some of our genetic cellular matter is open to changes during our lifetime, even in the womb. When certain conditions "run in your family," as we say, it may be partly due to certain genes. It can be equally due to the general environment and regional or family customs; particularly when it comes to food and lifestyle. This becomes amply evident when we see healthy immigrants arrive in a country like Canada; yet, a few years later their children (and sometimes the parents too) suffer excessively from metabolic diseases. Therefore, to look at your background will be helpful but it is not everything.

Looking Back

When you try to find out about your family health history reconstruct your family tree from a standpoint of health and disease. Remember that not always are your ancestors' health issues that obvious. Illnesses and conditions may have been misdiagnosed or simply have not been detected or reported. Still, family trends will become evident if you have an inquisitive mind.

The knowledge about many of these trends frequently is handed down in a roundabout way. Keep your mind tuned to remarks such as: "Weight problems always have been an issue in our family," or, "we always have been big people," "your father has a beer-belly just like his grandfather used to have," and so on. Cardiovascular problems may run in your family; you probably will be aware of those because of untimely deaths. Kidney disease runs in families too. Many of these factors may point to a possible history of undetected diabetes. Collect as much information as possible and enter it in *figure 3, Your Family Disease Tree,* which you find on p. 56.

Neuropathy and leg ulcers are other facts frequently known. Women often remember how cumbersome it was for their mothers and grandmothers having to bandage their legs day-in, day-out. Undiagnosed and uncontrolled diabetes may have played a role in their leg pain or fluid retention problems too. Then there are vision problems and the kind of loss of sight generally attributed to aging. While many vision problems may not relate directly to diabetes, others do. Keep an open mind and get a qualified health professional to help you sort things out!

If you have access to old photographs extreme weight loss over a fairly short period of time may be another benchmark for undetected diabetes; so is the proverbial beer-belly or "spare tire," an apple-shaped obesity with fat deposits around the midriff. An upper abdomen overhanging the belt-line almost always points to raised blood glucose levels or, at least, the start of insulin resistance.

The proverbial double chin too may indicate metabolic disease. In many women it may point to mineral imbalances, such as iodine and thyroid-related problems. As we shall see in the following chapters, conditions such as hypothyroidism may be predisposing factors for diabetes and other metabolic conditions. But then again, the double chin—particularly in men—may reflect testosterone imbalances with their own set of related issues: erectile dysfunction, lack of libido, and the likes.

Looking Ahead

While much of this genetic background information may serve you as an indicator of where you too may be heading there is no need to panic. Most and foremost, you want to develop your ability to listen to your own body. No need to become neurotic about any of these signs and symptoms. However, as you have seen in the introductory chapters, there is a near zero tolerance factor if you are serious about cutting your risk or even reversing already existing issues and maintaining your essential quality and span of life.

Here are a number of simple but telling initial questions you want to ask yourself:

⇨ What are my levels of stress?

⇨ Are there any recent changes in my night sleep patterns?

⇨ Do I frequently feel tired and need a short afternoon nap?

⇨ Does my body feel different in any way?

⇨ Do I experience high levels of thirst?

⇨ Have my bathroom habits changed?

⇨ Do I get irritable if I go any length without my water bottle or without food?

⇨   What do I eat and drink?

⇨   What are my daily dietary carbohydrate, calorie, and fat totals?

⇨   Do I get the shakes if I go past my regular mealtimes?

⇨   Has there been a change in the way in which my surroundings (family, partner, kids, and colleagues at work) respond to me?

In order to get a better grasp of what happens to your body, why, and when, let us now turn our focus to the early warning signs and symptoms in detail. As you will read through the following descriptions you may recognize the one or other issue as a problem of yours. Make note in the spaces provided therefore and remember that it is time to get a specific health check-up if you come up with at least three or four of the symptoms listed here.

Disease Starts with Your Mouth

Your mouth is where it all starts. So, any blemishes in your mouth are rather significant indicators. Every morsel of food and every sip of drink must pass through your mouth on its way to your digestive tract. But it does not stop there:

Questions of Oral Hygiene

Western medicine, along with many traditional and natural medicine systems, sees your mouth as a mirror of the biochemical processes going on in your body. These days, unfortunately, media commercials target your mouth as a possible cause of problems for other reasons. They advocate remedies that kill your natural bacteria, along with the regular use of tools such as tongue cleaners, bleach whiteners for home-use, and other frightening commercial trickeries. Of course, I too advocate impeccable oral hygiene, which includes brushing after every meal (not just once a day) and flossing. However, I am talking brushing your teeth and gums, not your tongue!

Your mouth does not make you sick; being sick makes your mouth go bad! If there are bad bacteria growing in your mouth they indicate gastrointestinal problems that need to be listened to—not suppressed. If you do experience issues with your mouth you must get them checked out in connection with your entire gastrointestinal tract, not as an isolated unpleasantry of your oral cavity! While your mouth directly reflects the state of your digestive system you cannot fix your gut by removing necessary bacteria and enzymes from your mouth. Your oral enzymes and bacteria are vital to help your saliva predigest your food and, specifically, your carbohydrates. This action is exactly what most mouthwashes are designed to undo. Not really helpful, as you shall see!

Brushing of your tongue coating deprives you of many necessary processes and, therefore, is abhorred among credible natural medicine professionals. But, while we are on the subject, have you checked the ingredient list of most commercial toothpastes and mouthwashes? It is not just the level of sugar that most of these products contain—sugar that may add to your glucose load if you are at risk of pre-diabetes or diabetes. They also contain an astonishing level of toxins that may aggravate many of your health issues.

The mucous tissue of your mouth easily absorbs anything that passes your lips. This includes those chemicals making up your mouthwashes, toothpastes, chewing gums, and all those other battle rams designed to kill your oral fauna. Once in your system these chemicals may act in unpredictable ways; one of which is to make you sick. Oh, and I forgot, yes you do rinse your mouth after using toothpaste—with more artificial mouthwash! Or, if you use water from your tap instead, it probably is still full of chlorine, high levels of sodium, filter residues, and a whole slew of other people's prescription drugs, many of which are known to add to your risk of diabetes.

In natural medicine we frequently use remedies of a modality called Homeopathy. Most of these remedies are produced in the form of oral drops or small round and coated pills (so-called globules) that you let melt under your tongue. The mucous tissue of your mouth directly absorbs these homeopathic remedies. This approach eliminates the remedies having to pass through your stomach or a possibly compromised gastrointestinal tract of yours in order to get to your blood, lymph, or other bodily tissues. One reason why these homeopathic remedies work so well is precisely because your mucous tissue very rapidly absorbs everything it comes in touch with. So, why should it not absorb those above mentioned toxins and other chemicals just as easily as it makes use of our gentle healing remedies?

If you meddle with nature in this first step of your digestive process you are doomed to pay the price with metabolic imbalances. The bottom line is that you must carefully watch what you push into your mouth—food and otherwise. Even sugar-free gum is no solution; it contains many other substances that do not benefit your health—substances that may not have to be declared. And, all that peppermint and menthol craze only serves to slow down your metabolism. Isn't that exactly the opposite of what we want? In short: diabetes avoidance—and illness avoidance in general—starts with your mouth!

1. *FACT Summary Oral Hygiene*

FAVOR	natural mouth and tooth care products without sugar and added chemicals.
AVOID	sugared and artificially flavored or colored foods and gums, toothpastes, breath fresheners, mouth washes, tooth whiteners, and other supposedly necessary (cleaning) substances that might contain unwanted toxins and additives—most major brand-names.
CONSULT	your nutritionist or natural healthcare professional and check all labels!
TEST	your toxin levels and pH value.

Your Personal Notes

Symptoms—Date(s) first noticed:

_____

Symptoms—Description:

_____

_____

Consultation Date(s) and with whom:

_____

Tests—Results:

_____

_____

Lifestyle Changes introduced:

_____

_____

Symptom Changes noticed:

_____

_____

Follow-ups:

_____

_____

5-Element Theory
according to Traditional Chinese Medicine

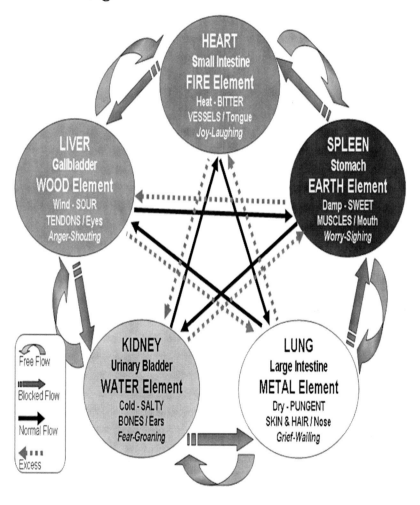

Figure 4 Five Element Theory According to Traditional Chinese Medicine

Increased Thirst or Dry Mouth

A fairly constant level of thirst is probably one of your first indicators that you may already be pre-diabetic and one of your last warning signs that you are heading towards serious metabolic problems and possibly diabetes. Thirst may indicate the beginning of kidney problems and likely points to moderate or severe glucose issues. The presence of thirst or a dry mouth usually happens during one of the last stages just prior to the diagnosis of elevated blood sugar. The diagnosis of full-blown diabetes is rarely far off. The sooner you become aware of your thirst or a constantly dry mouth the sooner you can get to the true source of your issues.

In the health care field we call them the "3 P's:" *polydipsia* (increased thirst), *polyuria* (increased amounts of urine), and *polyphagia* (increased hunger). Fluctuating and high blood sugar levels cause all three symptoms. When a healthy person drinks water or tea the thirst gets quenched almost immediately. But, for the pre-diabetic or diabetic person this may not be the case. All three symptoms clearly indicate that your blood sugar may be out-of-control.

If your blood glucose level is high it means that your blood sugar no longer can be moved out of your blood into your cells where it should be burnt off to produce energy. Instead, it overtaxes the filtering ability of your kidneys and spills over into your urine. This process requires additional water. Your body mobilizes the extra fluid either by dehydrating your tissues or by making you thirsty and forcing you to drink large quantities of liquids. At the same time, great hunger pangs are quite common because your cells no longer receive the necessary nourishment. The bottom line is, if you experience thirst despite drinking ample fluids it may be time for a visit to your medical professional for a battery of diabetes-related tests.

Particularly interesting is the approach of traditional Chinese medicine (TCM) to this phenomenon of increased but unrelieved thirst. TCM postulates specific and ever adapting interactions between the major body organs and their functions. TCM calls it the *Five Element Theory* (see figure 4, p. 63). This system of interactions was developed in China during the reign of the Yin and Zhou dynasties (between 1600 B.C. and 221 B.C.). As we shall see, this theory exemplifies the above described western interactions on many different levels.

According to the traditional Chinese medicine interpretation what is called the process of *T&T* (transport and transformation of nutrients in your digestive organs) takes place in conjunction with your *kidneys'* ability to produce the required energy. TCM uses the picture of a pot over a campfire: If the fire is too hot or if there is not enough liquid in the pot, the heat will dry up the fluid in the pot. If there is too much liquid in the pot, eventually the fire will go out and the food will not be cooked. This visual approach may all sound a bit strange or oversimplified until we replace the Chinese term *kidney* with our understanding of the function of our adrenal glands (see figure 5, p. 67). As you shall see, your adrenals play one of the most important roles in your body. Any level of stress can greatly impact on their health and ability to function properly. Read more about this in the chapter about *Adrenal Deficiency* (p. 183).

For now let us stay with our picture of the pot over the fire. Like western medicine, TCM makes a clear connection between how your body processes food and the function of your organs from stomach to pancreas (in TCM *spleen*), to kidney, liver, and heart. TCM and western medicine agree: You need well-functioning kidneys in order to regulate your body's water metabolism. Otherwise and over time, increased thirst will lead to a fluid imbalance in your body. Continued dehydration that affects your kidney function may influence your cardiac system and move you closer towards heart disease. These later stages already count among the so-called complications of diabetes. For further insights check out the sections about *Renal Deficiency* (p. 200), *Heart Disease* (p. 222), and *Kidney Disease* (p. 226).

You see, this is why we call diabetes a "disease complex." The workings of your body cannot be separated and isolated. Thirst is not the beginning of diabetes but a clear indicator that your body's ability to convert food into energy and to eliminate undesired byproducts has been compromised. When you experience constant thirst you do not wait for other signs before you get a thorough medical check-up.

Rivkah Roth DO DNM®

2. *FACT Summary Increased Thirst*

FAVOR	carbohydrate counts smaller than six grams per portion (not per declared serving size). Read the labels!
AVOID	sugar in any form and grain carbohydrates (turning to sugar) in excess of thirty grams a day.
CONSULT	your qualified mainstream or natural healthcare professional.
TEST	kidney and adrenal functions, blood sugar.

Your Personal Notes
Symptoms—Date(s) first noticed:

Symptoms—Description:

Consultation Date(s) and with whom:

Tests—Results:

Lifestyle Changes introduced:

Symptom Changes noticed:

Follow-ups:

Western Interpretation
of Processes Described by TCM Organ Theory

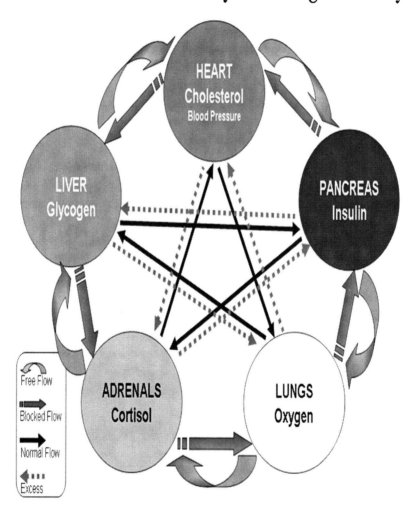

Figure 5 Western Interpretation of Processes Described by TCM Organ Theory

Rivkah Roth DO DNM®

Burning Tongue

The constant sensation of a burning spot a short distance back from the tip of the tongue is another sign reported by many pre-diabetic and diabetic patients. From a western medicine point of view this phenomenon can be explained via the lymph system, which runs through your tongue. While not fully understood yet, it is suspected that the burning spot is due to specific problems with your lymph drainage. The connection with a threat of diabetes is clear: Your lymphatic system is responsible not only for your immune system; it removes extra fluids from your body tissues and attempts to move fatty acids out of your system. Your small intestine is particularly rich in lymph vessels and, therefore, is most easily affected by food and other triggers. Yet, that same small intestine is also the part of your digestive system responsible for the absorption and processing of many of your essential nutrients, minerals, and vitamins.

In traditional Chinese medicine the tongue is understood to reflect the status of all your major body organs via the acupuncture meridian pathways that pass through your tongue. Chinese tongue diagnosis is a major tool employed in many a natural medicine practice. In fact, the burning spot according to Chinese medicine represents both the *lung* function and with it your body's oxygen exchange and the area of *T&T*. As we have seen, when we discussed the phenomenon of increased thirst (p. 64), *T&T* is the term used by TCM for the transport and transformation of nourishment and nutrients in your *stomach* and *spleen*.—The understanding of the *spleen* in traditional Chinese medicine is the equivalent to our western understanding of the function of your pancreas.— Keeping in mind that pancreas (insulin production) and liver (glycogen production) both fulfill ultimately important roles in your digestive process, it is no surprise that their levels of functionality according to TCM are reflected on your tongue in that *T&T* area.

Each of the three signs, thirst, dry mouth, or a burning tongue leads to a need to down larger than usual amounts of liquids. Closely connected to this craving for large amounts of fluids is an almost compulsive need experienced by many pre-diabetics and diabetics to add ice to all cold drinks. In a mistaken attempt to quench the burning sensation caused by excess sugar levels in your blood you add ice to everything in sight. Instead of giving you permanent relief these cold liquids, however, dowse the internal fire—speak energy of your metabolism. We have seen this graphically illustrated by the traditional Chinese medicine picture of the pot and the burner (p. 64).

In addition, cooled drinks obstruct the absorption of the essential nutrients and lead to cravings and hunger pangs—the third of the "3 P's" listed in the previous chapter. Ice physically slows down your metabolism and prevents the absorption of the essential iron, mineral, and vitamin supply to your body. Apart from an excess of sugar, a craving and need for ice most always indicates a lack of iron. Any long-term consumption of ice may result in anemia—particularly, if you are overweight or obese. If you are fair-skinned your doctor may pick up on anemic tendencies. However, chances are that your anemia will be missed if you are naturally dark-skinned. Anemic tendencies must serve as a solid warning sign for you that you may have developed pre-diabetes or full-blown diabetes.

We have mentioned that obesity often goes hand-in-hand with mineral deficiencies. To treat your weight issues in such a case rarely brings results. Weight-loss diets will not work for you because they rarely address the underlying causes. Even supplementing iron or vitamin B12 rarely brings relief if you are an "ice-addict." To help you reduce weight it would be far more beneficial for your healthcare provider to look for and correct the underlying cause or causes of your burning tongue. This may entail anything from a metabolic slow-down, intestinal malabsorption, hormonal imbalance (such as a cortisol deficiency or excess) and the resulting chronic acidification of your metabolism, and elevated blood sugar levels.

3. FACT Summary Burning Tongue

FAVOR	room-temperature drinks or hot teas and warm meals.
AVOID	adding ice to your drinks, refrigerated drinks and foods.
CONSULT	your qualified mainstream or natural healthcare professional.
TEST	mineral levels, iron deficiency, malnutrition, hormone levels, adrenal and kidney tests, blood sugar levels.

Your Personal Notes

Symptoms—Date(s) first noticed:

_____

Symptoms—Description:

_____

_____

Consultation Date(s) and with whom:

_____

Tests—Results:

_____

_____

Lifestyle Changes introduced:

_____

_____

Symptom Changes noticed:

_____

_____

Follow-ups:

_____

_____

Metallic Taste

Many diabetics report a metallic taste in their mouth. Other than it being a side effect of prescription medication or copper and other heavy metal toxicities this frequently is associated with a possible zinc deficiency. Among other essential minerals, zinc is one of the minerals most often found lacking in diabetics. For this reason you will find more about the pivotal role of the essential minerals in general and about zinc specifically in *Most Common Supplementing Needs for Diabetics* in *Part Three, Diabetes can be Controlled* (p. 300).

According to western medicine, sweet and salty taste receptors are found at or near the tip of your tongue, the sour receptors at its sides, and those picking up on bitter tastes towards the back of the tongue. Traditional Chinese medicine too assigns tastes—or lack thereof—to specific areas in your mouth representing organ function circles. According to TCM the sour taste is located on the sides of your tongue as well and belongs to the *liver* function cycle. Swellings or blemishes along the edges of your tongue may indicate *liver-* and *stomach*-related issues that western medicine would interpret as glycogen overproduction, accumulation of excess toxins, and other gastric issues; a good reason to look at your tongue on a regular basis. When we see such overlaps of different medical diagnostic systems there is a good chance for the information to be useful.

There is yet another way to look at these taste changes. The metallic taste—according to TCM connected with the *lung* cycle and the oxygen exchange of your body—sits in a band across the tongue about a centimeter behind the tip. TCM stipulates that the *lung* cycle interacts with your *spleen* cycle (pancreas in western medicine), and your *kidney* cycle. In western medicine too we know that the lung is responsible for reducing tissue acidity by its ability to exhale carbon dioxide with your breath. Likewise, your kidneys excrete acids and balance your body's bicarbonate levels, an important factor for achieving a more alkaline environment. This view ties together the interactions responsible in the development of diabetes: These are oxidative stress, the effects on insulin production or absorption, and the filtering ability of your kidneys.

In short, if you experience a metallic taste it is time to take a serious look at your metabolic functions and to get further check-ups.

4. FACT Summary Metallic Taste

FAVOR	individually balanced nutritional supplements, low-carbohydrate foods.
AVOID	one-sided nutrition, mineral-depleting foods high in carbohydrates, soft drinks, sugars.
CONSULT	your qualified mainstream or natural healthcare professional.
TEST	zinc and other essential mineral levels, pH levels, blood sugar and kidney values.

Your Personal Notes

Symptoms—Date(s) first noticed:

_____

Symptoms—Description:

_____

_____

Consultation Date(s) and with whom:

_____

Tests—Results:

_____

_____

Lifestyle Changes introduced:

_____

_____

Symptom Changes noticed:

_____

_____

Follow-ups:

_____

_____

Mouth Odor

Many diabetics experience quite a distinct mouth odor. It can range from what some individuals describe as garlic breath, to a sweet odor or a pronounced breath reminding of acetone. Short of indicating a parasite infestation, even that infamous morning breath might be an early warning sign of a major metabolic imbalance and of impending pre-diabetes or diabetes.

Mouth odor may have many different causes and needs to be carefully analyzed. Digestive issues are a most likely initial source. Many diabetics and individuals at risk of diabetes are overweight. Their digestive tract for one or another reason is working on a subnormal level or already is malfunctioning. If an *h. pylori* infection can be excluded, your health professional should consider a lack or excess of stomach acids, which too may cause unpleasant mouth odor.

Another major cause for bad mouth odors may be related to the function of your kidneys and, possibly, your liver. Problems caused by acidosis, a state of body acidity, usually lead to the typical acetone breath that many diabetics or their friends complain about. This type of breath may emerge as a fairly frequent problem. If it appears constantly or follows a sudden blood sugar spike episode (for instance after a meal too rich in carbohydrates) you should not take it lightly. You should see your mainstream medical doctor immediately.

The odor of your body and breath apparently changes well prior to an episode of an extreme blood sugar high (*hyperglycemia*), or also of low blood sugar (*hypoglycemia*). Both conditions, hyper- and hypoglycemia, may potentially be fatal if not detected and remedied quickly enough. Unfortunately, many individuals experience blood sugar highs and lows because they fail to control their blood sugar fluctuations. These days, some diabetics at risk use specially trained service dogs that are able to alert them to impending comatose situations. These dogs recognize changes to an individual's body odor and have the ability to warn their owners about twenty minutes before an imminent life-threatening episode. This is much earlier than any so-called scientific testing method available today is capable of detecting.

In the introduction to this section (p. 60) we have discussed the importance of choosing the right products and techniques to deal with some of the most obvious oral problems. In the following chapter we shall look in greater detail at the role of changes in your oral mucous tissues, teeth, and gums. It is important that you, and especially those around you, become more aware of any changes and that you learn to read your early warning signals since most of these signs and symptoms do follow distinct patterns.

5. *FACT Summary Mouth Odor*

FAVOR	frequent smaller low-carbohydrate meals to keep your blood sugar values steady and read your labels and serving sizes.
AVOID	blood sugar spikes and binges. Avoid cover-up treatments, see FACT Reminder # 1.
CONSULT	your qualified mainstream or natural healthcare professional.
TEST	kidney values and short and long-term blood sugar.

Your Personal Notes

Symptoms—Date(s) first noticed:

_____

Symptoms—Description:

_____

_____

Consultation Date(s) and with whom:

_____

Tests—Results:

_____

_____

Lifestyle Changes introduced:

_____

_____

Symptom Changes noticed:

_____

_____

Follow-ups:

_____

_____

Gum Disease

Your mouth is a mirror of your health. Periodontal disease, gingivitis, or other gum diseases are quite common in pre-diabetic and diabetic patients. Bad wound healing may be one reason. But, there is more to it. In past chapters we have seen how your tongue reflects the state of health of your entire system. The tongue is not your only mirror by which to judge what may be going on internally. Your entire mouth is a barometer of your metabolism. The condition of your mouth reflects many changes to your body chemistry at their very earliest stages, particularly those of your gastrointestinal system. A lack of intestinal absorption of the necessary nutrients will first of all affect all your various mucous tissues and will favor gum infections and receding gum lines.

A rather lengthy list of conditions such as viral infections, fungal infections, and several specific oral diseases, may affect the mucous tissue of your mouth. Bad breath may serve as your initial indicator. Your gums in particular are easily affected and may no longer be available to help you breakdown and digest the carbohydrates you eat.

Let us take a brief look at your digestive processes. In a simplified manner we can say that carbohydrates are digested in your mouth, proteins in your stomach, and fats in your small intestines. Our mothers were right when they reminded us to chew our food well. Intensive chewing produces sufficient amounts of saliva necessary for you to predigest the carbohydrates you eat. Your saliva fulfills an important function in the initial breakdown of these carbohydrates and in adjusting the acid environment of your digestive tract. Without proper chewing you do not produce enough saliva. Over time, and without sufficient amounts of saliva, your stomach acid levels drop. This plunge directly influences the digestion of your carbohydrates. Little wonder that many people who do not produce enough saliva are heading towards metabolic diseases such as diabetes!

If your digestion is poor, your ability to absorb vital nutrients from your food is even more meager. Without these nutrients the essential cell functions in your body stop working properly. Pretty soon, one or several of your organ systems will follow suit and may stop functioning correctly. Once any of your organ functions become compromised the speed with which changes take place will pick up and resemble an expanding downhill spiral; one organ system first, then another. Granted, these changes may be barely perceptible to you at first. But quickly, the downhill spiral will turn into an avalanche that—unless stopped in its tracks early on—will literally affect your entire body.

Sometimes oral inflammations point to an iron-deficiency related anemia, a lack of vitamin C, or insufficient levels of the B-group of vitamins. In many instances these problems are triggered or downright caused by excessive use of alcohol or smoking. Iodide and barbiturate drugs also might play a role in oral problems; as do hot foods and some spices. We already have seen that commercial toothpastes, mouthwashes, lipsticks, and other commercial products are known to be common triggers. Candy, chewing gum, soda drinks, and other sweets too tend to suppress your good and necessary natural body functions.

Low stomach acidity (lack of hydrochloric acid) is rather detrimental for the health of your gums and teeth. Stomach acids are needed to break down those carbohydrates that have eluded the digestive process initiated in your mouth and aided by your saliva. Low stomach acidity appears to be quite common among diabetics and those individuals at risk of developing diabetes. Future research will show if my suspicion holds true that, in correlation with chronic metabolic acidosis, low stomach acidity could serve as a specific early detection mechanism for people at risk of diabetes. We will look into the various underlying aspects leading to metabolic acidosis (p. 206) in the section about *Underlying or Predisposing Factors.*

6. *FACT Summary Gum Disease*

FAVOR	intensive chewing of your foods to provide sufficient saliva and hydrochloric stomach acid.
AVOID	alcohol and smoking; hot, spicy foods, soda drinks, candies, commercial mouth care products (see FACT Reminder #1).
CONSULT	your holistic dentist, qualified mainstream or natural healthcare professional.
TEST	iron-deficiency related anemia, vitamin B or C deficiencies, blood sugar levels.

Your Personal Notes

Symptoms—Date(s) first noticed:

_____

Symptoms—Description:

_____

_____

Consultation Date(s) and with whom:

_____

Tests—Results:

_____

_____

Lifestyle Changes introduced:

_____

_____

Symptom Changes noticed:

_____

_____

Follow-ups:

_____

_____

Mottling Teeth and Loss of Enamel

Several factors may play a role if you experience problems with thinning or loss (*dental attrition*) of your tooth enamel, tooth discolorations, and mottling. Good teeth are essential for the wellbeing of your entire body. Since your dentist deals with your teeth your medical doctor rarely is aware of what is going on in your mouth and may miss the most likely early risk indicators of pre-diabetes and diabetes. Keep a close eye on the condition of your mouth and ask your dentist to keep you informed about even the very slightest changes of your teeth.

The loss of dental enamel nearly always indicates problems with the way your carbohydrates are processed. Several factors play a role in this. The natural acidity level of your stomach is of utmost importance. Excessive tissue acidity quickly erodes your tooth enamel by a process that is looking to neutralize your acid-alkaline blood balance. For this purpose calcium, along with several other essential minerals, is leached from your bones and teeth. We will look closer at this process when we get to discuss in detail the implications of *Chronic Metabolic Acidosis* (p. 206).

Let me mention another very interesting fact. As we have seen recently, many concurrent type 1 and type 2 diabetes cases are surfacing. For several years, researchers have made a link between type 1 diabetes and gluten-sensitive enteropathy and one of its specific forms, celiac disease. Could it be that much of what applies to individuals suffering from gluten sensitivity also applies to many diabetics? We already know one link: diabetics and gluten-sensitive individuals share at least one DNA marker (HLA-DQ8), a factor presumably present in an astonishing 43% of the North-American population.

In my opinion it is entirely conceivable that the connections between diabetes and gluten-sensitivity do not end there. I have seen these tooth patterns in both gluten-sensitive patients and diabetics. Could it be that gluten-sensitivity precipitates any form of diabetes and that a gluten-free lifestyle actually might eliminate a slew of problems related to insulin production or resistance in individuals so pre-disposed, never-mind what type of diabetes? Or, is it more likely that metabolic acidosis simply is a predisposing factor for either disease?

One thing is certain: loss of tooth enamel is very common in celiac patients and in diabetics. For this reason many European healthcare environments use tooth enamel defects as a possible early indicator of gluten-sensitivity—even without a presence of the typical intestinal signs of atrophied vilii. Since the small intestinal section of the duodenum is involved in both disease patterns, maybe the same signs of enamel changes can serve as early risk detectors of gastrointestinal disease and the risk of pre-diabetes and diabetes? The chapter *Gluten-Sensitivity* (p. 215) in *Underlying or Predisposing Factors* will shed more light on such possible links or affinities.

7. *FACT Summary Loss of Enamel*

FAVOR	100% gluten-free diet.
AVOID	gluten and possibly lactose containing products.
CONSULT	your holistic dentist, qualified mainstream or natural healthcare professional.
TEST	potential gluten-sensitivity and related malabsorption and deficiency syndromes.

Your Personal Notes

Symptoms—Date(s) first noticed:

Symptoms—Description:

Consultation Date(s) and with whom:

Tests—Results:

Lifestyle Changes introduced:

Symptom Changes noticed:

Follow-ups:

Genitourinary Conditions Reveal

Whereas your mouth is the main portal through which nutritional elements—along with undesirable substances and toxins—enter your body, your genitourinary system is where either undesirable components leave it or the start of new life begins. Any changes in your daily habits may directly reflect changes to your body composition and state of health. In short, it pays to pay attention to what is coming out of your body!

Urinary Changes

Increased amounts of urine are directly connected to increased levels of thirst. We speak of polyuria when you frequently need to void large volumes of seemingly normal looking urine. Some of my patients call it their "Niagara-Falls syndrome." Voiding up to two and-a-half liters of urine per day is normal. Diabetics have been known to excrete easily twenty liters or more during the course of one single day. If you are not sure how much urine you are producing, collect all your urine during the course of a twenty-four hour period. You might be surprised at what you find!

Many individuals deny having urinary issues. Yet, I observe these patients using the clinic bathroom before and after every consultation. When I ask them about it—citing this evidence—they usually confirm it being normal for them to look for a bathroom on an hourly basis or at least very frequently. This very clearly is not normal. While this could have many other causes than diabetes, an involvement of your kidneys must be considered and you do want to get such issues checked out promptly and carefully by your doctor.

If not corrected in time, polyuria may lead to a mild or severe diabetic ketoacidosis. This is a condition whereby near-toxic levels of blood sugar and decreased insulin secretion cause an accumulation of ketone bodies. These are water-soluble bodies that result from the breakdown of fatty acids in your kidneys and liver and are used as an energy source in your brain and heart. An accumulation of ketone bodies brings about an electrolyte imbalance in your body; particularly the mineral ratio of your sodium (Na) and your potassium

81

(K) will be affected. An acidosis may develop slowly over time or quickly as an emergency. Remember: Your best way to be in control of what is coming out of your system is to manage what goes into it.

Your free fatty acid levels also contribute to this process of ketoacidosis. Free fatty acids are released from your adipose, speak fat, tissues. This puts additional stress on your liver once your insulin has lost its effect. Your oxidation mechanism is affected and contributes to, guess what again, acidosis. Nausea, vomiting, and abdominal discomfort or pain may accompany this condition. After an acute episode you may be overwhelmed by an irresistible urge to sleep. The typical acetone breath of many diabetics is a strong indicator of the presence of ketoacidosis and must not be taken lightly.

In ancient China the court physicians were not allowed to examine the emperor in person. If the emperor was ill his physicians were allowed only to check his tongue and pulse through a hole in a curtain. Other than this they had to rely on examining smell, color, and consistency of his urine and stool. The court physicians must have gotten it right. The Chinese emperors were famed for their health. Your sense of smell too is a valuable tool that you should learn to develop and use consciously. It will be of great help for a diagnosis if you can discern at least between no smell, the typical diabetic sweet odor, or the very strong odor reminding of horse urine or acetone that is connected to kidney related problems.

Color change in your urine is another indicator. Unless you are a heavy consumer of vitamins or are on specific prescription medications your normal urine color should be a pale yellow. Large amounts of clear, nearly colorless urine are as much a problem as is bright to dark yellow or brownish, sticky urine. Latter might indicate some level of infection or, once again, a prolonged involvement of your kidneys. You do not want to wait before getting such signs checked out.

Foaming urine is another issue that may relate—at least indirectly—to impending diabetes. It usually has to do with your protein absorption and it too is kidney-function related. You should be able to detect patterns between large amounts of foam and your consumption of certain foods. Just don't forget that grains too contain proteins. In fact more than meat proteins quite often an excess of grain carbohydrates results in foamy urine. Keep a log; what was good for the Chinese emperor should be good for you too! Remember, it is all about putting together the pieces of the puzzle.

If your healthcare provider suspects a genetic susceptibility to diabetes he or she will likely want to get your urine tested on a regular basis. Laboratory urine tests commonly measure also the specific gravity of your urine. Other factors like graininess, various sediments, and small amounts of blood also form part of a thorough urine analysis and allow your healthcare professional to rule out any lingering infections. In summary, any changes in your urine and your urine voiding patterns must be noted in conjunction with your kidneys' possibly being overtaxed from coping with long-term erratic or excess blood sugar loads.

8. *FACT Summary Urinary Changes*

FAVOR	immediate lifestyle changes, antioxidant-rich greens and light meats.
AVOID	unstable and excess blood sugar loads, soda drinks (diet or otherwise), alcohol, smoking.
CONSULT	your qualified mainstream or natural healthcare professional.
TEST	urine and blood sugar levels on a regular basis; sodium and potassium levels and ratios.

Your Personal Notes

Symptoms—Date(s) first noticed:

_____

Symptoms—Description:

_____

_____

Consultation Date(s) and with whom:

_____

Tests—Results:

_____

_____

Lifestyle Changes introduced:

_____

_____

Symptom Changes noticed:

_____

_____

Follow-ups:

_____

_____

Erectile Dysfunction in Men

Several recent studies of erectile dysfunction in men found strong links to diabetes or pre-diabetic stages. According to one study, men under the age of 45 years who experience erectile disorders may carry a sixty percent increased risk of developing type 2 diabetes. The outcome in the study group of those men aged 26 to 35 years, surprisingly, was even somewhat higher. These are truly scary perspectives!

If such a significant portion of our male population in their prime years experiences warning signs of pre-diabetes or diabetes in the form of erectile disorders this is not a positive omen for their future health—nor for that of any offspring of theirs. Even more so, this points to the importance of adopting necessary lifestyle changes early in life. Don't forget, early recognition of a possible risk is paramount when you consider the eight to fourteen year delay from the first signs to the actual diagnosis of diabetes! On the other hand, you benefit only if you are truly ready to take action and commit to the necessary lifestyle changes.

Let us see what TCM has to say about lack of libido. In traditional Chinese medicine a man's virility, and with it his erectile function, is directly tied to what TCM calls his *body fluids* and his *kidney* energy. Earlier, I explained that TCM assigns to its understanding of *kidney* energy what in western medicine views are your adrenals and other functions of your endocrine system. Adrenal deficiencies and imbalances affect your hormone levels from cortisol to testosterone. If you experience erectile dysfunctions you also may want to take a closer look at the following chapter about the impact of your testosterone levels.

The composition and amount of all body fluids, both in a TCM and a western medicine understanding—for instance through changes of certain hormonal levels—also affect your normal bodily functions. Unhealthy eating habits and a sedentary lifestyle along with stress, lack of sleep, and possibly several mineral deficiencies or imbalances all affect how your systems respond. In particular, all of these stressors affect your adrenals and the many hormones controlled by them. The implications on your health and future risks are considerable.

Therefore, here is my plea to all you younger men, and especially those in the 26- to 35-year-old group: If you experience less than satisfactory levels of libido along with at least two other signs and symptoms described in *Part Two, Figuring out Your Risk*, get yourself checked for testosterone deficiency and other hormone level issues along with adrenal and thyroid values in the context of possibly early stages of type 2 diabetes!

Most of all, I urge you to recognize that taking highly praised erection-supporting drugs or even similar natural compounds is not the solution. Erectile dysfunction is not the problem but the result of one of these other imbalances. And, in most cases, these underlying problems themselves can be produced by an unhealthy lifestyle and the wrong foods and drinks. Stop putting diesel into your gas tank and brake oil into your windshield washer container: Eat, drink, and live healthy from this day on!

9. *FACT Summary Erectile Dysfunction*

FAVOR	antioxidant-rich and low carbohydrate, low sugar foods; if you are overweight also low-calorie foods.
AVOID	unstable and excess blood sugar loads, alcohol, smoking.
CONSULT	your qualified mainstream or natural healthcare professional.
TEST	urine and blood sugar levels on a regular basis, PSH and testosterone levels, adrenal and thyroid values.

Your Personal Notes

Symptoms—Date(s) first noticed:

_____

Symptoms—Description:

_____

_____

Consultation Date(s) and with whom:

_____

Tests—Results:

_____

_____

Lifestyle Changes introduced:

_____

_____

Symptom Changes noticed:

_____

_____

Follow-ups:

_____

_____

Rivkah Roth DO DNM®

Low Testosterone in Men

Several studies and research projects are underway that are looking into the possible connection between low testosterone values and an increased risk of metabolic diseases. In fact, one third of all men diagnosed with type 2 diabetes have been shown to have low testosterone levels. And, men with low testosterone levels are three times more likely to develop hyperinsulinemia. An increased risk of cardiovascular disease and overall mortality in men over age fifty also has been stated in connection with testosterone deficiency.

Testosterone levels naturally decrease with age. One of the most recent such studies, albeit on men over seventy years of age, confirmed a strong correlation between lowered testosterone levels and a high body mass index. Allow me to put this into plain English for you: the more overweight these individuals, the lower their testosterone levels. Elevated numbers for body fat, short and long-term blood sugar, and the presence of inflammation markers turned out to be particularly indicative of a risk of diabetes.

Apart from being instrumental for your libido, testosterone plays an important role for your overall energy levels. It helps your immune system responses and even provides some protection against osteoporosis. Any use of anabolic steroids may be detrimental to your testosterone levels. These substances may prompt a condition called hypogonadism, and, thus, may affect your hormone production or your fertility, or both. This influences other of your endocrine glands too. Such a detrimental effect on your reproductive system should be good enough a reason to stay away from artificial muscle enhancers for good.

Hypothalamus or pituitary gland problems in many cases may be considered the underlying causes for lowered testosterone output. The hypothalamus regulates many of your pituitary hormones. It reacts to natural light and regulates your circadian clock as well as your body temperature. It plays a role in your immune system, your blood pressure, and your gastric reflexes. Most importantly—in our context of assessing your risk of diabetes—your hypothalamus plays a big role in controlling your food behavior. Hunger pangs may be directly related to problems with your hypothalamus and its indirect influence on your blood glucose levels.

If your testosterone levels are low most mainstream and some natural medicine professionals tend to increase your testosterone levels by synthetic or natural means. In my opinion this misses the mark. Instead, we need to look deeper into possible triggers and the complete workings of your endocrine system. Band-aid treatment approaches simply are not the answer for low testosterone levels. Read more about additional factors in the chapter about *Underlying and Predisposing Factors* (p. 197).

10. *FACT Summary Low Testosterone*

FAVOR	antioxidant-rich and low carbohydrate, low sugar foods.
AVOID	unstable and excess blood sugar loads, alcohol, smoking.
CONSULT	your qualified mainstream or natural healthcare professional.
TEST	testosterone, aldosterone, cortisol levels, adrenal and other endocrine system markers, and preventively urine and blood sugar levels on a regular basis.

Your Personal Notes

Symptoms—Date(s) first noticed:

Symptoms—Description:

Consultation Date(s) and with whom:

Tests—Results:

Lifestyle Changes introduced:

Symptom Changes noticed:

Follow-ups:

Rivkah Roth DO DNM®

Heavy or Painful Menses in Women

Heavy or painful and prolonged menses in your teenage years are no acknowledged indication that you may be developing diabetes later in your life. For now, research has not confirmed any possible links between a woman's early cycle problems and an increased likelihood of metabolic imbalances. However, in my natural medicine practice, it is stunning how many female diabetic patients in their teenage years have experienced moderate to severe issues with their menses. Could there, after all, be a metabolic connection that allows using the occurrence of heavy and painful menses in the younger years as a risk predictor of future pre-diabetes and diabetes?

Certain metabolic traits add to bloating, fluid retention, and increased pain around the time of your menses. These appear to be the same or similar underlying factors that form part of what we call the metabolic syndrome in connection with pre-diabetes and diabetes. I strongly suspect that this connection might turn out to be one of the very earliest indicators of an inherent risk of diabetes in women. We already know that women who recurrently suffer from severe menstrual problems are more likely to develop polycystic ovary syndrome and other similar conditions. Since these in turn have been linked to an increased risk of diabetes at least an indirect link already has been established.

Women who experience heavy or painful menses frequently tend to be heavier. Some of their weight and hormone problems may be related to adrenal and thyroid function changes. All of these concomitant factors too have been directly related to an increased risk of pre-diabetes and diabetes. It, therefore, stands to reason that we start looking at teens and young women more carefully with the objective of avoiding diabetes. And, if they do fit the profile of menstrual issues combined with some metabolic concerns—midriff obesity, lack of energy, or even hypertension—we immediately should institute diet and lifestyle changes.

Following the suggestions presented in this book and the *DIABETES-Series Little Books* has helped several of my female patients who suffered from heavy or painful menses. Simultaneously, it may have reduced their future risk of diabetes. So far the results are promising, but only time will tell.

If you are one of those female individuals suffering from severe monthly problems I would much like you to pay particular attention when you get to the chapters that deal with your metabolism, and especially with underlying metabolic acidosis (p. 206).

11. *FACT Summary Painful Menses*

FAVOR	antioxidant-rich and low carbohydrate, low-calorie, low sugar foods.
AVOID	unstable and excess blood sugar loads, alcohol, smoking; fatty and spicy foods, soda drinks.
CONSULT	your qualified mainstream or natural healthcare professional.
TEST	thyroid and estrogen levels, adrenal and other endocrine markers, urine and blood sugar levels on a regular basis.

Your Personal Notes

Symptoms—Date(s) first noticed:

_____

Symptoms—Description:

_____

_____

Consultation Date(s) and with whom:

_____

Tests—Results:

_____

_____

Lifestyle Changes introduced:

_____

_____

Symptom Changes noticed:

_____

_____

Follow-ups:

_____

_____

Polycystic Ovary Syndrome

Largely associated with overweight and insulin resistance, polycystic ovary syndrome (PCOS) may be a major and direct indicator of impending type 2 diabetes; or at least of a significant risk of diabetes. Nonalcoholic fatty liver disease too (see p. 203) has been shown to be closely related to PCOS, as well as to a risk of diabetes. Regular liver tests, therefore, are a must for anyone with polycystic ovary syndrome if you are even modestly overweight. And, what about that famed hip-waist ratio? Get suspicious if your hips keep packing it on.

As we have seen in the previous chapter, menstrual changes and problems may indicate future problems with polycystic ovarian syndrome. Other factors pointing to PCOS are a condition called *acanthosis nigricans* and sleep apnea (p. 133). Latter is probably mostly related to the excess weight and chronic metabolic acidification of your tissue, which also affects your oxygen balance.

Most commonly, polycystic ovary syndrome is the result of longstanding overall endocrine imbalances. These are largely the outcome of imbalanced and unwise food choices. Furthermore, it appears that increased rates of insulin production may prompt excess testosterone release in many women. First signs of such changes may include acne and—still more telling—the thickening of your hair.

Recently, even the diabetic community started to make that link between excess facial hair in women (prompting a condition called *hirsuitism*) and endocrine disorders and diabetes in particular. If you are a woman who grows more body hair and especially facial hair (upper lip), or if you show a male balding pattern, it is futile to go for repeat hair removal treatments. Instead, consider getting your doctor to work with you on establishing an acceptable hormone balance and overall endocrine system health.

Many mainstream treatments of hirsuitism and the prevention of polycystic ovary syndrome focus on blocking your testosterone. In our natural medicine practice we frequently isolate an underlying mineral imbalance. Once this imbalance is resolved, the newly found hormonal balance usually makes problems such as hirsuitism or polycystic ovaries disappear. Boron deficiencies are most common in these cases and may explain other concurrent issues such as bone loss, gastrointestinal problems, osteoarthritis, rheumatoid arthritis, and even fibromyalgia. Boron is one of your body's essential minerals and—in tiny amounts—may be able to boost and monitor your natural estrogen production.

A word of caution: only under the close supervision of a professional well versed in the mineral interactions and effects should you attempt supplementing with essential minerals or with vitamins and other supplements.

12. *FACT Summary Polycystic Ovary Syndrome*

FAVOR	antioxidant-rich and low carbohydrate, low sugar foods, boron and other essential mineral supplements.
AVOID	unstable and excess blood sugar loads, alcohol, smoking; fatty and spicy foods, soda drinks.
CONSULT	your qualified mainstream or natural healthcare professional.
TEST	estrogen and testosterone levels, boron and other essential minerals.

Your Personal Notes

Symptoms—Date(s) first noticed:

_____

Symptoms—Description:

_____

_____

Consultation Date(s) and with whom:

_____

Tests—Results:

_____

_____

Lifestyle Changes introduced:

_____

_____

Symptom Changes noticed:

_____

_____

Follow-ups:

_____

_____

Your Metabolism is Central

Your body's metabolism is not just figuratively at the center of your system. This is where it all happens. From food to drink, anything that you swallow is converted into energy by the highly fine-tuned interactions between your organs, glands, and tissues in a set-up more intricate than the wheels of a Swiss watch. Your metabolism is what drives you. However, your body works only as long as nobody throws it the proverbial monkey wrench. Without a working metabolism you cannot function.

And, it all comes down to what you eat. It is this simple. Yet, strangely enough, mainstream medicine mostly disregards food intake as a possible contributor to physical and functional problems. Isn't it interesting that every car mechanic first checks all the fluid levels in your vehicle and makes sure that you use only the best suited oils or additives to keep it running smoothly. So, in this section let us see what can go wrong if you feed the wrong fuels to your vehicle, speak your body. Most of the metabolic warning signs are "inward" except for:

"Ring Around the Collar"

No, it is not dirt! Far from it: that darkened and velvety stripe of skin at the base of your neck is a give-away. *Acanthosis nigricans* (AN), also called "ring around the collar," most commonly appears on your back at the base of your neck. But also in the armpits and the groins such hyper-pigmentations are a sure sign of insulin resistance. This connection with your insulin metabolism makes it a big risk marker of impending or existing diabetes. No surprise then, that obesity and—in women—polycystic ovary syndrome frequently go along with it.

The AN pigmentation marks are easier to be seen in individuals of darker skin color and should be considered a clear warning sign that you already are pre-diabetic and may be heading towards full-fledged diabetes. Older individuals have been known to tell about horror stories when their parents tried to remove their "dirt marks." When soap did not eliminate the marks bleaching was tried; unsuccessfully, needless to say. The discoloration of acanthosis nigricans takes place deep inside the skin. The only way to possibly get rid of it is by changing your insulin and glucose metabolism—from the inside out— through changes in food and lifestyle.

As soon as you notice such marks or changes you should insist on testing for diabetes. At the least, you should take this as an incentive for immediate lifestyle changes designed to eliminate blood glucose spikes and to avoid diabetes.

13. *FACT Summary Acanthosis Nigricans*

FAVOR	antioxidant-rich and low carbohydrate, low sugar foods.
AVOID	excess rubbing or bleaching procedures; unstable and excess blood sugar loads; alcohol and smoking.
CONSULT	your qualified mainstream or natural healthcare professional.
TEST	blood glucose and other diabetes related tests.

Your Personal Notes

Symptoms—Date(s) first noticed:

_____

Symptoms—Description:

_____

_____

Consultation Date(s) and with whom:

_____

Tests—Results:

_____

_____

Lifestyle Changes introduced:

_____

_____

Symptom Changes noticed:

_____

_____

Follow-ups:

_____

_____

Metabolic Interactions
Healthy Metabolism: Integrated Western & TCM View

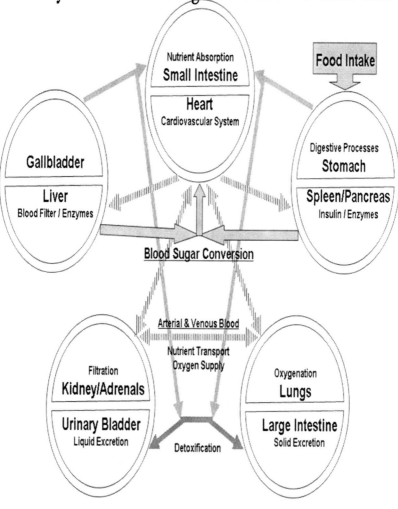

Figure 6 Metabolic Interactions - Healthy Metabolism

Overweight – Obesity

There is no such thing as being simply overweight. Two out of three North-American individuals are overweight or outright obese. This has triggered an entire industry around beauty and looks. Unfortunately, that entire weight and diet craze does shift away the focus from what is truly important. It is not the weight per se that is the problem, but the underlying lack of health that triggers your weight gain. You must start seeing weight gain as an expression of an internal imbalance or even a starting illness. People do not simply "get fat."

Have you gained weight around your waistline and cannot seem to get rid of it? Is your waistline no longer showing that desired hour-glass figure? Have you developed a beer-belly or a spare tire? Has your body started to turn an apple-shape? Or, are you packing on weight around your thighs and look like a giant pear? Did you know that during a lifetime an individual of average weight consumes 60 million kilocalories and more in food? Those are the numbers for a person without any extra weight; an individual who does not consume unneeded calories. Unfortunately, most overweight individuals consume considerably more than 60 million kilocalories in empty calories alone. And, to make matters worse, they expend less energy.

The medical books describe many causes for weight gain. Among them they list genetic factors, brain damage, endocrine system disorders, and prescription drugs. Environmental influences, socioeconomic status, psychological components (here the medical texts usually include binge eating and mid-night snacking) complement this list, along with excess food intake, large portion size, and a sedentary lifestyle. Mainstream medicine rarely looks at mineral deficiencies, adrenal and thyroid hypofunction, or food intolerances as causes of weight gain and obesity. But, before we consider some of these possible triggers, let us take a closer look at how the above-mentioned mainstream factors contribute to weight gain and obesity—and a future with diabetes—and how our natural medicine view differs in its assessment and approach to them.

1. Genetic Factors

Already according to the Merck Manual your heritability factor is considered to be no more than about thirty percent of all the influences that contribute to weight gain. Initial indications point to the fact that your genes mostly determine where the fat in your body is deposited, not how much fat your body packs on.

Research into the genetic factors of weight gain and obesity is ongoing and has led to other discoveries too. One of these discoveries is that of a protein called leptin. Leptin appears to be the link between adipose tissue (the body fat in which leptin is produced) and the brain cells that are responsible for your energy metabolism.

From a natural medicine point of view we do not like to connect inherited genes to problems such as weight gain. Instead, we look for underlying tendencies and family traits of malabsorption and adrenal or thyroid weaknesses as a possible starting point of "heavyset families."

2. Brain Damage

Mainstream medicine holds that a simple infection or tumors in the hypothalamus (one of your endocrine glands) may cause brain damage. An infection at this level may result in changes to the central nervous system in your brain. This is said to affect the body mechanisms that are controlled by such infected nerve cells.

Instead of simply blaming an infection for your problems, our natural medicine perspective tends to look at the cause of an infection for the origin of your issues. Everything in your body is connected; interactions between causes and responses are close. Foods are apt to trigger widespread inflammations. Excessive and long-term use of sugars and other refined and prepared (often toxin containing) commercial foods may easily lead to brain function problems. It does not take a tumor. In addition, sugar consumption may also lead to carbohydrate addiction; another important factor that we will discuss in greater detail in *Part Three, Diabetes can be Controlled* (p. 243).

We know that sugars block the absorption of many of the minerals in your body. A lack of certain minerals may result in imbalances and can promote your inflammatory processes even more. A natural medicine practitioner, therefore, will pay close attention to the levels of your essential minerals and the ratios between these minerals. Quite obviously, any missing minerals ought to be carefully replaced before you attempt any further reassessments.

3. Endocrine Disorders

Endocrine system disorders are probably part of the most notable causes of weight issues and obesity. Your endocrine system is comprised of a series of glands that typically are responsible for the production and function of your hormones. These hormones, once released into the surrounding tissues, are absorbed into your bloodstream where they are needed for the proper functioning of your body's many conversion processes.

We already have learned about the importance of your pancreas and your adrenal glands. The thyroid glands, parathyroid glands, and the pituitary gland in your brain also form part of your endocrine system and are responsible for the proper running of your body. In short, your endocrine system is responsible for much of your body's metabolism by secreting important hormones. A direct connection between endocrine imbalances and a risk of pre-diabetes and diabetes, therefore, is a given.

For this reason we will discuss in yet greater detail several of the thyroid conditions (p. 186), hypothalamus-pituitary disorders (p. 197), and adrenal deficiency (p. 183) in the chapter about *Underlying or Predisposing Factors*.

4. Prescription Drugs

Prescription drugs (among them corticosteroids) frequently are associated with weight gain. This is well known in mainstream medicine; yet, doctors continue to prescribe these medications even to individuals who are clearly at risk of weight gains and, thus, of mental or metabolic diseases such as depression and diabetes. Nothing is going to change in this practice unless you, the consumer patient, learn to question this practice and speak up. Remember, the doctor does not have to carry around your weight and become progressively less healthy; you do! So, make sure that you look for true solutions to your health problems and no instant band-aid cover-ups.

Pill-popping rarely offers lasting improvements, particularly not with weight problems. The list of drugs that name weight gain as a side effect is long; see *Part One, Drug-Induced Diabetes* (p. 40). Worst, some of the most dreaded prescriptions drugs that prompt weight gain (and potentially diabetes) are well-known anti-depressants and psycho-modulators.

Allow me to remind you again how stress can cause mineral deficiencies that, in turn, may trigger hormone imbalances, which lead to depression. Anti-depressants neither fix your hormone levels nor your mineral shortcomings or absorption problems. In fact, natural medicine professionals are well aware that these medications prompt intestinal problems and possibly launch a vicious cycle of more severe mineral deficiencies that is difficult to escape.

5. Environmental Influences

Environmental influences are a hot topic these days. Some rather disturbing reports are tying in our use of plastics with life- and health-altering changes.

These plastic compounds are all around you and include the dashboard of your car, building materials, furniture and carpets, plastics used to store foods, and many household items you use daily. It appears that these plastics release substances into the air and, most frighteningly, into your water sources. These substances may alter the way your hormones react. Needless to say, such undesired effects may appear out of your control. However, you do have a lot of input and choices. Some of these choices include how you buy your food, how you store it, and what you prepare it in.

Let us not forget the water you use for drinking and for showering or bathing in. Today, the purity of the drinking water in most towns and cities is greatly compromised. Plastic compounds are not the only undesirable substances that are not being filtered out. High levels of estrogen have been noted particularly in town and city drinking water sources and have been blamed on the widespread use of the birth-control pill and other prescription medications. While bacteria get filtered out and destroyed, hormones are not. Over time, these previously excreted hormones may directly affect your endocrine system and glands.

We already are noticing frightening changes in the physical development of today's youth. We have no idea how all these influences will affect us long-term. For now there is no denying it; these compounds affect your endocrine system. Since weight issues and diabetes-related problems are all connected to the proper functioning of your endocrine glands the implications may be huge. Do you see where I am going with this? Environmental pollutants may turn out to tip your scale towards disease far quicker than any of our medical texts and training programs have prepared us for.

What about carbon dioxide? I am going to skip on the larger environmental challenges our emission levels pose. Instead, I would like to draw your attention to our increasingly indoor-centered lifestyles. Much of the air you inhale is recycled air. Please bear with me if I take you a bit on a leap of faith in following my next thought. We will see in the chapter dealing with *Chronic Metabolic Acidosis* (p. 206) that a healthy individual of normal weight exhales 80 units of carbon dioxide for every 100 units of oxygen inhaled. However, an individual on a high-carbohydrate diet—fast-food, sandwiches, muffins, pizza, pasta, or rice—exhales up to 100 units of carbon dioxide for every 100 units of oxygen inhaled. This potentially represents a twenty percent increase of carbon dioxide in your indoor environment right there!

Think about it: How many individuals in your air-conditioned apartment, condo, or office buildings consistently complain of a lingering illness as soon as the fresh-air duct intake is being reduced in the heat of summer or the cold of winter? How many people in those building complexes are overweight and may contribute to increased carbon dioxide levels in the air? There may be considerably less oxygen in the air you get to breathe than what your body requires—a direct challenge to the building and systems engineers out there.

"Going green" is not just about preserving your surroundings—Mother Nature. Going green is even more important when it comes to preserving and revamping your own health and body. Read more about the role of the greens in your diet for your blood sugar regulation in the companion volumes to this book, the *DIABETES-Series Little Books.*

6. Socioeconomic Status

Much of the spread of obesity is being attributed to the socioeconomic status of a majority of those affected. It is being argued that decades ago physical labor and scarcity of foods kept those at risk lean and healthy. Today, people live a more sedentary lifestyle and, under time-pressure, they eat processed foods for convenience's sake.

The question whom to blame is not for us to answer here. It shows great progress that recently more and more schools ban the soft drink and junk food vending machines even at the cost of losing dearly needed corporate support. We need all public institutions to follow suit and establish criteria for healthy food choices. Become a trailblazer! Urge your kids' schools and your workplaces to provide healthier choices when it comes to snacks and cafeteria menus!

But, what about your home? More than simply blaming your environment, starting with your home, you may want to take action and take responsibility for your own body. Yes, the environment may put certain restrictions on an individual. But how come many of those affected manage to deal with the situation in a positive manner where others fail? We all have the ability to adapt. Our world does not stand still; it moves—so should we! Our health crisis is threatening to bankrupt the health account of your children. Do you realize that every one in your family must take responsibility for his or her well-being and contribute to positive choices for all?

There is no excuse for idly basking in destructive habits. The "I-need" attitude is not getting you anywhere. Enough of the "it-will-not-happen-to-me" attitude also; it just may happen to you or to your kids! It is understandable that change is challenging. The psychological impact involved in weight gain, therefore, earns great consideration.

7. Psychological Components

Psychological components may or may not tie in with socioeconomic factors. A high level of self-worth and purpose can protect you, but not always. Binge-eating and mid-night snacking may be enabled by stress in your personal life. Yet, it rarely is this simple.

As we shall see in *Part Three, Developing Healthy Eating Habits*, (p. 274) there may be chemical triggers involved in your binge eating, mid-night snacking, or your hunger pangs right after you have just finished an oversized meal. Wrong hormonal signals, underlying allergies, a lack of nutrients, or specific deficiencies of essential minerals may hide out at the root of your issues as much as the dreaded blood sugar spikes.

As you read on, many points will start sounding familiar to you. Write them down and mark those pages. Equipped with a set of clearly defined issues you will be more likely to get your healthcare provider to support you in a non-medicated, natural approach to beating your personal and very individual health challenges.

8. Portion Size

Then there is today's "double-size-it" trend. Aside from the marketing genius of our fast-food industry—once started on that track—a deficit in the necessary nutrients may make your body simply crave more food. Your gut cells are the closest things to your brain cells. Unfortunately, neither your needy gut nor your stubborn or untrained brain has learned to distinguish between helpful and destructive food intake. To reduce this equation to two terms: your body may be simultaneously "overfed and undernourished."

In this commercial and food-driven world of ours this is the legacy that you are about to impart to your children. The majority of commercial foods and fast-foods contain a large percentage of carbohydrates. Wheat is used as a binder in anything from so-called chicken fingers to meat patties—they should be called wheat-patties—and from soy sauce to many toothpastes and beauty products. The percentage of refined grains often exceeds that of any other ingredient.

Even our food guides promote grain carbohydrates as the number one food we are supposed to eat. However, grains (and that includes the much touted so-called healthy whole grains) are high in carbohydrates that all convert to sugar. Sugars in any form produce inflammation, as we have seen. In addition, grain-containing products also provide a high number of calories. And, since items made from flour are fairly tasteless by themselves, more sugar is added, more salt and—worst of all—more fat. Remember, fat is known as a flavor enhancer, but it comes with its own pitfalls.

Here comes the clincher: All these foods contain relatively few nutrients. The storing and milling process of your grains eliminates the majority of their natural minerals and nutrients. Fat, sugar, and salt also effectively displace many of the remaining nutrients and minerals. Your body soon becomes undernourished. It goes into its own hibernation and storage mode. Are you surprised that you desire ever larger portions? Increased appetite is a common early warning sign that points to malabsorption issues, actual mineral deficiencies, or an acid-alkaline imbalance of your system.

In addition, and as we mentioned earlier, many of these foods contain an actual addiction factor. These chemical triggers—literally—get you (and your brain) hooked. Carbohydrate addiction is real and does induce metabolic resistance. You learn more about food addiction in the chapter about *Gluten-Sensitivity* (p. 215) in *Underlying or Predisposing Factors*. So, remember, if you need more and more food to feel satisfied—I already assume that you are no longer an Olympic athlete who would be able to burn it off—it is time to get a check-up for possible signs of pre-diabetes or full-blown diabetes. Even more so, it is high time for drastic changes to your lifestyle and eating habits.

9. Sedentary Lifestyle

Sedentary lifestyle too may have reasons beyond the usually perceived boredom or laziness. Not everyone who leads a sedentary lifestyle becomes overweight or obese, and not everyone who feels tired and unmotivated will end up with diabetes. But, depression or simple lack of motivation may already be results of your sugar metabolism affecting your brain. They may be sure signs that you are heading down the path towards metabolic resistance and maybe even diabetes.

Don't misunderstand me, I am not handing you an excuse for avoiding exercise. But I want you to realize that biochemical processes may be behind the fact that you cannot find the enthusiasm to adhere to an exercise regimen. Essential minerals are your body's spark plugs. You may be deficient in one or several of them for whatever reason. As a result, your body experiences lack of absorption, increased tissue acidity, and lack of oxygen. Your body truly runs "out of air."

The biological processes involved in why-you-are where-you-are, when it comes to your state of health, are both complex and simple. Nutritional deficiencies need to be corrected before you can mentally cope with learning to look after your own body and health. It is a pity that today's healthcare (speak sick-care) system does not focus more on the many and widely available things that you can do to help yourself—before you start facing more severe health problems.

Putting Together the Pieces

There is yet more to this entire story of excess weight and obesity. Your body is subject to many associations and complex interactions. Remember: Everything in your body is connected. Your body reflects like a mirror what you eat or don't eat; literally from head to toe, from inside to outside. Traditional Chinese medicine always talks about this interconnectedness. Around it, TCM has developed its famous *yin yang* principle. It blames a lack of *yang* energy (western: adrenal function) and an excess of *yin* and *fluids* (western: pancreas, lack of circulation) for overweight and fat storing. To help the patient, traditional Chinese medicine has devised individually tailored treatment plans. Most importantly, it stresses the significance of proper food choices. With its system of interlinked diagnoses this is where TCM is a big step ahead of our western, allopathic approach. Its long proven understanding of successful prevention and treatment offers valuable insights that should perhaps be adopted by western medicine as well (see figure 7, p. 109).

Your weakest functional or anatomical link will be affected first. From there disease no longer progresses in a linear fashion. Every little imbalance triggers an exponential number of additional imbalances—some smaller, some larger. These in turn help to deepen your problem with weight issues. For this very reason the patchwork approach, practiced by mainstream medicine and even by many natural medicine practitioners, rarely helps. The most important step for you to get ahead in your battle against weight issues is for you to understand these connections and to find out how they relate to you. Remember, the best doctor is the patient, you!

According to mainstream medicine, weight issues have one most probable explanation, namely that you have developed insulin resistance. Insulin resistance puts you at direct risk of diabetes. And true, as you have learned in earlier sections of this book too, your beer gut publicly broadcasts that you quite probably are already pre-diabetic and that you truly are at risk of developing full-blown diabetes at some point in your future. However, insulin resistance never is your initial trigger. This is why, according to our natural medicine interpretation, your prescription medications mask but do not heal your diabetes. It is for this same reason of a symptomatic and not a causal approach that your weight-controlling meds help you reduce weight to a certain level only, and no further. Let us see how this plays out.

There is a chemical reason behind any accumulation of weight, call it tummy or beer-belly, spare tire, or anything else you like. Initially, it may take no more than an everyday event such as food, physical, or psychological stress to depress your adrenal function. Less than properly functioning adrenals prepare the ground for cortisol level imbalances. These reduce your body's ability to combat an inflammation in several of your tissues. Such an inflammation targets your brain and creates what is commonly referred to as "brain fog" (see figure 8, p. 118). No wonder you are having memory issues! Glandular imbalances also influence your body's functional processes and your essential mineral balances and imbalances. Many of your body's complex tissues and functions reflect these changes. For instance, changes to the walls of your arteries already represent your first step towards a cardiovascular event or an immune system problem.

Then there is the perhaps greatest impact, namely that of your gastrointestinal tract. Like it or not, your gut is connected to your brain in more ways than one. A majority of your immune system cells live in your gut. Biochemical imbalances in these cells, such as a lack of nutrients necessarily lead to inflammation in your intestines. Inevitably, you will experience bloating, flatulence, and a whole slew of other complications. Even the mildest chronic state of bloating (a persistent inflammation) results in what we call in natural medicine terms "leaky gut syndrome." We describe this in simplified terms as a condition in which proteins are being leaked through your intestinal cell walls into your bloodstream. These proteins are mildly or moderately toxic to your blood and quickly influence your blood gas composition. The bottom line is: inflammation directly causes oxidative stress. You literally are running out of air!

Where there is inflammation your body mobilizes your built-in health police, your macrophages (specialized killer cells). These rush to the scene in an attempt to eliminate the foreign intruders and quench any inflammation. Herein hides your biggest problem: Depending on what you eat and drink this is an event that occurs in your life daily. Following every meal, thus at least three times daily, your macrophages are called upon and become worn out; eventually, they stop responding altogether. Consequently, toxins and inflammations no longer are being removed from your body; instead they are being stored in your fatty (adipose) tissue. The result is obvious: If some of your cells are tired, so are you. Any persistent sign of tiredness is a signal that your cellular mechanism has become overloaded.

Have you ever experienced that after-meal urge to nap? It leaves no doubt in my mind that tiredness coupled with gastrointestinal symptoms is due to the above described biochemical chain. For this reason, I would never attribute it to laziness on your part if you suffer from a lack of motivation when it comes to regular exercise. It is rather expected that your desire or ability to commit to physical activity may vanish. Sleep issues and sleep apnea will probably be another factor in such a fatigue pattern as well. They provoke an ever-decreasing oxygen-carrying ability of your blood. Sadly, the entire process is a vicious cycle that repeats itself over and over, and slowly drives you ever deeper into your predicament.

Unfortunately, robbing you of your natural motivation is nature's greatest deception. Having said that, don't rejoice too early. Excuses such as "an expected lack of motivation" never lead to improvements. A lot of work is awaiting you. This is exactly why you want to find the cause and trigger of your very own personal vicious cycle. Lack of energy is how your body signals to you its need for nutrients. It is imperative that your healthcare provider identifies these deficiency issues correctly and helps you to remedy them systematically.

Unfortunately, until your system finds its internal balance this presents another giant trap: You feel hungry and develop cravings; sure signs of lack of nutrients—but not for lack of food. Until now, your pattern probably was to reach for that cookie jar because it is easy and seems to satisfy your cravings—at least short term. Guess what! If this is your approach you simply perpetuate the vicious cycle I described in this chapter about weight gain and obesity. Change of habits is definitely in order. Otherwise, with every additional repetition, your cycle will affect more tissues, organs, and body functions. And so, the destructive spiral grows. Soon enough your body reaches the stage we earlier called "overfed and malnourished" and your body turns acidic. This is the surest step towards diminishing your blood oxygen-carrying ability. The loop closes: your tiredness progresses. A heart event or kidney function lapse may not be far off. The avalanche towards diabetes and its serious complications has been set in motion.

Remember: act now and you can avoid all of this!

14. *FACT Summary Overweight, Obesity*

FAVOR	antioxidant-rich and low carbohydrate, low sugar foods, fresh water, green tea, exercise.
AVOID	fatty and fried foods, refined, carbohydrate- and sugar-rich foods, alcohol, soda drinks; sedentary lifestyle.
CONSULT	your qualified mainstream or natural healthcare professional.
TEST	inflammation markers, mineral deficiencies and ratios; blood glucose and other diabetes-, heart-, and kidney-related tests.

Your Personal Notes

Symptoms—Date(s) first noticed:

_____

Symptoms—Description:

_____

_____

Consultation Date(s) and with whom:

_____

Tests—Results:

_____

_____

Lifestyle Changes introduced:

_____

_____

Symptom Changes noticed:

_____

_____

Follow-ups:

_____

_____

Related Disease Processes
Western Pathology in TCM Graph Form

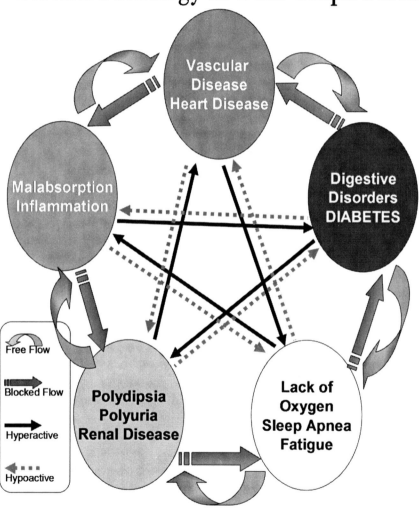

Figure 7 Related Disease Processes - Western Pathology in TCM Graph

Fat Cells Keep Water Out

Fat, or *adipose* tissue as it is called in medical lingo, is a form of connective tissue—the layer beneath your skin. It also surrounds your internal organs. How much extra fat your body contains largely determines how much excess weight you are bringing to the scale. Your healthy adipose tissue is a production site of hormones, such as the recently discovered hormone leptin. Unfortunately, your adipose tissue also stores any surplus lipids and toxins that your system has not been able to deal with at the time it was confronted with them.

Did you know that the body of an obese individual may contain five times the number of fat cells of that of an individual of standard weight? This extra number of fat cells is your very explanation why diets frequently don't work. No diet can reduce the number of these fat cells once your body has developed them. Dieting only succeeds in reducing the content of these cells. It does this by withholding anything that might translate into fats and by reducing your cell's ability to store these fats.

It probably is quite a revelation to you that dieting does not reduce the number of fat cells that you already have. You are right when you say that you should have known this earlier. In fact, the earlier you stop the development of additional fat cells the better; and, you always can prevent your existing cells from storing new fats. Excess fat interferes with your body's ability to use the insulin that your pancreas produces. Stored fat always has the potential of bringing you one step closer to a possible heart event and to diabetes.

Fat cells codetermine your insulin resistance factors and play a role in your free fatty acid and triglyceride levels. Most importantly, fat cells also keep out water. They affect the ratio between your body weight and your blood volume. Let me translate this into understandable terms: The more fatty tissue there is in your body the less blood your body contains per kilogram of body weight.

This harmful action of excess fat cells is significant for the following reason: The lower the percentage of blood that runs through your body, the lower the amount of oxygen it carries to your organs, nerves, brain, and other tissue cells. If your body carries less oxygen it will have available fewer antioxidants. Underlying inflammations arise and your body metabolism turns acidic. In other words, we have just returned to our vicious cycle of an acidic body environment that, by now, you are only all too familiar with.

Now you understand why beer-belly and midriff obesity are such obvious markers for a risk of diabetes and cardiovascular disease. Since insulin resistance places you already well on the road to disease progression it is important that you immediately start working on lifestyle changes and do not wait for other, additional signs to surface.

15. *FACT Summary Fat Tissue*

FAVOR	max. 1-2 teaspoons daily of extra-virgin olive oil or grapeseed oil, antioxidant-rich and low carbohydrate, low sugar and low calorie foods.
AVOID	fried, breaded, and otherwise fatty foods, any oil or fat sources other than the above, unstable and excess blood sugar loads, alcohol, smoking, other toxins.
CONSULT	your qualified mainstream or natural healthcare professional.
TEST	BMI (body mass index), blood glucose and other diabetes-, kidney-, and heart-related tests.

Your Personal Notes
Symptoms—Date(s) first noticed:

_____

Symptoms—Description:

_____

_____

Consultation Date(s) and with whom:

_____

Tests—Results:

_____

_____

Lifestyle Changes introduced:

_____

_____

Symptom Changes noticed:

_____

_____

Follow-ups:

_____

_____

Misleading Diet Recommendations

Here comes your next revelation. The fat you eat is not necessarily the only thing that makes you fat. In fact, most of the excess body fat you carry around stems from starches and sugars that your body has failed to burn up. These sugars have many sources. Your *Standard American Diet* (SAD) breakfast consists of orange juice, oatmeal or cereals and milk; it is a veritable sugar bonanza. Juice is sugar; oatmeal turns to sugar; milk is lactose, which is sugar. Such food choices may work for the skinny marathon runner next door, but they will not work for you. The cheese you eat will turn to sugar too. It is nearly entirely made up of lactose. Later—in the chapter about *Gluten-Sensitivity* (p. 215)—I will have some more to say about an addiction factor to casein, a component of lactose.

That tasty bagel, muffin, bread, the pasta, pizza, and that breaded chicken, all are starches waiting to be converted to sugar; they make your blood glucose shoot up sky high. If your body produces enough insulin to move these starches now-turned-sugars into your muscle cells these sugars can be burnt off into energy. However, this happens only if your activity level equals or exceeds your food intake.—Another one of those sentences that you should double underline!—If your activity level is less than your intake all these starches and sugars are stored as fat around your midriff instead of them providing you with energy. This is a simple mathematical equation and describes the process taking place in just about one in two individuals today and, unfortunately, includes your kids too.

True, your cells need a form of sugar in order to produce energy, and vigorous exercise can complete that job. But, you will not make headways as long as you keep feeding your body the foods that it cannot cope with. In computer slang we talk about "garbage in, garbage out." Your beautifully intricate plant called my body is no different from an average desktop or, as we have seen earlier, your car. In order to operate, your car needs the proper fuels and additives; your body requires the right foods and supplements. No difference!

Suggestions such as those presented by the food pyramid may work for an active, healthy person with a fast metabolism. But, for at least half of the world's population, the standard diet recommendations represent an intake level of carbohydrates (whole grains or not) and sugars (including your fruit) that far exceeds their body's ability to burn off. Have you noticed that most nutritionists and dieticians are of the fast-burn metabolic type? That is not you! Our healthcare systems have failed us. Why is it that most government recommendations for healthy eating and for the specialized diabetic diet still reflect such unreasonable amounts of carbohydrates in their intake recommendations? And, all of this despite it being obvious that it works for some of us and not for others to keep those sugar-turned-fats off!

Earlier, we have seen that your body metabolism is driven by a series of hormones. Some of them help your system; some of them impede your system. It all depends on the internal balance and the specific chemical interactions, many of which are driven by a large number of specialized enzymes and other of your essential tissue building blocks. If we consider that excess sugar has a direct effect on your mineral and trace mineral levels we start to understand the complexity of the problem. But, it should also make it crystal clear to you that you self-destruct any time you ingest a high-carbohydrate, high-calorie diet lacking of essential nutrients.

Much research into these mechanisms is still needed. However, a lot is known. *Part Three, Diabetes can be Controlled, Macro- and Micro-Mineral Supplements* (p. 307), will help you understand and sort through some of these processes.

16. *FACT Summary Misleading Diet Recommendations*

FAVOR	low-carbohydrate, low-calorie diet, e.g. Mediterranean diet, individualized supplements.
AVOID	deep-fried, processed, and other grain-carbohydrate foods and sugars in any form, excess calories.
CONSULT	your qualified mainstream or natural healthcare professional.
TEST	BMI (body mass index), blood glucose and other diabetes-related tests.

Your Personal Notes

Symptoms—Date(s) first noticed:

_____

Symptoms—Description:

_____

_____

Consultation Date(s) and with whom:

_____

Tests—Results:

_____

_____

Lifestyle Changes introduced:

_____

_____

Symptom Changes noticed:

_____

_____

Follow-ups:

_____

_____

_____

Diarrhea or Constipation

Any extraordinary event in your food elimination implies one or another kind of an ongoing inflammation. Just as increased urination might point towards a possible risk of diabetes, so might long standing episodes of loose stools, stools containing pieces of undigested foods, diarrhea alternating with the occasional constipation, ribbon-like stools, explosive or pasty stools, floating stools, and several other abnormal forms. You see, what may appear to be normal to you may not be desirable.

Naturally, food allergies—including gluten-sensitivity and lactose intolerance—must be eliminated as the root cause of your elimination problems before you try to connect any of these issues with a risk of pre-diabetes and diabetes. However, as we shall see, several of these gastrointestinal conditions may in fact accompany or facilitate a future risk of diabetes. I believe that many people could be spared a diagnosis of diabetes if their bowel-related issues were recognized early and addressed accordingly. Problems in the bathroom exceeding twenty-four hours are always indicative of issues with one or several of your organs or their function. It should not come as a surprise, therefore, that we find an above average number of diabetics among those suffering from irritable bowel disease and from colon cancer.

As I pointed out earlier, I would like to see research involving those individuals who display bowel and weight-related problems in tandem with pre-diabetes or diabetes. As with my patients, I would want to see these individuals being treated the way we approach celiac patients, namely, by putting them on a gluten-free and, in addition, low-carbohydrate diet. Since all three conditions (obesity, diabetes, and gluten-sensitivity) involve the duodenum section of your intestines such an approach might hold some promise. It is for this reason that I include in this book the following chapter about *Leaky Gut Syndrome*. It may yet turn out that diabetes in such a combination with intestinal issues and inflammation may be a mere symptom and not a root disease.

I highly recommend that you observe what your body eliminates and that you describe such during your next consultation with your healthcare provider. But—here comes a big and important warning—beware of the first-line response of most mainstream physicians wanting to prescribe a laxative for your constipation or something along the lines of Metamucil for your loose stools! It is highly unlikely that any of these medications will remedy the cause of your problem. In fact, such prescriptions frequently lead to a greater level of malabsorption and mineral deficiency and, thus, may aggravate your situation in the long run.

So, for now, keep insisting on wanting to find the actual organ-related cause of your irregular stools. For instance, you may find constipation to be tied to liver-related function issues, diarrhea to pancreas or spleen (lymph) problems, ribbon-like stools to adrenal and other endocrine deficiencies, and explosive or pasty stools to food sensitivities or allergies. In all these instances lasting results will always require addressing the underlying issues. And, to take this one step further, all of these complaints have one common trigger: wrong food choices.—But more about those later.

17. *FACT Summary Diarrhea or Constipation*

FAVOR	steamed or stir-fried vegetables, leafy greens, light proteins, and small quantities of olive or grapeseed oil, Mediterranean diet.
AVOID	mineral depleting foods such as sugar and processed foods or those you may be allergic to, soda drinks (diet and otherwise), alcohol.
CONSULT	your qualified mainstream or natural healthcare professional.
TEST	mineral levels including trace minerals, inflammation factors, CBC.

Your Personal Notes

Symptoms—Date(s) first noticed:

_____

Symptoms—Description:

_____

_____

Consultation Date(s) and with whom:

_____

Tests—Results:

_____

_____

Lifestyle Changes introduced:

_____

_____

Symptom Changes noticed:

_____

_____

Follow-ups:

_____

_____

Intestinal Inflammation
Affects Your Metabolism

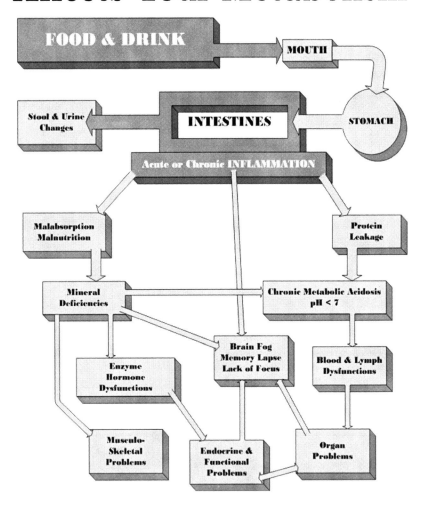

Figure 8 Intestinal Inflammation and Your Metabolism

Leaky Gut Syndrome

We have briefly touched on the leaky gut syndrome in the chapter about *Overweight and Obesity* (p. 98). A tummy containing swollen bowels may appear big—but it rarely does so due to excess fat. Instead, the proverbial large gut signals an ongoing inflammation of your bowels. Herein lays the problem and connection with a risk of diabetes down the road; and, quite a substantial risk at that.

⇨ A gut inflammation leads to protein leakage and upsets your blood composition.

⇨ A gut inflammation reduces or eliminates your nutrient and mineral absorption and leads to mineral deficiencies, imbalances, and cravings.

This is how it works: As a result of an allergic reaction your cell walls become porous. Triggers may be food allergies, medications, and even the wrong supplements. An initially local inflammation spreads quickly. Have you ever seen what happens to your green garden hose if left out in the heat or direct sunlight for too long? It goes all mushy, loses its elasticity, and is easily perforated—it starts to leak. This is exactly what happens to your gut when it develops leaky gut syndrome. Rather than being broken down properly and eliminated during your digestive process, proteins (mostly those from grains) leak through your intestinal cell walls. In time, these proteins end up in your bloodstream where they add to your oxidative stress and start to disrupt your endocrine and cell functions. Presto, there is your future with metabolic problems and possibly diabetes.

Many patients who come to my clinic for the first time believe that they have gained weight while, in effect, they suffer from an inflamed gut. Since their state of health (or ill-health) is all these individuals know they consider their condition as normal. No surprise then that they frequently miss out on the fact that they do have digestive problems. Nine out of ten patients flatly deny experiencing gastrointestinal issues; yet, they show all signs. Remember the Chinese emperors? They had their court physicians inspect their stool and urine daily. So, where does the hang-up in our society come from when it comes to discussing what our bodies discard? It is only gross if we eat and drink the wrong stuff! Do you know any dog lovers? They monitor their pet's do-doos without such hang-ups and adjust their feeding programs accordingly. Time to learn and follow suit!

Many of these same patients who deny intestinal issues also show up with puffy ankles, swollen lower arms and wrists; that too they think is ordinary. Since your kidneys play an important role in the elimination process, fluid retention is a definite warning sign of a possible kidney overload often due to excess levels of allergens. You will see this link between kidney issues and diabetes again and again. Unfortunately, recently I see this all too often already in infants and toddlers. Such swellings of the extremities may be direct signs of intestinal inflammation due to low-grade, persistent food allergies. Even infants still on mother's milk may be affected if the mother pumps herself full of unsuitable foods. Therefore beware: a pudgy baby with pasty stools already has issues!

Your gut has many functions before it gets to carry for you the five to ten pounds of waste destined for the toilet every day. Yes, this is the amount of stool that you do want to discard daily if you want to retain a healthy system! Your gut is your energy source and your body's power plant. If it is down, so are you. Your gut sorts out what needs to be absorbed into your system in order to drive your human body. It also eliminates what this same body needs to be protected from. Did you remember to double-underline these sentences?

Earlier, I mentioned that your intestines also contain a large number of your body's immune system cells. They are the link between intestinal weaknesses and a greater predisposition towards other organ malfunctions. Therefore, if these cells become inflamed they will no longer protect you from a long list of offenders. The short of it is that getting ill will be that much easier for your body.

An inflammation anywhere in your body indicates that something is amiss. Inflammations or fevers are designed to expel invaders or destroy bacteria. The positive side of any inflammation is that it points to a body that is still able to fight and is desperately trying to establish a viable balance. Inflammations are a natural built-in act of self-preservation aimed at creating a balanced body. A body that is in balance, in homeostasis, is able to function for a longer time and at a higher level of health. To establish a balanced system and keep your body in balance must be your health practitioner's goal for you and it should be your own goal too!

Food plays the dominant role in this process. You do not eat simply for something to do. You eat to live; more precisely, the cells that make up your body need to live. On average, your cells live between 105 to 125 days. Once they die off they need to be eliminated from your system. If there is proper nourishment available healthy new cells replace the old ones. Over the course of the next three to four months you need to properly nourish these new cells in order for them to function correctly. If your nutrient level remains deficient these new cells will reflect this imbalance. Your body deteriorates and moves a step closer to illness. If your nutrient level is sufficient these same new cells will be healthier than the ones they replace. Your body moves a step closer towards healing.

All the food and drink you ingest affects your gut. From there it is directed to the rest of your entire system and to those new cells in need of nourishment. If you put destructive foods into your mouth your various body parts lack the necessary fuel and stop functioning properly. It is that simple! Sometimes, even by eating the best foods, your gut may become inflamed. Intestinal inflammations also may be triggered by the use of antibiotics, NSAIDs (non-steroidal-anti-inflammatory drugs), and other prescription drugs. Alcohol consumption, smoking, recreational drugs, and many of the environmental factors too are known to kill off healthy intestinal bacteria. Any of these unnatural interceptors are sure to deprive your body of its essential nutrients and to lead to leaky gut syndrome.

Gut problems affect everything—including your skin. Allergies, acne and other skin issues are directly related to your intestinal problems. Show me a teenager or an adult with skin problems who does not have some intestinal issues! Many western medicine elements still consider it farfetched to connect skin diseases with certain inflammatory gut processes. Traditional Chinese medicine, on the other hand, has long acknowledged such a link. In its meridian pathway system traditional Chinese medicine connects the *large intestine* meridian with the *lung* meridian and calls the skin their shared surface organ. The simplified version of the theory goes something like this: The inflammation (they call it *heat*—we call it intestinal toxins) must vent. One of these vents is your skin, which we know is the largest organ of your body.

Let us sum up: A lack of essential nutrients by itself (either by malabsorption or by malnutrition) is enough to cause your weight gain and to lead to loss of bone mass and even muscle atrophy. If your body is of the storing-type it senses that it will not be able to meet its nutritional requirements and goes into a self-preservation mode. It starts storing unburnt sugars and starches as fat. Even an excess of protein eventually can be turned into sugar and be stored as fat.—Steaks bigger than the size of your palm (not including your fingers) are out!—We have called such a body that lacks its essential building blocks "overfed and undernourished."

An inflamed bowel often is the first actual symptom that your nutrient-energy transfer works considerably below par. For this reason, several theories claim that we may have to look at diabetes in a new light and consider

121

classifying it as an inflammatory disease. No matter what theory, full-blown diabetes does not surface at the beginning of your issues but towards the end. Therefore, "go with your gut!" Become proactive, and start feeding your body (and gut) in a way that keeps down the inflammation and builds healthy cells. Start reading *Part Three, Developing Healthy Eating Habits,* (p. 274) to find more specific answers.

18. FACT Summary Leaky Gut Syndrome

FAVOR	antioxidant-rich and low carbohydrate (possibly gluten-free), low sugar foods, Mediterranean diet.
AVOID	fried, breaded, and otherwise fatty foods, unstable and excess blood sugar loads, alcohol, smoking, many prescription drugs.
CONSULT	your qualified mainstream or natural healthcare professional.
TEST	BMI (body mass index), colonoscopy, IgA, blood glucose and other diabetes-related tests.

Your Personal Notes

Symptoms—Date(s) first noticed:

_____

Symptoms—Description:

_____

_____

Consultation Date(s) and with whom:

_____

Tests—Results:

_____

_____

Lifestyle Changes introduced:

_____

_____

Symptom Changes noticed:

_____

_____

Follow-ups:

_____

_____

Review

Historically, the diabetic person was known to lose weight and generally be of slight stature. In many of these slender individuals (except for their beer-belly) the functions of pancreas and liver are compromised; often overactive. For these individuals dehydration is a major problem. On the other hand, today, the majority of overweight diabetic patients retains water, stores fat, and shows all signs of an inflamed gut. Their systems quickly turn toxic and trigger chronic metabolic acidosis. From there, it is but one step to hormonal imbalances, insulin resistance, increasing obesity and diabetes.

How do you know the difference between a healthy gut and one with an ongoing inflammation? A healthy gut has an easy time staying regular. There is no yo-yo guesswork between diarrhea and constipation. There is no burning at the anus. There are no internal or external fissures, hemorrhoids, and no itching. There are none of those in-a-hurry moments.

On the other hand, an abdomen that houses swollen intestines looks and feels flabby. When you lay on your back the entire area below the diaphragm may feel like a large balloon covered by lax and soft muscles. Everything inside such a tummy seems to be movable and soft. Contrarily, in a slender individual with little or no bowel inflammation, but with possible insulin resistance (particularly after ingesting a meal too rich in carbohydrates), the enlarged tummy has a rigid feel to it. In such a lean person with elevated blood sugar the abdominal wall itself feels like an additional layer of tissue has reinforced it. These individuals seem to be wearing a solid armor.

If gut issues appear to be part of your pattern you are well advised to abstain from grains, possibly to the same degree a person sensitive to gluten would have to eliminate grains. This brings us to another interesting point: These days, a large number of excessively obese patients resort to gastric bypass surgery. In order to reduce their ability of eating large meals around two thirds of the stomach of these individuals is stapled shut. In a Y-like shape the remaining upper part of their stomach then is being reconnected to their small intestines, by-passing the upper intestinal portion called the *duodenum*. According to the latest numbers, it has been shown that ninety percent of these surgery patients who have been diabetic prior to their stomach reduction no longer are suffering from diabetes after their surgery. Mainstream medicine considers these patients "cured from diabetes" and advocates surgery whenever there is real excess weight. Ask a natural medicine professional: how can surgery cure? Such a result to us indicates nothing but deterrence.

So, how does it work? I believe that, in time, we may find out that once again the possible connection between obesity, diabetes, and gluten-sensitivity or celiac disease may come into play. It is precisely the *duodenum* and *jejenum* section of the small intestine that is most severely affected in celiac disease and that is being bypassed in bariatric surgery procedures in diabetics. Therefore, these patients may find that their insulin response normalizes because they no longer confront this section of their gut with inflammation-producing grain products. In addition, let us not forget that the duodenum is the part of your gut that is most strongly involved in the absorption of calcium. Interestingly enough, I see similar levels of calcium deficiency in diabetic and celiac patients when I interpret their hair tissue mineral analysis results. This then might explain the similar findings with regards to changes of the calcium metabolism in overweight individuals, diabetics, and celiac patients.

Time will show if my suspicion bears any merit and if there really is a tighter link via inflammatory gut symptoms produced by various levels of gluten-sensitivity and apparent diabetes (see figure 9, p. 126). Until then, you may simply want to experiment with a gluten-free diet—just remember that as little as one gram of gluten may retrigger intestinal inflammations if you are so predisposed. It is rather likely that this approach will help clear up many of your gut (and weight) issues.

For now, you will find a lot more information that applies to your specific and non-gut related issues in the following pages.

The Toxic Trigger Loop
Your Road to Inflammation

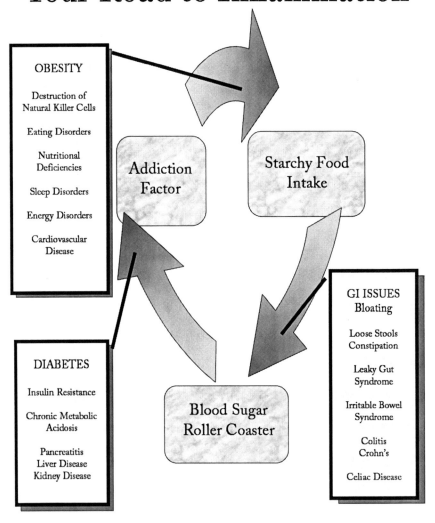

OBESITY

Destruction of
Natural Killer Cells

Eating Disorders

Nutritional
Deficiencies

Sleep Disorders

Energy Disorders

Cardiovascular
Disease

**Addiction
Factor**

**Starchy Food
Intake**

DIABETES

Insulin Resistance

Chronic Metabolic
Acidosis

Pancreatitis
Liver Disease
Kidney Disease

**Blood Sugar
Roller Coaster**

GI ISSUES
Bloating

Loose Stools
Constipation

Leaky Gut
Syndrome

Irritable Bowel
Syndrome

Colitis
Crohn's

Celiac Disease

Figure 9 The Toxic Trigger Loop – The Road to Inflammation

Brain Fog has Reasons

Brain fog can have many reasons. One such trigger that we have just finished looking at are intestinal problems. An inflamed gut nearly always triggers brain fog, memory lapses, and loss of focus because it interferes with your nutrient absorption. If these are some of the symptoms you experience keep a very close eye on your digestive system. You will see that you may return to where you started, namely with inadequate food and lifestyle habits. Brain cells are very demanding; they need a substantial amount of nutrients and oxygen. An acidic system starves your brain. Among the lifestyle habits none contribute more to brain fog than several of your sleep disorders.

Difficulties Falling or Staying Asleep

Sleep disorders are a growing problem among adults and youths alike. In fact, in the USA, there have been reportedly 18 million people with some form of diagnosed sleep disorder. At least 8 million of these individuals are using prescription medication every single night. The number of individuals using over-the-counter drugs presumably is considerably higher but is unknown. Some of you recognize the potential problem of addiction to these drugs. As soon as you stop taking these sleeping aids or tranquilizers you may experience withdrawal symptoms. Understandably, you will misinterpret such withdrawal episodes as renewed periods of insomnia. In professional terms we call them the rebound effect.

Natural medicine offers many good ways around this. However, it is not as simple as going to the health food store and picking up a sleep-inducing herb. The causes for sleep problems are too manifold and only a specialist professional has the training and experience to help you solve your individual issues and causes without triggering other problems in the process. Most types of sleep disorders are not isolated problems. When it comes to sleep we often find ourselves confronted with the chicken or egg question. Intimately related to your daytime activities and your biochemical body processes, sleep problems may be the cause as much as they may be the result of deeper imbalances. In our natural medicine approach, therefore, we always look for possible triggers, feedback loops, and vicious cycles. It is in the nature of many serious conditions that, in time, they may spiral out of hand. Most sleep issues reflect such states.

Interestingly, many diabetics and people at risk of diabetes suffer from a variety of sleep disorders. One internal imbalance causes another dysregulation that, in turn, triggers a never-ending cycle. All of these problems have a direct connection to your daytime habits, your lifestyle, and your eating patterns. Once you recognize these links you should quite easily be able to control and eliminate your sleep disturbances.

Let us look at several recurring sleep issues cited frequently by pre-diabetic and diabetic patients.

Waking Up in the Middle of the Night

Waking up in the middle of the night may be related to your body's water metabolism. We already discussed these issues when looking at how increased blood sugar prompts more frequent visits to the bathroom. Even so, most individuals find it easy to get back to sleep after a quick trip to the bathroom.

However, waking up in the middle of the night and not being able to return to sleep may be related to the function of your liver. Over the course of a day each one of your function cycles and organs goes through active and passive periods. For instance, the most active period for your liver happens to fall into the very early morning hours. This liver activity frequently prompts another problem common to many diabetics: Diabetics report higher blood sugar values in the morning despite not having eaten since the previous night. This is called the "dawn phenomenon." Theoretically, your sugar values should drop the longer you are without food. This, unfortunately, is not the whole truth. Roughly four hours after your last meal your blood sugars are starting to drop below what your system considers acceptable. Your cells, however, need continuous nourishment even during the night. Your liver monitors this situation. If your blood sugar levels drop for any length of time your liver releases glycogen and prompts your pancreas into increased insulin release. Up goes your blood sugar and produces said "dawn phenomenon."

No, I am not making a case for midnight snacking! I am making a case for more consistent blood sugar control by avoiding sugar spikes and drops during the day. This is the only approach that gets rid of your nightly hypoglycemic episodes and curbs your increased liver activity. Therefore, lower your carbohydrate intake, up your lighter proteins! Nightly episodes of hypoglycemia can be fatal. They must be prevented—preferably not by emergency-snacking on sugar cubes or extra chocolate. It is important that you understand this: You do not fix the nightly episode by what you eat at midnight. You fix it by how you eat during your entire day. If you eat a high-carbohydrate breakfast consisting of cereals, orange juice, and milk a midnight hypoglycemia episode is nearly guaranteed.

Better than downing that nightly rescue sugar cube, chocolate, or candy that keeps you on the roller coaster of blood sugar imbalances, deficiencies and cravings, consider spreading smaller protein portions throughout your day. In addition, follow some of the suggestions we will discuss in *Part Three, Diabetes can be Controlled* and in the companion volumes, the *DIABETES-Series Little Books*.

19. *FACT Summary Sleep Disturbances*

FAVOR	low carbohydrate, low sugar foods, light proteins.
AVOID	sugar spikes, midnight snacking.
CONSULT	your qualified mainstream or natural healthcare professional.
TEST	urine and blood glucose, and other diabetes-related tests.

Your Personal Notes

Symptoms—Date(s) first noticed:

_____

Symptoms—Description:

_____

_____

Consultation Date(s) and with whom:

_____

Tests—Results:

_____

_____

Lifestyle Changes introduced:

_____

_____

Symptom Changes noticed:

_____

_____

Follow-ups:

_____

_____

Sleep Environment

Many factors other than illnesses may play a role in the quality of your sleep. Some of them are external—and we shall touch on them only briefly—but, nevertheless, sleep disturbances may be the underlying causes of your fatigue, daytime sleepiness, restlessness and other symptoms.

First and foremost, forget sleeping with a nightlight on; and don't let your kids fall into that habit either! If you need to visit the bathroom during the night do it in the dark or use a dim light only. Only completely dark surroundings will allow the necessary body rhythms and biochemical processes to become active. You may have heard of a hormone called melatonin. Produced by your pineal gland (brain), in your retina (eyes), and in your intestines (but only if you are surrounded by complete darkness), melatonin plays a major role in your circadian clock. Not spending enough time in total darkness not only affects your sleep patterns, it directly affects the total health of your cells, your immune system and—most poignantly—your mood.

It also does not help if your mind cannot shut off. If your mind keeps racing, because you are worried about forgetting certain chores for the next day, simply put paper and pen beside your bed and jot down your thoughts as soon as they surface. Within a few nights you will start feeling relaxed because you no longer worry about forgetting any of your important to-dos. Stress and worries can rob your sleep, and affect your adrenals. A lack of certain essential minerals too can keep you awake. Many individuals at risk of developing pre-diabetes and diabetes are already low on essential minerals. And, for that reason, worries are very common in people dealing with diabetes or pre-diabetic symptoms.

Traditional Chinese medicine always connects mood with some organ dysfunctions (see figure 4, p. 63). TCM considers it possible for the *spleen* (western medicine: pancreas) to be injured by constant worries, your *kidneys* (adrenals) by fright, and the *liver* by anger. Now, if that is not an incentive to look for mind-calming alternatives such as meditation, low-impact exercise, and properly individualized essential mineral supplements (and a pitch-black bedroom)!

20. *FACT Summary Sleep Environment*

FAVOR	low-impact exercise, meditation, proper eating, pitch-black sleeping environment.
AVOID	night lights, stress.
CONSULT	your qualified mainstream or natural healthcare professional.
TEST	hormone levels, mineral and trace mineral levels.

Your Personal Notes

Symptoms—Date(s) first noticed:

_____

Symptoms—Description:

_____

_____

Consultation Date(s) and with whom:

_____

Tests—Results:

_____

_____

Lifestyle Changes introduced:

_____

_____

Symptom Changes noticed:

_____

_____

Follow-ups:

_____

_____

Snoring and Sleep Apnea

Snoring and sleep apnea may become an issue mostly for overweight and obese pre-diabetics and diabetics. During your sleep your airways become obstructed. In obese persons snoring is three times more common than in people of average weight. Most individuals are not aware that they experience repeated episodes of snoring; even less that they suffer from sleep apnea. Snoring may be further aggravated by the use of antihistamines, tranquilizers, sleep medications, or alcoholic beverages. Snoring often is a precursor to episodes of sleep apnea.

Sleep apnea affects men more than women. Most patients who experience phases of sleep apnea tend to sleep on their backs. In this position it is possible for your tongue to fall back against your throat and to effectively seal off your air passages. Over time, this may lead to mucus build-ups, which in turn lead to nasal blockages and the obstruction of your airways during sleep. Periods of sleep apnea may last for as little as ten seconds or as long as two minutes. During one single night there may be a couple to several hundred instances when your breathing actually stops. During these times, little or no oxygen reaches your airways and your lungs. It is rather obvious that this may result in a serious decrease of the levels of your overall blood oxygen and cell health.

An episode of sleep apnea may lead to interrupted sleep and to sudden awaking and gasping for air, even to sudden waking due to a coughing attack. The bottom line is: if you experience sleep apnea or snoring you likely will not feel rested the following day. Daytime drowsiness, hypertension, morning headaches, and cardiac issues may result from recurrent sleep apnea. To make matters worse, obstructive sleep apnea poses a major risk for fatal strokes.

Ask your family members to observe your sleep and breathing patterns from time to time—especially, if you are overweight or show any of the signs mentioned above. It is best for you to become familiar with other signs that may be pointing to possible snoring or sleep apnea episodes. Let us explore those most commonly observed in the following chapters.

21. *FACT Summary Snoring or Sleep Apnea*

FAVOR	antioxidant-rich and low calorie, low carbohydrate, low sugar foods.
AVOID	super-size meals, fried, breaded, and otherwise fatty foods, unstable and excess blood sugar loads, soft drinks, alcohol, smoking.
CONSULT	your qualified mainstream or natural healthcare professional.
TEST	BMI (body mass index), blood gas levels, blood glucose and other diabetes-related tests.

Your Personal Notes

Symptoms—Date(s) first noticed:

_____

Symptoms—Description:

_____

_____

Consultation Date(s) and with whom:

_____

Tests—Results:

_____

_____

Lifestyle Changes introduced:

_____

_____

Symptom Changes noticed:

_____

_____

Follow-ups:

_____

_____

Lack of Energy or Tiredness

We have seen how the increased need to consume large amounts of liquids and the passing of equally large amounts of urine may deplete your body's electrolyte balance. Many of your body's organs and functions depend on the right and precise level of positively and negatively charged particles, your electrolytes. You may have heard about the sodium-potassium balance, an important cofactor in a variety of complications from heart disease to kidney dysfunctions.

The interaction between sodium and potassium is but one example of a possible electrolyte imbalance. Ratio imbalances are frequently found in individuals with a tendency towards diabetes. Electrolyte imbalances suppress a row of negative or positive charge-dependent body functions. Most importantly, they directly affect your level of energy production. This makes your electrolyte ratio an obvious culprit when it comes to the levels of tiredness many diabetics experience.

Electrolyte imbalances are not the only cause of energy lows, however. Several times already, over the course of the previous pages, we have pointed to the role of your hormones. Hormonal issues, in particular adrenal deficiency or hypothyroidism, too can prompt anything from lethargy to depression in a person at risk of pre-diabetes or diabetes. We shall explore these links in greater detail in the section about *Underlying or Predisposing Factors* (*Adrenal Deficiency*, p. 183, and *Hypothyroidism*, p. 186).

Exhaustion is directly related to your food intake. Malnutrition is common among individuals who experience blood sugar imbalances. It is due to insufficient intake of essential nutrients or malabsorption and, nearly always, results in fatigue, lack of motivation, or downright exhaustion. In *Part Three, Developing Healthy Eating Habits* (p. 268) we shall look at this mechanism of malnutrition in greater detail.

While tiredness is to be expected, it is important that you understand that sudden or chronic fatigue without an apparent cause does not need to be accepted. Sudden or gradual loss of energy is a big warning flag for a possible risk of pre-diabetes and diabetes; and, you quickly want to get to the root of your lack of energy. It may be one of your very first signs that you are heading towards diabetes.

Bring up your issues with tiredness during your next visit with your doctor and have your natural healthcare practitioner help you identify your specific causes of lack of energy.

22. *FACT Summary Lack of Energy*

FAVOR	antioxidant-rich and low carbohydrate, low sugar foods.
AVOID	any mineral depleting processed foods, soft drinks, alcohol.
CONSULT	your qualified mainstream or natural healthcare professional.
TEST	electrolyte levels, adrenal and thyroid tests, essential mineral levels, blood glucose and other diabetes-related tests.

Your Personal Notes

Symptoms—Date(s) first noticed:

_____

Symptoms—Description:

_____

_____

Consultation Date(s) and with whom:

_____

Tests—Results:

_____

_____

Lifestyle Changes introduced:

_____

_____

Symptom Changes noticed:

_____

_____

Follow-ups:

_____

_____

_____

Daytime Sleepiness

Do you need to nap after a meal? Did your doctor diagnose you with hypersomnia? Most likely your blood sugars are going through the roof. Excessive carbohydrate intake will prompt your insulin levels to rise too quickly. Subsequently, your blood glucose levels crash and so do you. The catnap after lunch or dinner is a major warning flag and proves that you are likely pre-diabetic—if you are not already suffering from full-blown diabetes.

When your body does not get enough hours of night sleep, when your sleep is disrupted, or when your sleep environment is less than ideal, your body cannot get its minimum level of rest. Uninterrupted rest is needed for your body to perform a long line of necessary functions that result in anything from physical to mental energy the following day. Morning and daytime tiredness are direct reflections of lack of nighttime sleep. In a majority of overweight and obese individuals the need for daytime napping may also be related to sleep apnea or other nighttime sleep disruptions. As we have seen, snoring or sleep apnea will result in the reduced intake of oxygen. Oxidative stress (reduced blood gas levels) might well be another cause of your overall fatigue.

Your knowledgeable healthcare professional should be in a position to help you determine if factors such as the following may be involved in your specific situation: hypoglycemia or hyperglycemia, hypothyroidism, adrenal deficiency, anemia, electrolyte imbalances, or nutritional deficiencies. Once the cause of your issues has been properly identified, your doctor will be able to address and remedy the source of your daytime fatigue directly and, in most cases, quite effectively.

No matter what turns out to be the cause of your tiredness, look for the symptoms related to it and remain vigilant. To be tired on an ongoing basis is not normal. And, coffee or other tonics are no solution because they are prompting another crash as soon as their effect is worn off. Instead, look for the underlying biochemical imbalance and understand tiredness as a possible risk indicator of metabolic problems.

23. *FACT Summary Daytime Sleepiness*

FAVOR	Night: quiet, dark environment, a regular unwinding routine, maybe meditation or breathing exercises. Day: cause-specific; low carbohydrate diet.
AVOID	Night: noisy, lit sleep environments, late bedtimes, carbohydrate or fatty snacks prior to bedtime, heavy exercise, stress, commercial sleeping aids. Day: sugar and high carbohydrate foods or drinks.
CONSULT	your qualified mainstream or natural healthcare professional.
TEST	adrenal and thyroid tests, blood glucose and other diabetes-related tests, mineral levels.

Your Personal Notes

Symptoms—Date(s) first noticed:

Symptoms—Description:

Consultation Date(s) and with whom:

Tests—Results:

Lifestyle Changes introduced:

Symptom Changes noticed:

Follow-ups:

Crankiness

It is a small step for your imagination to figure out that any chemical imbalances in your system—coupled with perhaps a lack of sleep—might affect your mood. You might not notice it yourself but your friends and acquaintances quite likely will be acutely aware of an unusual shift in your behavior.

I don't know of any studies into this precise subject of mood patterns in pre-diabetic or diabetic individuals: However, from my personal experience, I can state that I know of no diabetic among my family, friends, acquaintances, and patients who does not, to some level, exhibit periods of increased emotional tension. For some reason this seems to happen especially during the evening hours between 9 p.m. and 11 p.m.

Should you encounter a similar pattern among your friends—diabetic or not—at all cost avoid any confrontation or arguments with them around that time of night. At best, your questions, comments, and contributions may prompt intense and passionate discourses and explanations from their side. Their responses may come across atypically forceful, and authoritative. Their voice may carry a somewhat cranky and pressed note. Any of your questions may trigger your diabetic friend to pick a friendly or not so friendly argument. Bottom line though, he or she will be in an intense mood and take everything highly personal. At worst, the diabetic may resort to verbal or even physical aggression. Most abuse situations reach crisis proportions around that same time of the evening. Could there be a correlation? Could many irrational acts be attributed to uncontrolled sugar levels that prompt hormonal imbalances?

At any rate, it is best for you to be prepared. Try not to let these patterns escalate. If you can, schedule some quiet activity during that time and gently steer away from discussing topics that might elicit a strong and passionate response—from daytime plans to personal beliefs, politics, or social engagement.

24. *FACT Summary Crankiness*

FAVOR	quiet times, meditation, reading, writing.
AVOID	potentially aggravating discussions and situations, TV.
CONSULT	your qualified mainstream or natural healthcare professional.
TEST	blood glucose and other diabetes-related tests.

Your Personal Notes

Symptoms—Date(s) first noticed:

_____

Symptoms—Description:

_____

_____

Consultation Date(s) and with whom:

_____

Tests—Results:

_____

_____

Lifestyle Changes introduced:

_____

_____

Symptom Changes noticed:

_____

_____

Follow-ups:

_____

_____

Depression

Many individuals develop a tendency to depression prior to developing diabetes. These physical and emotional components of depression frequently are triggered by adrenal and thyroid imbalances. Interestingly, these hormonal imbalances may be caused by the same mineral deficiencies that eventually will set off your blood sugar problems. Such mineral deficiencies may be more pronounced if you are taking suppressive prescription medication. In addition, in *Part One, Drug Induced Diabetes* (p. 40), you have seen that several of the prescription medications used to alleviate depression actually may cause diabetes. If you turn out to be at risk of developing pre-diabetes and diabetes this link between prescription medications and diabetes alone should be a pretty good reason for you to look for alternatives to anti-depressants!

It is important that you learn to address the real cause of your droopiness and that you abstain from suppressing your system with prescription medications. If, in addition, snoring and sleep apnea are part of your pattern, understand that the resulting lack of oxygen will quickly affect your level of mental clarity and produce brain fog. In fact and unfortunately, it is more likely that such symptoms may prompt a mainstream medicine diagnosis of depression rather than a more accurate assessment of reduced oxygen intake or turnover.

Thinking clearly relates directly to the amount of oxygen delivered to your brain cells. In turn, your oxygen intake relates to the way you breathe. But this is only one part of the equation. Your food intake also influences the oxygen carrying ability of your blood. You will find out more about this process in the chapters about *Chronic Metabolic Acidosis* (p. 206) and *Lack of Oxygen* (p. 211).

By now you recognize the widespread consequences triggered by one single biochemical factor that is out of balance. Chain reactions are easily begun throughout your body. Blood cells that carry less oxygen affect your immune system reaction too and open the door to deficient antioxidant responses. Without adequate antioxidant levels inflammations in one or the other tissues of your body may follow. As we have seen, newest research surrounding the pancreatic beta cells indicates such an inflammatory process as a possible cause of diabetes.

Therefore, do not take brain fog lightly, do not brush it of as, "I am getting older," or, "I am not that smart." Most importantly, do not let the mainstream medical system stamp you as "depressed" and put you simply on suppressive—and, might I say, additionally acidifying—medication. Insist that the cause of your issues be identified—from intestinal or other inflammations to blood sugar fluctuation, mineral deficiencies, hormone imbalances, or sleep apnea. It should not be this way but, if you feel depressed, you or your family might be well advised to do some homework first before agreeing to a quick solution with possible side-effects from addiction to deeper depression and even suicidal tendencies.

25. *FACT Summary Depression*

FAVOR	antioxidant-rich and low carbohydrate, low sugar foods.
AVOID	inflammation producing foods, soft drinks, alcohol, smoking.
CONSULT	your qualified mainstream or natural healthcare professional.
TEST	electrolyte and blood gas levels, blood glucose and other diabetes-related tests.

Your Personal Notes

Symptoms—Date(s) first noticed:

Symptoms—Description:

Consultation Date(s) and with whom:

Tests—Results:

Lifestyle Changes introduced:

Symptom Changes noticed:

Follow-ups:

Musculoskeletal Complaints

When we look at diabetes, musculoskeletal issues rarely come to mind as possible initial warning signs of a metabolic disease. However, there are several quite important conditions that may serve as important warning beacons. Many of your musculoskeletal symptoms may have to do with your blood composition and blood circulation levels. For instance, elevated blood sugar levels affect the viscosity of your blood. The thicker your blood, the less blood flows through the fine capillaries.

Sticky blood affects anything from wound healing to the function of your eyes and that of your nerves. Eye problems and neuropathies, therefore, are common complications of diabetes. However, it is important to recognize the early changes. The sooner you become proactive, the better your chances to avoid further blood sugar imbalance and cell damage.

Also, because of the changes to your blood, your extremities (hands and feet, elbows and knees, shoulders and hips) appear to be affected most easily. As you will see in this chapter, problems with your legs, feet, or wrists too may be important early indicators of an increased risk of diabetes and must not be ignored.

And then there is the all important loss of bone density. Particularly women simply expect to show decreased bone density scans with increasing age. However, loss of calcium may be a possible indicator of gastro-intestinal issues and a direct reflection of reduced mineral absorption.

Tendons too can suffer. Feeling increasingly stiff, or a tendency towards tendon injuries, also indicate mineral deficiencies and absorption challenges. They too may serve as possible indicators of early blood sugar imbalances and need to be looked at in the context of a metabolic risk.

Let us now take a closer look at some of these conditions and what they can teach us about avoiding diabetes.

Restless Legs Syndrome

Jumpy or jerking limbs on trying to fall asleep appear to be a rather common complaint among individuals who experience blood sugar spikes. Newest statistics find restless legs syndrome in up to ten percent of the general population. Allopathic medicine considers it an issue mostly experienced by those fifty and older. In my patient work I have encountered restless legs syndrome in younger individuals too. From the feedback I receive, it particularly appears to affect persons suffering from the precursors of impaired glucose transport.

Western medicine still lacks the rationale for restless legs syndrome and, to date, does not offer a cure. For now, the common approach is to make a connection with neuropathic issues and to put people on prescription medications that affect their nerve and brain function. Some of these medications have rather significant side effects. Natural medicine is not looking to medicate the affected system (nerve transmission) but is looking for a possible cause as a starting point for changes. This is what may be taking place:

We have learned that insulin is supposed to transport glucose into the cells in order to produce energy. In many pre-diabetics and diabetics, as well as in kidney disease patients, this mechanism has become disturbed. Maybe you have ingested a larger than acceptable glucose load with your latest evening meal and, for some reason or other, your system cannot handle the absorption of the additional glucose molecules. As a result, and if there is a lack of insulin production or an insulin resistance, the sugar cannot enter your cells where it should be converted to energy. Instead, it remains in your blood vessels for too long and reduces the ability of your blood to carry oxygen to your tissues including your nerves and your extra-cellular fluid. Your blood figuratively turns sticky. At the time of falling asleep many patients report a sensation of humming or tingling in fingertips, toes, and calves. Your body's tiny nerve endings literally feel frazzled. Rapid, jerky, mostly involuntary movements of your limbs appear to bring some short-lived release, but they are not the answer.

Deeper seated mineral deficiencies may trigger enzyme and vitamin shortcomings. Among them the B group of vitamins and iron play a role. In fact, we quite commonly find slightly depressed iron levels in many patients who complain about restless legs syndrome long before they are diagnosed with anemia by western medicine. Carbohydrates require B6 vitamins for their conversion into glucose. B1, B2, B3, B5, and biotin are later needed for glucose to be converted into energy. In addition, excess proteins too are converted into

145

glucose. These amino acids require B6, B9, B12, and more biotin for this process (see figure 16, p. 273). Making sure that you get the right amounts of the necessary B vitamins, therefore, is paramount. And, since many minerals are needed for your vitamins to become absorbed, your health professional also may want to carefully assess possible underlying mineral deficiencies.—A likely problem, particularly if you are affected by intestinal issues.

We have seen how sugar highs can prompt a dangerous period of subsequent low blood sugar. These same excess sugar levels also affect the fine endings of your nerves and interfere with the normal signal transmission in your body—in addition to eventually plunging you into a hypoglycemic episode. If you counteract such a hypoglycemic phase with another sugar boost you catapult yourself back on the hyperglycemia-hypoglycemia roller coaster. The result of such an approach is predictable: your symptoms—namely wakefulness, humming or tingling nerves, and jumpy legs—worsen. It is best to prevent such incidences in the future by avoiding glucose peaks. Pay attention to what you have eaten prior to your occurrence of restless legs syndrome. Maybe you choose to keep a detailed food journal until you have become well acquainted with your body's response patterns.

If you are affected by restless legs syndrome it is important that you discuss these issues with your specialized healthcare provider who can assist you with your body's trace mineral, vitamin, and nutrient balance. Remember: your body attempts to preserve itself! At times, not being able to fall asleep restfully may be one of the ways that your body uses to protect and warn you. You will find out more about the natural approach in *Part Three, Most Common Supplementing Needs for Diabetics* (p. 300) and in the companion volumes, the *DIABETES-Series Little Books*.

26. *FACT Summary Restless Legs Syndrome*

FAVOR	essential fatty acids, antioxidant-rich and low carbohydrate, low sugar foods, B group vitamin supplements.
AVOID	blood sugar roller coaster, soft drinks, alcohol.
CONSULT	your qualified mainstream or natural healthcare professional.
TEST	mineral, iron and vitamin B levels particularly vitamin B6, blood glucose and other diabetes-related tests.

Your Personal Notes

Symptoms—Date(s) first noticed:

_____

Symptoms—Description:

_____

_____

Consultation Date(s) and with whom:

_____

Tests—Results:

_____

_____

Lifestyle Changes introduced:

_____

_____

Symptom Changes noticed:

_____

_____

Follow-ups:

_____

_____

Leg Cramps

Another predicament for many individuals with metabolic issues is their sometimes nightly battle with leg or foot cramps. These dreaded charley horses range from mild to severe and usually come on out of the blue. Cramps can be extremely painful. In a worst-case scenario the muscle cramping may be strong enough to partially misalign a small toe joint or even cause mild to severe muscle strains.

Remedies include practical approaches. Electrolyte imbalances should probably top your list of items to address. Not drinking enough fresh water throughout the day or drinking too much coffee, which is known to have a diuretic effect on your system, can be significant triggers. Dehydration is a common reason for leg cramps because a dehydrated body builds up extra lactic acid—a condition that is experienced by many individuals who are at risk of developing diabetes. Drinking a glass of spring water (avoid tap water if you are on a water softener system!) at the first signs of muscle spasms has instantly helped many of my patients. You would be surprised how quickly this works.

Western medicine often cites calcium imbalances in connection with muscle spasms. According to our natural medicine understanding, a calcium deficiency is directly related to a chronic state of metabolic acidosis—the very reason why you experience the lactic acid build-ups that I mentioned earlier. Remember, excess sugar in your blood turns your blood acidic. Consequently, your body mobilizes calcium from your bones in order to balance your increasingly acidic blood pH value. Apart from the lactic build up, I suspect that redeposits of leached-out calcium in your soft tissue also may contribute to the dreaded cramps.

Sometimes magnesium or adequate amounts of vitamin D3 are needed first in order to support your calcium absorption. However, taking extra calcium and magnesium tablets is not always effective because of the inefficiency of your gut (*duodenum*). Your natural healthcare practitioner may suggest a homeopathic equivalent or another form of supplements that use the mucous tissue of your mouth for quicker absorption, and in order to bypass your already compromised gastrointestinal system.

Some individuals make a connection between eating red meat for dinner and a greater likelihood of waking up with muscle cramps. Red meat supplies a different and easier absorbable form of iron than do other natural sources of iron, including vegetables. An excess heme-iron boost (iron from a meat source) may lead to a temporary effect on the mineral balance and, in particular, the iron to copper ratio in the blood supply to your muscles. This reduces your blood oxygen levels and, thus, aids in your muscles' cramping up.

There is yet another explanation. Zinc and copper are known iron antagonists. With quite some likelihood these minerals will already be significantly deficient if you are diabetic or at risk of diabetes. Again, the impact of a sudden heme-iron boost will create an even greater imbalance in your essential mineral ratios. This imbalance is apt to trigger a more violent response of your musculoskeletal system.

As for some first response suggestions: try putting weight on the affected limb by stepping on it or by pushing it against a hard surface at the first signs of cramping. You may find the cramps rescind quicker if you step on a cold floor. An old Swiss folk remedy had us wear a copper penny in our bed socks and between the insoles of our day-shoes to avoid muscle cramps. If the chemical reaction between the body's perspiration and the copper was enough to influence the trace mineral balance in our body may be debatable. It worked; that was all that mattered!

Today we understand why the copper penny may work, namely because iron and copper are antagonists. Allow me to caution you from buying a copper supplement of any kind (other than using a copper coin in your shoes or a copper bracelet)! Copper can be highly toxic to your body; and, there are other and safer ways to bring up your essential mineral balances, which we will discuss in *Part Three, Most Common Supplementing Needs for Diabetics* (p. 300). Therefore, once again, consult a knowledgeable natural medicine practitioner before you get yourself on any possibly dangerous supplement regimen.

27. *FACT Summary Leg Cramps*

FAVOR	plenty of fresh, clean water, balanced diet, mineral supplements as per tests.
AVOID	diuretics, calcium deficiency, large amounts of red meat, soft drinks, blood sugar spikes.
CONSULT	your qualified mainstream or natural healthcare professional.
TEST	iron or copper levels, blood gases, blood glucose and other diabetes-related tests.

Your Personal Notes

Symptoms—Date(s) first noticed:

Symptoms—Description:

Consultation Date(s) and with whom:

Tests—Results:

Lifestyle Changes introduced:

Symptom Changes noticed:

Follow-ups:

Easy Bruising

According to our standard medical texts easy bruising is mostly attributed to fragile vessels and is not considered a serious condition. Period! If you bump into an object and you get a bruise that is considered normal. In a couple of days the affected area will turn all colors of the rainbow. A few days later the bruise is supposed to have disappeared.

For the diabetic and the individual at risk matters are a bit more complicated. It is a sign of deeper imbalances when you find new bruises on your arms and legs without remembering having hit a hard object. Seldom, do these bruises heal within a couple of days. In fact, some bruises even may end up as open sores and wounds. Bruises in diabetics and already in individuals at risk of diabetes tend to be persistent. Bad wound healing—in addition to pointing to sugar level fluctuations—may indicate deep underlying nutritional malabsorption or malnutrition issues. It is part of the big picture presented by an essential mineral deficiency and by the reduced oxygen-carrying ability of your blood.

The association between bad wound healing and diabetes is well known. The problem, however, is common among most patients who suffer from a malabsorption process, be that diabetes, celiac disease, irritable bowel disease, or any other gut-related functional disturbance. Before jumping on the diabetes bandwagon, therefore, eliminate all these other conditions as possible causes. The danger is that the common tendency towards malabsorption shown by individuals who are affected by any of these conditions easily predisposes you to secondary problems. Over time, your nervous system may also suffer and lead to a gradual loss of sensation. The bruises may go undetected, may open into ulcers, and prompt more serious problems—such as the ones we will address in the chapter about *Amputations* (p. 233).

Bruises are a result of leaking capillaries and may be consistent with blood loss and some level of anemia. Iron deficiency and vitamin B12 deficiency present additional known challenges to the pre-diabetic or diabetic individual. These deficiencies must be dealt with swiftly in order to stop further tissue damage. Unfortunately, it is not as simple as snacking out on vitamin B12 tablets or iron pills. In fact, such indiscriminate supplementing habits might lead to additional and unwanted consequences. For this reason I always advise against supplementing without prior consultation with a knowledgeable and responsible health professional.

28. *FACT Summary Easy Bruising*

FAVOR	balanced diet, mineral supplements as per tests.
AVOID	unstable and excess blood sugar loads, soft drinks, alcohol, smoking.
CONSULT	your qualified mainstream or natural healthcare professional.
TEST	iron, vitamin B, and other mineral levels, blood gases, blood glucose and other diabetes-related tests.

Your Personal Notes

Symptoms—Date(s) first noticed:

_____

Symptoms—Description:

_____

_____

Consultation Date(s) and with whom:

_____

Tests—Results:

_____

_____

Lifestyle Changes introduced:

_____

_____

Symptom Changes noticed:

_____

_____

Follow-ups:

_____

_____

Muscle Pain

Muscle pain is quite common in the diabetic or the person at risk of diabetes. The good thing about muscle pain is that it indicates that you still can feel. Alterations in your glucose absorption mechanism are the primary source of this phenomenon. As we have seen, your cells need blood sugar to produce energy. Insulin resistance or lack of insulin production may block this absorption and conversion process. Consequently, more blood sugar remains in your blood stream and, in turn, reduces the oxygen-carrying ability of your blood and allows for lactic acid build-up. This hinders the blood circulation through your muscle tissue. Your muscle tissue no longer receives its essential nutrients. As a result, your muscle tissue produces less energy. Over time, you find yourself losing muscle tone. In a lean person this will be noted as atrophy. In an overweight or obese person you may more likely observe your muscles going flabby.

Because your muscles no longer are properly nourished you will soon experience unrelieved pains and perhaps much increased stress on your now unsupported and weakened joints. Many of your body's essential building blocks are known to be chronically deficient in diabetics. We have pointed to this many times and will discuss it in greater detail in *Part Three, Most Common Supplementing Needs for Diabetics* (p. 300). However, rather than being simply caused by a lack of nutrients, your muscle pain may also be a result of a process that actually demineralizes your musculoskeletal system; this is directly connected to your blood composition and supply within your tissue.

Your blood needs to maintain a constant acid-alkaline balance slightly on the alkaline side. If it tends to the acidic side it immediately remedies this by dissolving existing building blocks from your body. Calcium and magnesium are some of the first substances affected in this manner. The main reason for their depletion is that they are easily available through extraction from your skeletal system, and that they are able to rapidly balance your blood pH level. We already have mentioned how these minerals are re-deposited as plaque in your arteries, thus making less blood flow available to your tissues and possible putting you at risk for a cardiac event. Deposits also can target your joints and lead to calcifications and arthritis. Or, they may target your soft tissue and cause painful conditions such as rheumatism and even lead to fibromyalgia.

My clinical work has taught me to carefully look at any chronic muscle pain in the context of metabolic acidosis; and, since this includes the demineralization of your bones, to consider considerable mineral deficiencies and a possible long-term risk of diabetes. Do not underestimate, therefore, what your muscles may try to tell you and seek the advice of your knowledgeable health professional.

29. *FACT Summary Muscle Pain*

FAVOR	water, green or white tea, balanced, mostly alkaline diet containing ample green vegetables.
AVOID	acid-producing, processed foods, fatty meats, soft drinks, alcohol, smoking.
CONSULT	your qualified mainstream or natural healthcare professional.
TEST	pH value, blood glucose and other diabetes-related tests.

Your Personal Notes

Symptoms—Date(s) first noticed:

_____

Symptoms—Description:

_____

_____

Consultation Date(s) and with whom:

_____

Tests—Results:

_____

_____

Lifestyle Changes introduced:

_____

_____

Symptom Changes noticed:

_____

_____

Follow-ups:

_____

_____

Diabetes-Related Foot Problems

Now that you understand how your unstable blood sugar values affect the oxygen and nutrient supply of every cell in your body it should become easier to see why those body parts further away from your trunk may be affected first. High blood sugar, combined with its effect on your blood's oxygen-carrying ability, seems to affect the viscosity of your blood. Quite obviously, this reduces the circulation rate and the availability of essential nutrients to the more distant parts of your body. Blood circulation to your feet, in particular, is even more reduced if you are not very physically active.

With too much sugar in your blood your nerves no longer receive their necessary nourishment either. You gradually lose sensation in your extremities. This is when matters can become dangerous because you no longer feel properly. Your feet have to work even harder if you happen to be overweight—as are many individuals at risk of diabetes. In such a case, your weight distribution may be less than ideal. Build-ups of thickened skin on your soles are common results; so are injuries that may go undetected. You should take seriously any corns, ingrown nails, blisters, or those thick patches of hard skin on the side of your foot or on the sole between your toes. If you are overweight your tummy gets in your way when you try to check your feet. You no longer may be able to lift your feet to a level where you can inspect them properly and daily. Injuries to the sole of your foot and between the pads of your toes, therefore, are easily missed; particularly if you have lost sensation. Your feet consequently become infected and abscessed. Proper and timely treatment is absolutely essential.

What you wear is important! Many diabetics or individuals at risk of diabetes may think that their shoes fit—when in fact they don't. You must avoid pressure points at any price. Special orthopedic insoles or shoes are available for people with diabetic and other foot problems. Make use of what is available and keep checking regularly with a foot care expert who is especially trained to deal with diabetes-related issues.

Remember, any undetected injuries may become infected. Any repeat foot problems and bad wound healing are obvious warning signs of uncontrolled blood sugar spikes. Without someone cleaning up these infections quickly and lastingly, ulcers and eventually gangrene may settle in and, in a worst case scenario, necessitate amputation. This, unfortunately, is an all too common complication of diabetes. I should not have to stress that foot problems are entirely avoidable with proper care.

30. *FACT Summary Foot Problems*

FAVOR	fitting shoes or diabetic shoes or inserts, daily visual checks and carefully dried feet and toes after every shower or bath.
AVOID	barefoot walking, ill-fitting or open-toe shoes, pressure points.
CONSULT	your foot care specialist regularly.
TEST	blood glucose and other diabetes-related tests.

Your Personal Notes

Symptoms—Date(s) first noticed:

_____

Symptoms—Description:

_____

_____

Consultation Date(s) and with whom:

_____

Tests—Results:

_____

_____

Lifestyle Changes introduced:

_____

_____

Symptom Changes noticed:

_____

_____

Follow-ups:

_____

_____

_____

Fungal and Bacterial Infections

Fungal and bacterial infections too are common among individuals with diabetes. If you are not already diabetic when you develop such infections for the first time, they may serve you as an important warning sign of a possible risk of pre-diabetes. To make matters worse, fungal infections can lead to deep cracks and ulcers in your skin, and create the ideal conditions for secondary bacterial infections.

Oral thrush and even vaginal overgrowth frequently are also related to starting high blood sugar levels. Don't let your health professional simply shrug off such issues as *Candidiasis*, a fungal infection common to individuals with gastrointestinal issues. Your candida symptoms may be indicative of more serious issues: blood sugar imbalances and starting kidney problems.

Most foot conditions—from strong foot odor to infections and even swollen ankles—are linked with insufficient kidney function. It goes something like this: Hyperglycemia (high blood sugar) reduces your blood circulation. In addition, and over time, high blood sugar levels contribute to a deficient immune system. This in turn allows an environment conducive to skin infections, such as fungus in the spaces between your toes.

Fungal infections, no matter in what tissue they surface, are hard to eradicate. Western medicine "treats" them by suppressing them. Needless to say, this approach rarely proves successful long-term. Again and again, suppressed infections return along with unpleasant itches, rashes, and burning. Topical dressings may protect from additional infections. But, no reliable results can be achieved long term unless the root cause is addressed, your blood sugar related problems. Otherwise, there is always the danger that the infection may move deeper and start to affect the bone leading to what we call osteomyelitis.

Fungal infections are particularly persistent if you experience underlying chronic signs of metabolic acidosis—our ever-recurring baseline for individuals prone to blood-sugar imbalances. It is best to emphasize alkaline foods and avoid acid-producing foods such as grain carbohydrates, processed foods, soft drinks, and alcohol. In addition, impeccable personal hygiene is important. It is good practice, after every shower or bath to make it your habit to dry your feet thoroughly—especially in-between and around your toes—in order to prevent fungal infections. Therefore, once again, depending on your condition keep up that running biweekly or monthly appointment with your foot care specialist. Once a year is simply not enough!

31. *FACT Summary Infections*

FAVOR	dry, clean feet, daily visual inspections, alkaline diet.
AVOID	wet feet, open sores, acid producing foods.
CONSULT	your foot care specialist and natural medicine professional.
TEST	blood glucose and other diabetes-related tests.

Your Personal Notes

Symptoms—Date(s) first noticed:

_____

Symptoms—Description:

_____

_____

Consultation Date(s) and with whom:

_____

Tests—Results:

_____

_____

Lifestyle Changes introduced:

_____

_____

Symptom Changes noticed:

_____

_____

Follow-ups:

_____

_____

_____

Bunions

An interesting phenomenon seems to be common to many people with diabetes and to those individuals with celiac disease. As a structural osteopath, I frequently see patients who experience recurring issues with an unstable pelvic or sacroiliac alignment. One leg frequently appears longer when these patients are resting on their back on the treatment table. Many of these same patients also suffer from a foot condition called hallux valgus, or bunion.

Bunions affect predominantly one foot: the one that carries increased weight. I find that, most often, the reason for uneven weight-bearing is the above mentioned misalignment of either the sacrum or the pelvis, or both. In quite a number of patients it is easily possible that such misalignments have existed since birth.—A valid reason for us structural osteopaths or chiropractors to suggest that you have your babies checked during their first year of life.—If any misalignments are present, your body weight increasingly may fall towards the inside of your foot. Many overweight individuals show this with a knock-kneed stance in younger years. In this condition it is hard to properly roll your feet when you walk; not least, because a collapsed arch often goes with this position. After a while, the impact on the joint of the big toe may lead to a local inflammation. In its initial, inflammatory stage this tends to be rather painful.

However, the swelling of the big toe joint is not the whole problem. In time, the uneven weight distribution leads to an angle change of your big toe. Calcium deposits around the joint edges are common too. The big toe starts to point towards the midline or even the outer edge of your foot rather than pointing straight ahead. Soon enough, your big toe joint becomes unstable and forms an angle with the long (*metatarsal*) bones of your foot. In elderly patients this always entails the possibility of a total joint luxation (dislocation). These changes must be caught in time; otherwise, the base of the toe may start to push through the skin of your foot. Open wounds and infections are bringing you a sure step closer to future amputations. Surgery may be necessary to prevent the base of your big toe from rolling out of its joint to avoid causing more problems. Thus, take care of it in the earlier stages.

It is important to understand that—unless the cause (such as a misalignment of your sacrum or your pelvis) is corrected—no surgical procedure that attempts to correct your bunion will offer true and lasting relief. In the upcoming chapter *Complications, The Largely Avoidable "After" Facts* (p. 233) we will talk more about your feet. Proper daily care and a maintenance program with a diabetes foot specialist, hopefully, will keep you safe from these complications.

32. *FACT Summary Bunions*

FAVOR	well fitted shoes and a good spinal, postural maintenance program.
AVOID	badly fitting shoes or quick fixes of supposed uneven leg length by means of sole and heal lifts.
CONSULT	your chiropodist and your qualified structural osteopath or chiropractor.
TEST	blood glucose and other diabetes-related tests.

Your Personal Notes

Symptoms—Date(s) first noticed:

Symptoms—Description:

Consultation Date(s) and with whom:

Tests—Results:

Lifestyle Changes introduced:

Symptom Changes noticed:

Follow-ups:

Carpal Tunnel Syndrome

Less known than any of the above described foot problems, yet high on the list of suspected warning signs for possible pre-diabetes, may be signs of carpal tunnel syndrome in your wrists. It is generally accepted that repeat motion injuries, extreme tension, rheumatoid arthritis, or neuropathy (a complication of diabetes) may cause carpal tunnel syndrome. Carpal tunnel syndrome in these cases is the result of the narrowing of the nerve duct at the base of your wrist. This narrowing and constant pressure exerted on the sheath of the nerve may lead to inflammation and to temporary or permanent nerve damage, extreme pain, and reduced range of motion.

From my clinical experience—and, as a former pianist—I can state that it is rather unusual to find repeat motion triggered carpal tunnel syndrome simultaneously in both wrists. But, this is precisely what we are seeing in many a diabetic or pre-diabetic person. A small 2006 English study found that at least thirty-five percent of those individuals diagnosed with carpal tunnel syndrome might already be affected by metabolic changes. In plain English, these individuals found out that they were pre-diabetic when they were diagnosed with carpal tunnel syndrome. The nerve damage leading to carpal tunnel syndrome in these individuals may quite easily be explained by the known damage of high blood sugar levels on the fine nerve endings, particularly those of your extremities. Most importantly, these findings confirm that a lot of physical and functional damage occurs to the body well before you become aware that you are showing signs of pre-diabetes or even full-blown diabetes. The earlier you recognize a possible risk the more you can do to counter it.

My experience leads me to believe that future studies might confirm these findings especially in individuals who display pain or full-fledged carpal tunnel syndrome in both wrists. For more than a quarter of a century I have been working with patients who looked me up for help with constant pain in both wrists or individuals who came to see me after they had undergone bilateral surgery for carpal tunnel syndrome. I find it remarkable that many of these individuals kept complaining about continued and unchanged pain long after their surgery. Since most of these individuals also happened to show early warning signs pointing to probable pre-diabetic changes I routinely put them on my "urge-to-change lifestyle" regimen. In those who followed my recommendations the wrist pain-related problems soon disappeared.

I am, therefore, not at all surprised at the findings of the above-cited study. It provides lots of food for thought and, you too can help unravel the many questions we still have about our hugely growing threat of diabetes: Keeping an open mind and advising your healthcare professional of possible signs and connections between carpal tunnel syndrome and pre-diabetes is but such a first step.

33. *FACT Summary Carpal Tunnel Syndrome*

FAVOR	essential fatty acid and antioxidant-rich, low carbohydrate, low sugar foods.
AVOID	inflammation producing foods, soft drinks, surgery as a first line of action.
CONSULT	your qualified mainstream or natural healthcare professional.
TEST	blood glucose and other diabetes-related tests.

Your Personal Notes

Symptoms—Date(s) first noticed:

_____

Symptoms—Description:

_____

_____

Consultation Date(s) and with whom:

_____

Tests—Results:

_____

_____

Lifestyle Changes introduced:

_____

_____

Symptom Changes noticed:

_____

_____

Follow-ups:

_____

_____

Skeletal Instabilities

High or fluctuating blood sugar levels directly affect your nerve impulses. Needless to say, sugar hikes also affect many other biochemical processes in your body. Whatever the actual trigger or missing prompt may be, the absorption of your essential cell- and tissue-building blocks becomes compromised once your glucose levels are out of control. It is assumed that a value of 7 mmol/L or 126 mg/dl presents the threshold above which cellular damage becomes possible. Such internal blood sugar instabilities directly affect your skeleton because they raise the acidity level of your system. As we have seen, calcium, magnesium, and other elements may need to be mobilized from your bones and teeth in order for your body to adjust the acid-alkaline balance of your blood. As a side effect, this results in bone loss and weakens your structural support system.

Your skeleton may be affected also indirectly. If your tendons, muscles, and other surrounding tissues receive less than their share of essential nutritional substances and oxygen they will fail to support your spine and joints. No longer will they be able to protect your hip and shoulder joints, or keep the blood flow to your extremities intact. Remember our traditional Chinese medicine *Five-Element* chart (p. 63)? TCM stipulates: When the *spleen* (western: pancreas) no longer functions properly your muscles fail to receive their necessary nourishment. Such patients are said to suffer either from a *deficiency* that we would call "muscle weakness," or an *excess*-condition we might call "muscle cramps."

Directly linked to your food intake and TCM's *spleen* "transport and transformation" function is also the function of the *liver* according to traditional Chinese medicine. TCM believes an imbalance in the *liver* to affect your tendons, which, it says, may ail from a *deficiency* (weak joints, loss of strength) or an *excess* condition (rigid, stiff joints). Wandering pains are common in people with metabolic syndromes. In TCM wandering pains too are associated with the function of the *liver*. Muscles (*spleen*), tendons (*liver*); *liver* and *spleen* (or pancreas) are responsible for your metabolism and are linked to the state of health of your musculoskeletal structure. Doesn't it rather astonish that, already thousands of years ago, the Chinese recognized this connection and directly tied it in with your food intake and lifestyle?

According to my experience, individuals at risk of diabetes and full-blown diabetics alike tend to show similar patterns of musculoskeletal problems. A malposition of the sacrum tops this list. Pelvic or sacroiliac misalignments lead to low back discomfort and are probably also connected to mineral deficiencies and unbalanced mineral ratios. As we have seen in a previous chapter, these structural imbalances nearly always end up being reflected in the position of your feet where they prompt more or less severe changes.

Stitches between the shoulder blades too are a common complaint of diabetics—as well as female heart disease patients. In western medicine we speak of *dermatomes* when we look at the skin zones, which are supplied by particular nerves that exit in pairs from between your vertebrae. This theory of the *dermatomes* and the traditional Chinese medicine theory of the *back-shu points*, both draw a connection to your internal organs. Each spinal segment with its related pair of nerves is believed to influence one of your organs. What always amazes me is how both theories (western mainstream medicine and traditional Chinese medicine) are in full agreement as to which spinal area reflects and influences which organ function. It is interesting that these aforementioned stitches, indicating system weaknesses, often occur either at the level of the heart point or that related to diabetes, according to TCM.

The possible musculoskeletal warning signs of metabolic changes are many. Neck problems too may be indicative of a metabolic risk. Neck pain, blockages, and misalignments may point to sleep apnea, tooth grinding, and other aspects we have discussed earlier. Furthermore, any chiropractor or osteopath will acknowledge a direct structural connection between neck problems and low back misalignment or discomfort.

It is hard to isolate one body part from another. Especially along your spine there are many links and interconnections. You should, therefore, pay close attention to any issues and problems that your musculoskeletal system seems to indicate. Both, western anatomical knowledge and traditional Chinese medicine theory agree on this. Keep your structure sound and your internal organs and functions may work better!

34. *FACT Summary Skeletal Instabilities*

FAVOR	good posture and exercise, essential fatty acid and antioxidant-rich, low carbohydrate, low sugar foods, individual exercise plan.
AVOID	bad lifestyle choices, procrastinating, back tension.
CONSULT	your qualified osteopath or chiropractor and your mainstream or natural healthcare professional.
TEST	X-rays, blood glucose and other diabetes-related tests.

Your Personal Notes

Symptoms—Date(s) first noticed:

_____

Symptoms—Description:

_____

_____

Consultation Date(s) and with whom:

_____

Tests—Results:

_____

_____

Lifestyle Changes introduced:

_____

_____

Symptom Changes noticed:

_____

_____

Follow-ups:

_____

_____

Deteriorating Vision

Eye disease due to diabetes is one of the leading causes of blindness in North America. According to mainstream medicine full-fledged eye disease is considered a complication of diabetes. We, therefore, will discuss it in greater detail in the chapter about eye disorders under *Complications, The Largely Avoidable "After" Facts* (p. 236). However, it is very important that you realize how significant early vision changes are. They may alert you well prior to other signs and can point you into the direction of approaching diabetes. Vision changes ought to prompt you into immediate lifestyle changes.

⇨   Are you experiencing difficulties reading?

⇨   Are you misreading numbers?

⇨   Is your vision blurred?

⇨   Is night-driving becoming increasingly stressful?

⇨   Can you read smaller type on your computer screen but you can no longer read your newspaper?

⇨   Are you considering getting a new prescription for eyeglasses?

Think again; it may not simply be natural aging that is affecting your vision. It may well be the first signs that the fine blood vessels and nerve endings that supply your eyes are affected by chemical imbalances and, in particular, by blood sugar fluctuations.

You better schedule a visit with your medical doctor before you spend your money on new glasses as soon as you notice three or more of the signs and symptoms described in *Part Two–Signs and Symptoms, The "Before" Facts*; particularly so, if these signs and symptoms go along with any of the vision changes listed above. Once you experience these vision problems, chances are that you no longer are properly regulating your blood sugar levels.

As with many of the other early warning signs and symptoms, if you don't pick up on them in a timely manner—or if you delay or resist making the necessary lifestyle modifications—you may be faced with more serious complications later. Let your eyes guide you to a healthy lifestyle!

35. *FACT Summary Deteriorating Vision*

FAVOR	essential fatty acid and antioxidant-rich, low carbohydrate, low sugar foods, specific mineral and vitamin supplements, bright lighting.
AVOID	oxidative stress, processed foods, soft drinks, alcohol, lack of exercise, insufficient lighting.
CONSULT	your qualified eye doctor and mainstream or natural healthcare professional.
TEST	eye tests, blood glucose and other diabetes-related tests, mineral levels.

Your Personal Notes

Symptoms—Date(s) first noticed:

_____

Symptoms—Description:

_____

_____

Consultation Date(s) and with whom:

_____

Tests—Results:

_____

_____

Lifestyle Changes introduced:

_____

_____

Symptom Changes noticed:

_____

_____

Follow-ups:

_____

_____

Summary of Diabetes Risk Indicators

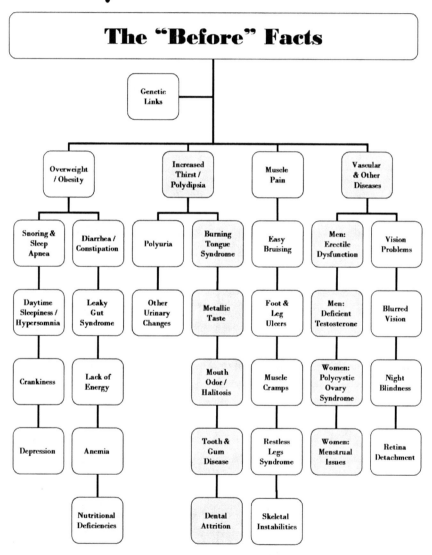

Figure 10 Diabetes Risk Indicator Summary

Knowing Underlying or Predisposing Factors

After we have looked at some of those "Before" conditions whose possible link with pre-diabetes and diabetes is frequently missed, let us now move on to those that show a clear and obvious link with diabetes. Many of these are major illnesses by themselves and may surface long before you are diagnosed with diabetes. Unfortunately, western medicine tends to look at these conditions as separate and unrelated problems. It rarely associates them with an increased future risk of diabetes, despite research indicating a clear link. This is probably a major reason why diabetes does not get diagnosed until very late in the game (see also p. 29).

Thyroid conditions, for instance, are widespread; as common as overweight and obesity are and which they seem to be related to. Your thyroids are part of your endocrine system, but are no more than one determining factor for your health and wellbeing. Your adrenals too play an important role. For some reason, few mainstream primary care physicians look at adrenal deficiencies for a possible connection to a risk of diabetes. Stress has long been a buzzword and has been related to diabetes. But, most importantly, stress directly affects your adrenal system. Without your adrenals working properly your entire hormonal system falls out of line, including your thyroids. Since diabetes is a hormone-related disease it should be obvious that adrenal and thyroid imbalances may directly affect your risk of turning pre-diabetic and diabetic.

Stress can cause additional problems: a wide range of addictions. Individuals under stress are more likely to smoke, drink, or over-eat. Smoking and alcohol-related problems are generally considered risks for your lungs and liver. Yet, daily smoking and alcohol consumption have also been linked to an increased risk of developing pre-diabetes and diabetes. Why is the public not informed about this negative effect of smoke exposure on your liver and your pancreas and its ability to produce insulin?

Smoking and drinking acidify your tissues and organs; so does over-eating, eating the wrong foods, and not eating the right foods. An acidic system is open to any onslaught from within and from without. Since your body is a network of tightly interacting processes and reactions it will respond to any "wrong

170

input" with a function decline. Nothing remains without an effect on parts or the whole of your system. For this reason, natural medicine professionals will always consider all functions of your body and not simply a single system. This is where mainstream medicine, unfortunately, misses out much of the time. For example, when you show elevated blood pressure most doctors may treat you for hypertension and vascular disease and not for the causative factors of smoking, alcohol consumption, and tissue acidity. The implications are obvious. We cannot separate what is done to the body (or what is omitted) from how it functions.

Many of us natural medicine practitioners are trained to check for possible links between these seemingly "unrelated" problems. But, even in our environment, the awareness about possible indicators of a future risk of diabetes still needs to be raised. At any rate, whenever any of the symptoms and syndromes discussed in the following chapters surface you always (emphasis on *always*) should keep a close eye on the possibility of an increased risk of pre-diabetes and diabetes; especially, if you have come up with another one or two conditions out of our list of "Before" facts.

Smoking

Smoking plays a significant role in the development of diabetes and drastically increases your risk of hypertension (p. 176). You don't smoke? That does not mean that you are risk-free. Even if it is downplayed, that same risk of smoke inhalation exists for exposure to second-hand smoke too. Smoking or exposure to second-hand smoke affects both your liver and your pancreas. Any changes in their function over time will affect how your body produces and uses its insulin. It is but one small step from these pancreatic function changes to an increased risk of pre-diabetes and diabetes.

Secondly, and very directly, smoking affects the oxygen-carrying ability of your blood and ups your chances of developing chronic metabolic acidosis, an almost certain predictor of diabetes or cancer. We will look into these implications in greater detail at the end of this section (p. 206). The bottom line is that lack of oxygen in your many tissues and functions will as severely impact your body's function as a dirty carburetor will reduce your car's performance.

Thirdly, there are other considerations if you smoke or are exposed to second-hand smoke: Smoking builds up unacceptable levels of toxins in your body and brain, such as cadmium, lead, and many other addictive substances. Most of these toxins are stored in your fatty tissue—indefinitely. Since they are cumulative your increasing toxin levels will contribute to a general slow-down of healthy body functions. Most importantly, these toxins break down your body's immune system response. It is simple, the longer you smoke—or are exposed to someone who smokes—the lower becomes your body's ability to fight disease.

The bottom line is that smoking influences the way your body absorbs its nutrients. It plunges your body into an overall state of nutrient deficiency. Minerals are among these nutrients and they should be one of your built-in mechanisms that could help remove toxins from your tissues. If toxins build up faster than they can be removed your minerals burn out and never get a chance to do what they are designed for, namely to promote your hormone and enzyme production. Little wonder, that hormone-related problems, such as erectile dysfunction (p. 85), low testosterone levels (p. 88), and infertility are becoming so wide-spread and are being linked to smoking and other lifestyle factors.

If you smoke—or someone you know smokes—get help to stop. But realize that stopping to smoke should go hand-in-hand with other lifestyle changes, especially when it comes to food choices, an individualized supplement regimen, and exercise.

36. *FACT Summary Smoking*

FAVOR	exercise in fresh air, antioxidants, balanced diet high in minerals and vitamins, personalized natural detox supplements.
AVOID	smoking, second-hand smoke and other environmental dangers.
CONSULT	your qualified mainstream or natural healthcare professional.
TEST	blood gas levels, toxins and mineral deficiency levels, blood glucose and other diabetes-related tests.

Your Personal Notes

Symptoms—Date(s) first noticed:

_____

Symptoms—Description:

_____

_____

Consultation Date(s) and with whom:

_____

Tests—Results:

_____

_____

Lifestyle Changes introduced:

_____

_____

Symptom Changes noticed:

_____

_____

Follow-ups:

_____

_____

Alcohol

Alcohol consumption too may precipitate your diabetes. Alcohol directly turns to sugar and considerably raises your blood glucose levels. Regular alcohol consumption will also put you at risk of developing hypoglycemia (low blood sugar) because it provokes increased insulin secretion from your pancreas. In addition, alcohol impinges on your liver. It does not take long for your liver function to be affected, particularly, if you consume alcohol (even in smaller quantities) on a regular basis.

From beer to vine to hard liquor, they all impact on your physical system; and, the less compatible the drink, the sooner you will be facing trouble. A lower alcohol content does not necessarily make for fewer problems. There may be additional, hidden dangers in drinks such as in beer. The mineral and toxin profile of many beer drinkers shows unacceptably high cobalt levels—possible remnants from beer brewed in the traditional copper kettles. Cobalt is accumulative and toxic in larger amounts. Beer drinker's cardiomyopathy is but one of the possible heart health threats.

Furthermore—and not directly related to its alcohol content—one of the ingredients used for the production of beer is malt. Malt is derived from barley, a gluten-containing grain. The malt content of beer may well be the root cause of your inflamed gut. This is especially true if you are one of those individuals that tend towards gluten-sensitivity, intestinal inflammation, and bloating. If that is you, even one beer now and then is not acceptable. The beer-belly says it all!

Grain-based liquors too may trigger these same issues with gluten; needless to say, a good reason to stay away from any of these drinks. What about red vine, rum, or some similar gluten-free option? While some supposed health benefits of grapes are making headlines, the sugar content of even one glass of vine is no less than the allowance for a whole meal for the person at risk of diabetes. Wouldn't you rather eat some nutritious and satisfying food instead? Needless to say, rum and other similar—albeit grain-free, mostly fruit-derived—liquors are even higher in their sugar content and, therefore, are not an option either.

When it comes to metabolic threats, as you see, there is some truth to that talk about the "beer" belly. At any rate, if you or one of your friends develops a beer-belly you should carefully, and at regular intervals, check into an impending threat of pre-diabetes or diabetes.

37. *FACT Summary Alcohol*

FAVOR	water, green or white tea, roiboos tea, and high-antioxidant, low-sugar fruit drinks— such as pomegranate juice diluted with spring water.
AVOID	unstable and excess blood sugar loads, beer, liquors of any kind including whiskey, vodka, possibly wine, especially white wine.
CONSULT	your qualified mainstream or natural healthcare professional.
TEST	enzyme levels, BMI (body mass index), blood glucose and other diabetes-related tests.

Your Personal Notes

Symptoms—Date(s) first noticed:

_____

Symptoms—Description:

_____

_____

Consultation Date(s) and with whom:

_____

Tests—Results:

_____

_____

Lifestyle Changes introduced:

_____

_____

Symptom Changes noticed:

_____

_____

Follow-ups:

_____

_____

_____

Hypertension

When your blood pressure starts climbing above 140 mm Hg (*systolic*) and 90 mm Hg (*diastolic*) you are said to experience raised blood pressure or to head towards a condition called hypertension. If you are found to suffer from diabetes and if at the same time your blood pressure goes above 130/85 mm Hg you are considered at high risk. Many general practitioners will want to start preventive treatment, speak prescription medication.

We already have seen that smoking may lead to hypertension. Other causes for hypertension are excess salt use—something we will yet be looking at in greater detail. Impaired kidney function or existing insulin resistance may prompt hypertension too; and, even chronic acidity may play a role. Blurred, vision, head aches, facial flushing along with dizziness and fatigue are common symptoms.

Unlike mainstream medicine, natural medicine considers hypertension and vascular disease both complex, not singular, conditions. We know that several biochemical processes play a role in the development of high blood pressure. Before we look at some of them in more detail, I want you to consider the following: Your red blood cells live between 105 to 120 days. This gives you the minimum time frame within which natural choices and lifestyle modifications can become effective. Therefore, improved lifestyle choices will show positive results in as little as three to four months. A small effort for making a huge difference to your life, wouldn't you say!

The sooner you realize that your blood pressure is too high the better. If, however, you already are in immediate danger you may not be able to avoid prescription medication. These prescription medications generally are considered "for life." If you do not eliminate the underlying metabolic acidosis by adopting immediate lifestyle modifications your downhill slide has begun; never mind improved lab results thanks to your prescription medications. From the moment your doctor puts you on any of these prescription medications you will figure in the medical records as one of the moderate to high-risk mortality patients. It is largely up to you if you end up becoming one of those statistics or not. Even on prescription medication you have a choice and the opportunity to change the medical statistics (and your health) in your favor.

If you are determined to eliminate the triggers and sources of your hypertension by eliminating your destructive food habits it is important that, right from the get-go, you discuss this with your physician. If your doctor understands that you are seriously committed to stringent lifestyle modifications there are ways to work with the prescription medications as temporary solutions only. Just be aware that few health professionals will be prepared to stick out their neck for you. You better be credible and prove willpower in battling the acidification and early decay of your body by controlling what you eat and drink.

We will be looking in detail at how this acidification comes about in the chapter about *Metabolic Acidosis* (p. 206). The downside of the process of metabolic acidification is that you have calcium float around in your blood vessels, looking to deposit itself in any of your body tissues—including the walls of your blood vessels. In many overweight people the minerals drawn from your bones contribute to the deposits along the walls of your arteries. In time, this solidifies into plaque build-up. Once plaque has built up on the walls of your arteries these will become either less pliable (hardened arteries), or the diameter available for your blood to circulate freely simply becomes diminished (plaque build-up). In both instances your blood pressure rises. This very mechanism puts you at risk for stroke and heart disease; and, it also may point you towards a future with diabetes.

The calcium, magnesium depletion of your bones is not the only process that causes high blood pressure. Excess sodium chloride (as contained in table salt) coupled with deficient potassium intake also fundamentally contributes to blood pressure problems. If you want to maintain the natural mineral balance of your body—and, in fact, this is what health is all about—you want to consume on average no more than one part of sodium to five parts of potassium. In North America most people consume at least ten times more sodium than potassium (p. 312). Way out of balance! Your body pays for this imbalance without delay!

If your blood pressure is above the acceptable range most physicians and dieticians will recommend that you restrict your salt intake. This is the correct approach if you consume too much salt either by adding it tableside to everything you eat or by consuming high levels of hidden sodium when you eat processed foods and salted snacks. Remember, salt is a traditional preservative and is beng added to anything in brine, such as pickles and, of course to roasted nuts, chips, and other snack foods.

However, many of the more health-conscious patients may fall into the opposite trap of stopping their salt intake totally. They are then highly surprised when such an approach fails to make the desired difference to their sodium-potassium balance. From a natural medicine standpoint, the idea of restricting your salt intake to reduce hypertension may fail to bring the desired results unless you drastically increase your potassium levels or address any underlying hormonal problems.

Just allow me to caution you: it is not as simple as eating more bananas and potatoes to bring up your potassium levels. In fact, their extra starches may prompt other problems that your body may pay for dearly, such as producing temporary sugar spikes. Therefore, once again, I cannot stress enough how important it is for you to seek the advice of a knowledgeable health professional. It is important to set up an individualized program before you make changes to your eating regimen or spend money on maybe the wrong supplements.

When we look at the sodium-potassium imbalance the idea of having to increase one element in order to lower another (less desirable one) is not new. Unlike with their recommendation to restrict salt in order to lower your sodium levels, these days the medical community advocates that you should raise your good cholesterols in order to reduce your bad ones. Finally, we are getting one step closer to an agreement on a treatment approach between mainstream and natural medicines! Now mainstream medicine needs to apply the same principle to your electrolyte balance as well.

I have always been curious to find out why so many pre-diabetics and diabetics tend to consume higher amounts of salt. Natural medicine reasons as follows: Due to your malabsorption syndromes the essential mineral balance in your body systems is off—as we have explained. This results in an impaired function of your taste buds. It also prompts your body to signal that it lacks some essential minerals. Salt (or sugar) being the most easily available substance, therefore, usually is the first that comes to mind and is craved.

Your healthcare practitioner can help you identify what specific minerals you need to supplement, when, and for how long. Since the functions of most minerals are interconnected in some way or another you do not want to self-medicate. This could quite quickly make your imbalance and overall condition even worse.

38. *FACT Summary Hypertension*

FAVOR	antioxidant-rich and low carbohydrate, low sugar foods, specific and individualized supplement regimen.
AVOID	acid producing and fatty, processed, and high-carbohydrate foods, soft drinks, alcohol.
CONSULT	your qualified mainstream or natural healthcare professional.
TEST	electrolyte and essential mineral levels, BMI (body mass index), blood glucose and other diabetes-related tests.

Your Personal Notes

Symptoms—Date(s) first noticed:

_____

Symptoms—Description:

_____

_____

Consultation Date(s) and with whom:

_____

Tests—Results:

_____

_____

Lifestyle Changes introduced:

_____

_____

Symptom Changes noticed:

_____

_____

Follow-ups:

_____

_____

_____

Vascular Disease

In the previous chapter we looked at what elevated blood pressure can do to you. Long-term effects of high blood pressure may lead to vascular disease. Vascular disease is categorized into micro-vascular disease (such as in changes to your eyes), and into macro-vascular disease (such as in general heart problems and specific heart diseases). High blood pressure is just one of the possible shifts in your system. Elevated cholesterol, lipid, and triglyceride levels are other possible imbalances that affect the biochemical processes of your body. All of them contribute to vascular disease.

Vascular disease is most closely connected to diet, sedentary lifestyle, obesity, hypertension, hyperglycemia, and smoking or alcohol. Even mainstream medicine suggests that individuals with diabetes should pursue healthy eating habits in order to control their blood glucose levels. This mostly involves restriction of refined carbohydrates and alcohol. In addition, your physician will suggest a regular exercise regimen and will strongly discourage smoking and alcohol intake in order to avoid further build-ups along your blood vessels.

Along with your vascular system your liver and pancreas are most strongly involved in regulating the metabolic processes that lead to vascular problems. Your liver plays a particularly important role in the removal of unwanted lipids. Your lipoproteins are classified as very low density (VLDL), low density (LDL), and high density (HDL). High triglyceride and low HDL-cholesterol (the "good" ones) values are the most common undesirables.

As soon as your laboratory report shows these values outside their acceptable range your doctor will probably want to put you on statin or other drugs. These drugs are designed to improve your laboratory test results. Once this happens it will be difficult to get your system turned around for good. The medication will immediately start doing your body's job. And true, the results in most cases will appear to be positive. However, don't forget, as long as you are on medication, better lab reports do not mean that you are in better health! No different from when we discussed hypertension, the problem here too is that the prescription medications do not change what has led to your condition in the first place. The medication in your system will block your body's ability to alert you to your imbalances. Your body will consider its own defense system superfluous and may shut down its built-in coping mechanisms. Without drastic changes to your lifestyle, your system hits a downhill slide; soon you will need higher doses and additional prescription medications to counteract the side effects of the earlier ones.

During an initial consultation with a new patient I routinely ask about their history of high blood pressure, hypertension, or possible initial signs of vascular disease. It happens surprisingly often that these patients deny experiencing even the slightest issues. Yet, short, rapid breaths, flushed cheeks, a reddish nose tip, and sometimes even a multitude of small red capillaries showing in the white of their eyes are a sure sign give-away; as are these patients' slightly eruptive and overly assertive mannerisms. Naturally, we must guard against mistakenly interpreting the flushed cheek signs of allergies as those of hypertension or vascular disease. But, to the trained health professional the distinction should be clear. So, why do many (especially younger) patients with obvious initial signs of hypertension and vascular disease fall through the cracks of our mainstream health screening system?

Even if your laboratory results show highly elevated lipid or cholesterol levels it does not mean that your doctor will warn you about the risks you are in for. Overworked doctors have failed to call back such patients and to discuss their immediate need for lifestyle changes. Male patients with above margin lab results, in particular, seem to fall through the cracks of the system. Worse, when told about their high cholesterol and lipid levels these "tough guys" tend to brush off the results as not important. Denial is no solution! The "bad boy" pride is totally out of place when it comes to an imbalance of your lipid levels. Plate-sized steaks and fries don't make you appear more "manly." In fact, your libido will probably already have paid the price and, with certainty, keeping up such an approach will move you a step closer to becoming an emergency statistic. The bottom line is: You do not want to wait for this to happen. You want to start with your lifestyle changes long before you develop lipid problems and other vascular changes!

39. *FACT Summary Vascular Disease*

FAVOR	immediate and thorough lifestyle changes including food, drink, and exercise.
AVOID	unstable and excess blood sugar loads, high-fat foods, soft drinks, alcohol, smoking.
CONSULT	your qualified mainstream or natural healthcare professional.
TEST	blood glucose and other diabetes-related tests.

Your Personal Notes

Symptoms—Date(s) first noticed:

_____

Symptoms—Description:

_____

_____

Consultation Date(s) and with whom:

_____

Tests—Results:

_____

_____

Lifestyle Changes introduced:

_____

_____

Symptom Changes noticed:

_____

_____

Follow-ups:

_____

_____

Adrenal Deficiency

We looked at the traditional Chinese medicine approach to how your body creates energy when, in *Part Two, Figuring out Your Risk*, we discussed the symptom of increased thirst (p. 64). There, we drew the parallels between the traditional Chinese medicine understanding of the *kidney* element and our western medicine knowledge of the function of the adrenals. According to our western interpretation your adrenal glands are responsible for the production and control of some fifty of your body's hormones. Among those are the well-known stress hormone cortisol (a *glucocorticoid*), DHEA (*dehydroepian-drosterone*), and aldosterone.

As we have seen earlier, distressed levels of cortisol may lead to increased insulin sensitivity and may disturb your conversion mechanism of carbohydrates, fats, and proteins. This is a very important point to remember. Cortisol production in a healthy individual reaches its low around midnight and its peak in the early morning hours. In the diabetic individual this natural cortisol-high frequently is not present. We already have mentioned this condition as the "dawn syndrome" experienced by many diabetics as a reaction of the liver's need to produce increased amounts of glycogen. Such an increased glycogen output usually follows a nightly period of hypoglycemia. Insulin sensitivity is an inevitable result.

While these processes affect much of your neuromuscular function, cortisol deficiency also reduces your ability to cope with stress and your resistance to infections. Frequently disregarded by mainstream medicine practitioners, adrenal deficiency is one of the conditions opening the door to many serious diseases. Aside from illnesses, real or perceived stress of physical or mental origin is one of the major inducers of adrenal deficiency.

Let us recap the most common signs related to adrenal deficiency:

⇨   Unmotivated to exercise or exhausted after moderate exercise.

⇨   Unable to get out of bed early morning.

⇨   Cannot get going but improves towards lunchtime.

⇨   Energy trough around two o'clock in the afternoon followed by a short energy-high early evening.

⇨   Easily tired but too exhausted to sleep, and waking up every couple of hours.

⇨ Reduced immune system function leading to frequent allergy attacks or colds.

There are other indicators too that may alert you to a possible battle with adrenal deficiency. These include repeat cravings for sugar, salt, caffeine, or codeine-containing colas. If you make it a habit of repeating, "I just need that cup of coffee to get going," you need to strengthen your adrenals to get you going! The coffee, coke, or extra sugar, or salt do nothing but give you a short-lived pick-up followed by an even greater crash. These substances, in fact, will increase the stress on your adrenals by causing inflammatory responses throughout your body and depressing your cortisol levels even more. When it comes to your adrenals light initial stimulation over time turns into full-fledged burnout. Surely, this is not the way to go; yet, this is exactly how coffee, cola, sugar, and salt affect your body's energy exchange system. Time to look at the real cause and get away from these band-aid solutions!

Think of it this way: You experience the warmth of a nice campfire. When you walk away from it your body perceives the surrounding cold as even colder. So, you return to the fire and add another log or two to warm up your body. At some point it gets too hot for you to sit close to the fire. You again move away a little ways only to get shivering even worse. In fact, you may end up turning up that heat even more until your entire surroundings catch fire.

Autoimmune diseases, fibromyalgia, confusion, anxiety, depression, and a variety of other symptoms also find one of their causes in adrenal deficiency. Most importantly, in *Part One, The Basics* (p. 19), we pointed to the role of cortisol imbalances in the early development of diabetes and hypoglycemia. You, therefore, don't want to wait until you are diagnosed as a diabetic before you start working on your stress-induced adrenal deficiency.

There are several different approaches towards balancing and strengthening your adrenals. They largely depend on your body's essential mineral and electrolyte balance. Only your knowledgeable natural health practitioner can help you avoid mistakes and find the most effective route.

40. *FACT Summary Adrenal Deficiency*

FAVOR	antioxidant-rich and low carbohydrate, low sugar foods, supplements according to your test results.
AVOID	stress, acidifying foods and drinks, soft drinks, alcohol, caffeine.
CONSULT	your qualified mainstream or natural healthcare professional.
TEST	hormone, electrolyte and mineral levels, thyroid levels, blood glucose and other diabetes-related tests.

Your Personal Notes

Symptoms—Date(s) first noticed:

_____

Symptoms—Description:

_____

_____

Consultation Date(s) and with whom:

_____

Tests—Results:

_____

_____

Lifestyle Changes introduced:

_____

_____

Symptom Changes noticed:

_____

_____

Follow-ups:

_____

_____

_____

Thyroid Dysfunctions

If you are at risk of diabetes one underlying cause may be that your thyroid glands function below par or are burdened with too great a toxic load. Your thyroid glands form an important part of your endocrine system. They produce and control a large number of hormones that, in turn, regulate your various body functions. Your thyroids provide a function somewhat comparable to that of your car's spark plugs.

Thyroid and other endocrine dysfunctions may influence your diabetes risk directly, as in hypothyroidism or hyperparathyroidism, or in a more round-about way, such as via thyroid toxicity. In our natural medicine practice we are not satisfied with simply remedying your present problem, that is, your risk of diabetes. We like to get to the root of your issues, in this case the condition of the organs that provide the drivers and regulators known to be weakening or supporting your body's metabolism.

Hypothyroidism

For decades, hypothyroidism was considered a condition present mostly in post-menopausal women. This view is changing rapidly. Men too and much younger women now seem to be affected by it; even teenagers and young school age children. Many of those affected by hypothyroid disorder are overweight. And many of those overweight do not realize that they may be affected by some stage of a thyroid condition because their lab results still fall within the "acceptable" range.

In the natural medicine community many of us wonder how much of this rapid spread of hypothyroid conditions might be attributed to the high toxin levels present in our environments and our city and town water. Phenols, PCBs, PBBs, dioxins, perchlorates, and a long list of additional chemicals are considered "good" to "strong" contributors to hypothyroidism. Dioxins, along with several other offenders, have been directly linked to the development of diabetes. Any of these toxins do affect your endocrine system and, therefore, influence the production, levels, or function of your natural hormones.

Hormones play a major role in your digestive process. They affect your carbohydrate, protein, and fat metabolism as well as the way your body is able to use many of the vitamins. Your thyroids not only affect your digestive processes, they also are involved in the way your body uses oxygen. They help activate your nerves and influence your muscle action. It is obvious that any damage—be it caused by the environment or by internal stress and imbalance—must result in an ailing state of your thyroids.

The following two forms of hypothyroidism are of particular interest with regards to their potential role in the development and progression of diabetes. Possible underlying factors for the secondary development of diabetes are:

1. a failure of your pituitary glands that leads to the secretion of insufficient amounts of TSH (thyroid-stimulating hormone)

2. a malfunction of your hypothalamus that prompts the secretion of insufficient amounts of TRH (thyrotropin-releasing hormone).

Intimately connected with the proper functioning of your thyroids is the essential mineral iodine. Iodine deficiency is on the rise despite the governments of North America and some other countries iodizing most of our commercially available table salts. It is interesting to note that several of my "salt-addicted" patients with high sodium levels show low iodine levels. If supplementing of salt with iodine were effective would we not expect iodine levels to rise with increased salt intake?

There are several other minerals that appear to affect the health of your thyroids. The fluoride added to your town drinking water and your toothpaste also may play an active role in the development of your hypothyroidism. Fluoride supplementation may decrease your calcium and magnesium levels, which are mediated by your endocrine glands—despite the supposed function of fluoride of assisting in the absorption of calcium.

You will easily recognize the signs and symptoms of hypoactive thyroid function if they are part of your pattern:

⇨ overall low body temperature

⇨ cold intolerance

⇨ slow but steady weight gain

⇨ difficulties losing weight

⇨ a puffy morning face with droopy eye lids

⇨ a somewhat swollen tongue in the morning

⇨ fluid retention (no, it is not fat!)

⇨ some levels of constipation.

In fact, higher sodium levels in your body will lead to greater water retention in your tissues. This fluid, therefore, no longer is available for excretion via the action of your intestines and kidneys and to help you clear your body of debris and toxins. The consequences are:

⇨ diminished energy levels

⇨ fatigue

⇨ brain fog

⇨ a tendency to depression

⇨ muscle aches

⇨ muscle cramps and joint pain

⇨ infertility and low sex drive

⇨ premenstrual syndrome

⇨ elevated cholesterol levels.

Frequently, hypothyroidism leads to dry skin and hair. Your hair may feel coarse and fall out; your nails may become brittle. Much of your skin may turn whiter because of a general level of anemia. However, occasionally the palms and soles of your feet turn a shade of orange, This happens because your body no longer is able to convert beta-carotene into vitamin A.

As we have seen repeatedly, many diabetics experience not only hyperglycemia (high blood sugar) but also many episodes of hypoglycemia (low blood sugar). Hypoglycemia and low blood pressure commonly relate to the hypo-function of your thyroid glands and, therefore, might point to hypothyroidism as an underlying condition. Rectifying your hypothyroid condition quickly and effectively might improve your problems with diabetes.

Together we have gone step-by-step through a detailed list of possible signs and symptoms of risks that may indicate a pre-diabetic or even diabetic stage. When you compare the above printed list of hypothyroid signs and symptoms with your typical diabetes-related issues does it not sound all too familiar? It may pay to start by addressing a possible thyroid function disturbance simultaneously with or even prior to dealing with symptoms of diabetes.

41. *FACT Summary Hypothyroidism*

FAVOR	antioxidant-rich and low carbohydrate, low sugar foods, supplements as specified by test results.
AVOID	hypoglycemia and blood sugar fluctuations, processed foods, exposure to environmental toxins.
CONSULT	your qualified mainstream or natural healthcare professional.
TEST	thyroid and adrenal tests, iodine and other mineral levels including iron, blood glucose and other diabetes-related tests.

Your Personal Notes

Symptoms—Date(s) first noticed:

_____

Symptoms—Description:

_____

_____

Consultation Date(s) and with whom:

_____

Tests—Results:

_____

_____

Lifestyle Changes introduced:

_____

_____

Symptom Changes noticed:

_____

_____

Follow-ups:

_____

_____

_____

Thyroid Intoxication

Your environment is toxic. Countless substances that influence your hormonal equilibrium surround you. These particles are present in everything from the air you breathe and the water you drink and bathe in to the food you eat, the clothes you wear, the mattresses you spend a third of your life sleeping on, the houses you live in, the carpets you walk on, and the offices or shops you work in. Many toxins need to be processed by your thyroid glands daily, hourly. The chicken or egg question holds true value here. It is hard to establish if toxins shut down the function of your thyroids after initially overtaxing them or if your thyroids are already previously weakened to the point that they fail to counteract these toxins.

In this context I want to mention no more than a couple of the most common and widespread of these toxic offenders. Among them we find mercury, chloride, and fluoride. Astonishingly enough, all three of them are elements many of you are in contact with every day. Their deposits in the body are cumulative and can have major implications for your health. Let us start with mercury:

Mercury finds its way quickly into your brain tissue and is still commonly found in your tooth fillings. It is also part of a substantial number of prescription medications such as some diuretics, laxatives, antiseptics, antifungals, and antiparasite remedies. From its widespread use in pesticides, mercury easily finds its way into the food chain and especially affects grains along with some of the animals that eat these grains. Via water run-off mercury finds its way into the algae that serve as a food source for smaller fish. These small fish then are eaten by larger fish, fish that in due course end up on your dinner table.

Mercury accumulates in your body at an estimated daily rate of 0.5 milligram of which one tenth is deposited in your brain where it blocks out the essential mineral zinc. This is an important fact: as we shall see in *Part Three, Macro- and Micro-Mineral Supplements* (p. 319), zinc is one of the most important essential minerals for your gastrointestinal health. Zinc also may have a significant role to play in the avoidance of diabetes. Other nutrients that have the ability to counteract mercury are vitamin E, selenium, and niacin (but please remember our earlier warning about niacinamides, p. 40).

While mercury is a straightforward toxin, chloride and fluoride do have an important role to play in the proper functioning of your body. They form part of your body's electrolyte system that also includes your sodium and potassium interaction. Hydrochloric acid, for instance, an important chloride-containing component of your stomach juices helps balance your blood pH and your elimination process and is highly essential to good health (in the right amounts).

If your natural fluoride and chloride levels are too low you may experience a greater likelihood of intestinal or sinus inflammations. On the other hand, excess amounts of chloride can result in raised blood pressure and iron deficiency anemia; all conditions that, once again, we frequently find in individuals diagnosed with diabetes and in those who are over-weight and obese (most of whose thyroids are affected). Chloride and fluoride also appear in the environment in their less humanly compatible forms as chlorine and fluorine. These are toxins and their widespread use negatively affects you very directly and by several avenues.

For instance, if you are on town or city water, you inhale considerable cumulative amounts of chlorine while you enjoy your morning shower or clean your house and wash your laundry. Remember you don't just breathe chlorine-filled air; you also absorb it directly through your skin. Last but not least, you ingest it after washing your store-bought vegetables in town water or after watering your supposedly natural herb-garden. Lately, chlorination is being widely considered as a possible cause for reduced male fertility, increased rates of urinary bladder and colorectal cancer, as well as for Hodgkin's lymphoma. But for the pre-diabetic and diabetic person its possibly harmful influence on your gastrointestinal tract and your body's pH value is of even greater concern.

No, I don't intend to send you into a panic mode. But, for quite some time now, the natural medicine community has suspected close links between our growing environmental crisis and the out-of-control spiraling occurrence of metabolic diseases such as diabetes and chronic gastrointestinal disorders. We see fewer cases of metabolic disease in people who are on their own well water— except where they treat it regularly with, guess what, chlorine and use salt to counteract its natural hard minerals.

Let us look at one more such toxin: fluoride. Fluoride initially was thought to help your teeth and bones. Consequently, it has been widely supplemented to daily necessities such as your drinking water and many commercial types of toothpaste. It is assumed that fluoride works by neutralizing in your mouth certain enzymes that play a part in the carbohydrate digestion. Unfortunately, fluoride may deactivate also many of the necessary enzymes. It is suspected that fluoride plays a role in the increased incidence of gastrointestinal lesions and that it hinders your glucose breakdown. For quite some decades already we have known that too much fluoride in your system—instead of hardening your bones—in fact, demineralizes them. Many studies, some of which quickly were contradicted by several government press releases, indicate that long-term supplementation with fluoride may significantly raise your risk of bone fractures and possibly even lower your IQ.

Our discussion of the negative impact of mercury, chloride, fluoride represents but a list of few examples. The catalog of toxins and natural or manmade compounds with the potential of overloading your thyroids is long and exceeds the scope of this book. Simply keep in mind that your body is made up of organic compounds. It is a system of highly intertwined and interrelated checks and balances, which directly and indirectly influence each and every action of your body's functions and processes.

To date, we have no way of foreseeing how your body will deal with each and every synthetic substance it is being confronted with for any length of time. Nor can we predict the short and long-term influence of the onslaught of what I call "recycled hormones" and "recycled prescription medicine cocktails" that are not yet being filtered out of our city water sources. Just as natural medicine looks at every individual as an indivisible system, so we cannot separate man from nature or nature's influence from man's health. But, at the same time, nature has given us all those substances that help us build a healthy body. To avoid what hurts us and to seek out what helps us should be our goal—always!

42. *FACT Summary Thyroid Intoxication*

FAVOR	organic, antioxidant-rich diet, a regular natural detox regimen according to your healthcare professional's suggestions.
AVOID	environmental and food toxins.
CONSULT	your qualified mainstream or natural healthcare professional.
TEST	thyroid values, toxic minerals, blood glucose and other diabetes-related tests.

Your Personal Notes

Symptoms—Date(s) first noticed:

_____

Symptoms—Description:

_____

_____

Consultation Date(s) and with whom:

_____

Tests—Results:

_____

_____

Lifestyle Changes introduced:

_____

_____

Symptom Changes noticed:

_____

_____

Follow-ups:

_____

_____

Hyperparathyroidism

It is your parathyroid gland—a group of small endocrine glands—that enables the demineralization of your bones and teeth. These tiny glands are located behind your thyroid glands on either side of your throat. Do you remember our discussion of fluoride in the previous chapter? Your parathyroid glands are one place where we suspect excess fluoride levels to play havoc. Any dysfunction of your parathyroid gland raises your alkaline phosphatase levels, an enzyme that works in an alkaline environment and is present in all body tissues, especially in your liver.

We distinguish primarily two imbalances leading to the hyper-function of your parathyroid glands: In your primary form of hyperparathyroidism high parathyroid hormone (PTH) levels prompt high serum calcium values, but low phosphorus levels. Since calcium levels affect your nervous system, many nervous disorders are part of this condition. High serum calcium levels may also promote stone formation and contribute to kidney ailments.

On the other hand, in your secondary hyperparathyroidism the PTH is low while high serum phosphorus levels may point to kidney disease. As you see, it comes back to mineral imbalances. Maintaining your body's calcium to phosphorus ratio of 2.5 to 1 is imperative. There is a much you can do about this: Save the environment and your own system; stop buying and drinking soda drinks of any kind.

Some of the most common symptoms of hyperparathyroidism are:

⇨ lack of energy or fatigue

⇨ depression

⇨ headaches

⇨ decreased sex drive

⇨ thinning hair

⇨ gastric esophageal reflux disease (GERD)

⇨ abdominal pain

⇨ hypertension

⇨ heart palpitations

⇨ kidney stones

⇨ bone pain and osteoporosis.

Demineralization is usually a sign of a chronic underlying metabolic acidosis. Most commonly caused by indiscriminate eating habits and drinking soft drinks daily, chronic metabolic acidosis can lead to a slew of gastrointestinal complications. Worst, it may culminate in full-blown diabetes. For this reason the proper functioning of your parathyroid gland is indirectly yet ultimately instrumental in avoiding a risk of pre-diabetes and diabetes. Therefore, keep in mind the list of symptoms and seek out the advice and support of a capable health professional.

43. *FACT Summary Hyperparathyroidism*

FAVOR	antioxidant-rich and low carbohydrate, low sugar foods.
AVOID	self-supplementing, processed foods, soft dinks and other carbonated drinks.
CONSULT	your qualified mainstream or natural healthcare professional.
TEST	PTH and other thyroid tests, mineral levels, blood glucose and other diabetes-related tests.

Your Personal Notes

Symptoms—Date(s) first noticed:

_____

Symptoms—Description:

_____

_____

Consultation Date(s) and with whom:

_____

Tests—Results:

_____

_____

Lifestyle Changes introduced:

_____

_____

Symptom Changes noticed:

_____

_____

Follow-ups:

_____

_____

Hypothalamus-Pituitary Disorder

Your hypothalamus consists of, some of the smallest structures in our brain. It links your endocrine system to your nervous system. It regulates and controls the connection between mind and body. Parts of your hypothalamus act as your body's pleasure and reward centre. Eating, drinking, and other primary drives rely on—or damage—the proper functioning of your hypothalamus. In particular, your hypothalamus regulates your appetite and assists in maintaining your normal body temperature. Obesity may be directly related to the functioning of your endocrine system. Excess appetite and extreme body temperatures most commonly indicate issues with your hypothalamus-pituitary-adrenal axis.

In the earlier chapters of *Part Two, Figuring out Your Risk*, we saw that polyuria (voiding large amounts of urine, p. 81) and polydipsia (feeling thirsty, or a fluid intake in excess of the average two liters of water a day, p. 64) are some of your earliest warning signs that your body may have reached a pre-diabetic state. So far, we have looked at an impaired kidney function as a possible cause. However, a disorder of your hypothalamus-pituitary function may cause polyuria as well.

These endocrine glands of yours may become deficient in the anti-diuretic hormone vasopressin (ADH). When vasopressin levels become low your blood sodium levels rise. This may constrict your blood vessels and result in kidney problems and hypertension. Along with it, as we shall see, excessive urine output and thirst may result in diabetes. Vasopressin does not act alone. Other hormones are involved too: for instance, in the fluid balance of your body the hormone aldosterone. Latter is produced by your adrenals. We briefly discussed it in the chapter about *Adrenal Deficiency* (p. 183).

It is particularly interesting to note that the following stimulate the release of vasopressin (ADH):

⇨   Exercise

⇨   Stress

⇨   Hypoglycemia

⇨   Beta-blockers and angiotensin medication

⇨   Prostaglandins.

On the other hand, these interfere with the release of vasopressin:

Rivkah Roth DO DNM®

⇨ Alcohol

⇨ Glucocorticoids

⇨ Alpha-blockers.

In summary, there are two possible connections between a hypothalamus-pituitary disorder and the development of diabetes:

1. A lack of vasopressin released to your kidneys may result in your near compulsive need to drink huge amounts of fluids. This most likely will result in insulin dependent diabetes.

2. Your kidneys fail to properly respond to the vasopressin release. This in turn will lead to type 2 diabetes. It also may prompt vision problems, nerve deafness, and the reduced muscle tone of your urinary tract and your bladder—a common reason for those uncontrolled and embarrassing in-a-hurry moments.

It almost certainly points into the direction of a vasopressin deficiency if you feel dizzy and queasy any time you do not have access to enough fluids for any length of time. As we have seen earlier, such a deficiency influences your glucose mechanism and predates the development of chronic kidney disease. This condition needs to be properly treated; otherwise it may snowball into a full-fledged complication, namely kidney failure and the need for dialysis.

According to western medicine problems involving vasopressin (ADH) are acknowledged to trigger temporary or permanent diabetes. As in most conditions, medication may bring about temporary relief. But, these drugs do not eliminate the cause of your biochemical imbalance. Natural medicine believes that by removing the cause and triggers we can help your body revert to a better state of health before such problems lead to permanent tissue damage. Needless to say, any symptoms that indicate the improper functioning of your endocrine system ought to be brought to the attention of your healthcare professional immediately.

44. *FACT Summary Hypothalamus-Pituitary Disorder*

FAVOR	according to symptoms and underlying causes.
AVOID	acid-alkaline imbalance, mineral deficiencies and ratio imbalances, processed foods, soft drinks, alcohol.
CONSULT	your qualified mainstream or natural healthcare professional.
TEST	aldosterone and vasopressin levels, kidney and urine tests, blood glucose and other diabetes-related tests.

Your Personal Notes

Symptoms—Date(s) first noticed:

_____

Symptoms—Description:

_____

_____

Consultation Date(s) and with whom:

_____

Tests—Results:

_____

_____

Lifestyle Changes introduced:

_____

_____

Symptom Changes noticed:

_____

_____

Follow-ups:

_____

_____

Renal Deficiency

Full-blown kidney disease is a frequent and incapacitating complication of diabetes that we will deal with in greater detail in a later chapter in *Complications, The Largely Avoidable "After" Facts* (p. 226). Your kidneys are significantly involved in filtering your blood, conserving or excreting water, and maintaining your acid-base balance. Renal or kidney imbalances and deficiencies may surface much sooner and in a less obvious manner then in fully developed kidney disease.

Mainstream medicine rarely mentions renal deficiency directly. Yet, according to natural medicine, and well before the other and more prominent signs of fullblown kidney disease show up, you may be heading towards a pre-diabetic or diabetic state when you show these signs of deficiencies. It is important for you to recognize kidney and bladder-related weaknesses as potential early warning signs. One such symptom we mentioned when we discussed polyuria, which can be caused by a deficiency of vasopressin (ADH) or a lack of response to it in your kidneys—we linked it to an underlying adrenal and stress issue.

Kidney-related symptoms may not surface until about the same time or even after your diabetes has become obvious. Yet, when looking at the intake questionnaires of patients given a clean bill of health by their general practitioner, I quite frequently can spot tendencies of impending problems by recognizing the mere accumulation of their many minor signs and symptoms. If you can use these early signs as nudges towards a healthier lifestyle—and, by that I mostly understand healthy eating and drinking habits—many of the known and logic consequences of stressed kidneys may never have to materialize. Recognizing these connections emphasizes the importance of you taking responsibility for how you treat your body. As long as you remain vigilant you quite likely will be able to avoid unpleasant complications and possibly diabetes itself.

External signs such as frequent urination or puffy and swollen ankles and legs are rather obvious. But, let me give you an example of how other kidney or bladder-related problems may be used as a predictor of diabetes in a natural medicine environment: Urinary tract infections have become all too common in today's society. More women appear to suffer from UTI than men. Your mainstream doctor prescribes antibiotics already while you wait for the laboratory test results. It you have ever found yourself in this situation you may be well aware how common it is for these test results to come back negative, indicating that there—supposedly—was no UTI. In the meanwhile, you have gone through excruciating pain every time you need to visit the washroom. More so, you have taken unnecessary antibiotics, thereby potentially reducing your body's response mechanism for when you really will need them. Yet, your mainstream doctor just shakes his or her head and mumbles something to the effect of "paranoia" or "pretending."

It is heartbreaking to see many of these patients thus labeled start to develop self-doubts. Needless to say, this adds to their already significant stress levels. In my practice I too have encountered many patients complaining about recurrent UTI-like symptoms combined with negative test results and no effective response to the customary mainstream medical treatment with antibiotics. Upon further investigation, quite frequently, I find a connection to excess potassium deposits. At the same time these patients show deficient levels of chromium, magnesium, manganese, sometimes sulfur, and some vitamins of the B group. Once these minerals are balanced the symptoms of their supposed urinary tract infections disappear. However, since the very same mineral imbalances may also be implicated in diabetes, I always suggest a thorough workup on these patients. Many of them are highly surprised to find that they are already well on their way to pre-diabetes.

This example of how UTI-like symptoms in a round-about way may lead to a suspicion of diabetes is not the only possible connection. Many natural medicine practitioners talk about Candida infections as another warning sign. Candidiasis, or Candida as it is called in short, is an opportunistic fungal overgrowth that can affect your entire system from mouth to gut to genitals. From what you have read in the chapter about *Leaky Gut Syndrome* (p. 119) you understand that such an overgrowth quite directly reflects a breakdown of your gastrointestinal health. In addition, there is always a possibility of secondary infections, such as a bacterial infection. Is it not interesting that the first recommendation for Candida is to avoid all sugars and many starches along with many other foods that also can have a negative impact on your blood sugar levels? When you will read the *DIABETES-Series Little Books,* the companion volumes to *At Risk?,* you will see much similarity with the tried and tested dietary recommendations for our *Natural Medicine Centre* diabetes patients.

These two examples don't exhaust all possible organ-related warning flags for early risk recognition. If I have opened a new approach to thinking of your body as "one indivisible whole," I have no doubt that you or your natural medicine practitioner will pick up on any possible connections much sooner than mainstream medicine tests will be able to indicate potential problems.

45. *FACT Summary Renal Deficiency*

FAVOR	antioxidant-rich and low carbohydrate, low sugar foods, supplements according to test results.
AVOID	stress, unstable and excess blood sugar loads, alcohol, smoking.
CONSULT	your qualified mainstream or natural healthcare professional.
TEST	adrenal hormones, levels of potassium, chromium, magnesium, manganese, sulfur, B vitamins, blood glucose and other diabetes-related tests.

Your Personal Notes

Symptoms—Date(s) first noticed:

_____

Symptoms—Description:

_____

_____

Consultation Date(s) and with whom:

_____

Tests—Results:

_____

_____

Lifestyle Changes introduced:

_____

_____

Symptom Changes noticed:

_____

_____

Follow-ups:

_____

_____

Nonalcoholic Fatty Liver Disease

Nonalcoholic fatty liver disease (NAFLD) is spreading particularly in the more affluent countries and among our young. When we discussed polycystic ovary syndrome (p. 92) we already encountered a link with nonalcoholic fatty liver disease. The link between diabetes and some forms of liver disease is not new either. A significant majority of those affected by nonalcoholic fatty liver disease suffer from metabolic syndrome and are likely to develop full-blown type 2 diabetes. Your serum ferritin levels appear to play a major connection between nonalcoholic fatty liver disease and diabetes. Chromium deficiency may be a determining factor in this.

Nonalcoholic fatty liver disease seems to be the result of inflammation and, due to excess fat accumulations, possibly fibrosis. These are all results of your high triglyceride levels. According to standard medical texts decreased levels of fatty acid oxidation or increased levels of free fatty acids may be among the first triggers of nonalcoholic fatty liver disease. Therefore, watch your triglyceride levels!

It is of particular interest that high carbohydrate intake has been connected with nonalcoholic fatty liver disease to a significantly greater degree than fat intake has been. This does not come as a surprise to many of the natural medicine professionals who long have recognized the biochemical processes associated with carbohydrate conversion. Fats do not make you fat to the same degree as carbohydrates do. Many diabetic patients do better on a low-carbohydrate diet, contrary to what most endocrinologists, diabetes educators, and nutritionists still recommend.

Insulin resistance versus the liver's glycogen producing function is another probable explanation that connects nonalcoholic fatty liver disease with diabetes. Both conditions tend to cause weight gain. In both conditions lifestyle changes are the most recommended approach towards disease control. The presence of nonalcoholic fatty liver disease, therefore, immediately should raise suspicion of a likely future with pre-diabetes and diabetes. Take NAFLD as a big red flag when it comes to your diet and lifestyle. Its message to you is that of a call to immediate and proactive change.

46. *FACT Summary Nonalcoholic Fatty Liver Disease*

FAVOR	max. 1-2 teaspoons daily of extra-virgin olive oil or grapeseed oil, antioxidant-rich and low-carbohydrate diet (max. 30 grams of grain carbohydrates per day), low sugar foods.
AVOID	fried, breaded, and otherwise fatty foods, any oil or fat sources other than the above, unstable and excess blood sugar loads, alcohol, smoking.
CONSULT	your qualified mainstream or natural healthcare professional.
TEST	liver enzymes and other liver tests, hormone levels, blood glucose and other diabetes-related tests.

Your Personal Notes

Symptoms—Date(s) first noticed:

Symptoms—Description:

Consultation Date(s) and with whom:

Tests—Results:

Lifestyle Changes introduced:

Symptom Changes noticed:

Follow-ups:

Your Food to Disease Avalanche

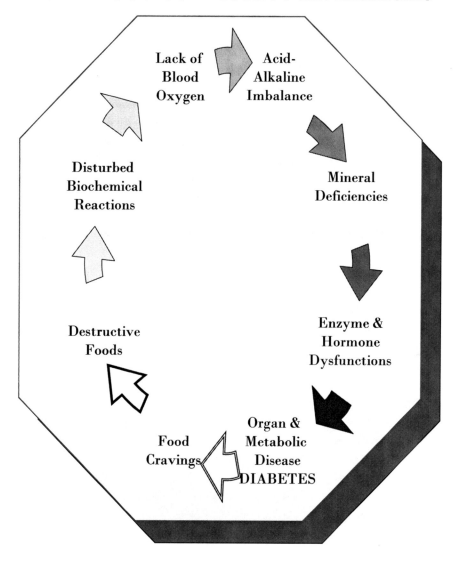

Figure 11 The Food to Disease Avalanche

Chronic Metabolic Acidosis

Temporary or chronic stressors exert a direct influence on your body chemistry and your body's citric-acid cycle, also called the Krebs Cycle.—This is your body's energy production mechanism during which CO_2 (carbon dioxide) for elimination from your system is being produced.—Such stress triggers include physical and mental stressors along with destructive food, exercise, and sleep habits. Any single one of them can cause mineral or hormonal deficiencies, which in turn may lead to significant imbalances that disrupt your body's homeostasis (internal balance). Ratio imbalances or deficiencies of essential minerals, along with other factors, may cause an excess of lactic acid in your system. This process is called "acidosis." Body acid values smaller than (<) pH 7 represent an acidic, those greater than (>) pH 7 an alkaline or basic metabolism.

As a result of metabolic acidosis the energy production from your calorie intake may be reduced by as much as eighty percent; allow me to put this in numbers: 80% of energy reduction! No car engine runs on a mere twenty percent of its typical octane requirements. Neither can a human being run on a mere fifth of its energy requirements. Yet, these days, statistics put the rate of people with metabolic imbalances at one out of every two. Pretty terrifying considering a possible future of a whole avoidable slew of illnesses from cancer to diabetes, wouldn't you agree!

As you shall see, metabolic acidosis may hold the answer for those cravings, fatigues, and other ailments of yours. All these symptoms clearly indicate that you are well advanced on your path towards conditions such as diabetes and, if the state of acidosis remains uncontrolled for any length of time, possibly even organ failure. Apart from speeding up your aging process, prolonged acidification of your body directly leads to a lack of blood oxygenation. An acidic body environment increases the number of free radicals in your system. In our natural medicine practice we call this an "acidic terrain," and we always treat it as a serious warning sign for things to come—unless immediate preventive action is being taken by the patient; such action being healthier lifestyle choices.

Metabolic acidosis may be implicated in many diseases, even in heart and vascular disease. Recognizing metabolic acidosis early is your first defense against plaque build-ups and serious cardio-vascular problems. This is how it happens: Your blood needs consistent and predictable levels of all of its components. Blood acidification causes calcium and other minerals such as magnesium to be extracted from your bones and teeth in order to rebalance your blood pH value. On one hand, this demineralization leads to bone loss and consequences such as osteoporosis. On the other hand, it may result in the hardening or narrowing of your blood vessels and in plaque build-up, which brings you one step closer to a major cardio-vascular event.

Hormones too are involved in this process of demineralization of your bones. The endocrine gland that enables calcium and magnesium loss from your bones and teeth is your parathyroid gland. We already have taken a closer look at the mechanics of this process in the chapter about *Hyperparathyroidism* (p. 194).

According to mainstream medicine two basic mechanisms may cause metabolic acidosis: One, your kidneys fail to excrete dietary hydrogen; in plain English, the liquid ingested with your food and drink. Two, your kidneys or gastrointestinal tract do not function properly and lose bicarbonate. If this happens, your body no longer is able to balance the blood pH value of pH 7.41 for your normal arterial blood and pH 7.36 for your venous blood. Herein lays the problem: Western medicine confirms a diagnosis of metabolic acidosis only once your blood pH values and your bicarbonate levels drop below acceptable levels. At that point, however, the imbalance becomes life-threatening and your blood no longer can find its homeostatic balance without outside interference.

It is for this reason that western medicine considers metabolic acidosis a complication of underlying conditions such as diabetic ketoacidosis or acute kidney failure. In short, allopathic medicine treats metabolic acidosis as an "additional" disease. In treating metabolic acidosis mainstream medicine, therefore, starts by medicating the condition which it considers to have caused metabolic acidosis, such as diabetes or kidney disease.

Starting from a distinctly different premise, natural medicine tends to see beginning levels of chronic metabolic acidosis as the determining and underlying factor in the development of the above mentioned conditions and not simply (in its severest form) as their consequence. In addition, natural medicine looks at metabolic acidosis as the slowly developing outcome of a variety of disturbed biochemical reactions that result in an imbalance of your body's acid-alkaline balance. According to this view, such imbalances lead to a slew of mineral deficiencies. These, in turn, influence anything from enzymatic reactions to other more complex hormonal and biochemical effects (see figure 11, p. 205).

The natural medicine approach appears to make sense since even mainstream medicine acknowledges that metabolic acidosis can take on a milder, yet chronic form. Nevertheless, according to our natural medicine view, even a low-grade acidosis must be understood as a clear warning sign of the possible unpleasant things to come. This point of view changes the entire approach towards dealing with the acid-base balance of your body in particular and with your state of health or disease overall. For this reason, natural medicine does not wait until metabolic acidosis becomes evident before it decides to intervene. Such an intervention, if it wants to be effective, preferably takes place at a much earlier stage of your imbalance. It, therefore, shows significantly greater promise towards complete reversal and rectification of many of the symptoms and, in fact, of diseases such as type 2 diabetes, celiac disease, and many other progressive, mostly gastro-intestinal and metabolic conditions.

It is pivotal to keep the acid-alkaline balance of your body stable. This entails many beneficial lifestyle and diet recommendations that all must be individually tailored to you. For this reason, you should consult a knowledgeable healthcare practitioner. Do not attempt to solve by yourself this million-piece puzzle of your state of health!

Let us look at metabolic acidosis yet from another, very timely aspect: carbon dioxide emission levels. It is not only our environment that experiences global warming; our bodies too are undergoing similar changes. Increased levels of blood acidity reduce your body's ability to carry oxygen. As we will see in the following chapter, carbon dioxide emission levels of a body in a state of chronic metabolic acidosis too are significantly on the rise. Now, without sufficient levels of oxygen your nerves don't function properly; nor do your organs and all your essential biochemical processes.

Remember, in the first paragraphs of this chapter we mentioned that metabolic acidosis could reduce your energy output to a mere twenty percent. Such a reduction does not even leave you enough energy to deal with your next meal—never mind, any other processes for which oxygen is vital.

47. *FACT Summary Chronic Metabolic Acidosis*

FAVOR	essential fatty acids, antioxidant-rich and low carbohydrate, low sugar foods, alkaline-based diet.
AVOID	processed foods, soft drinks, unstable and excess blood sugar loads, alcohol, smoking.
CONSULT	your qualified mainstream or natural healthcare professional.
TEST	blood gas levels, electrolyte balance, mineral deficiency levels, blood glucose and other diabetes-related tests.

Your Personal Notes

Symptoms—Date(s) first noticed:

_____

Symptoms—Description:

_____

_____

Consultation Date(s) and with whom:

_____

Tests—Results:

_____

_____

Lifestyle Changes introduced:

_____

_____

Symptom Changes noticed:

_____

_____

Follow-ups:

_____

_____

Oxygen is Essential
For Tissue & Organ Health

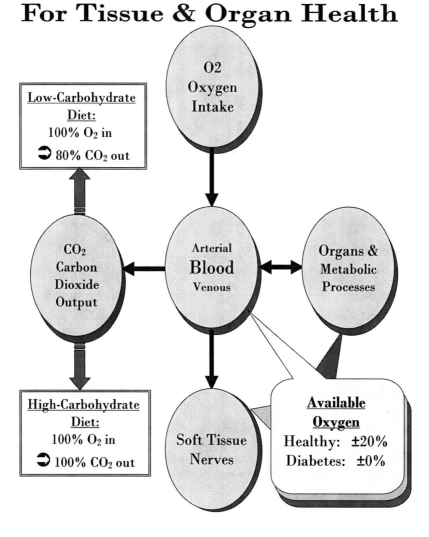

Figure 12 Oxygen for Tissue & Organ Health

Lack of Oxygen

"Show me and I believe you!" How often have we cited this expression! Yet, this principle of needing to see something in order to believe its existence fails when we pose the most fundamental question about what you ultimately require for survival. Your body needs water in order to hydrate and function. You can see and touch water. Much more so, your body needs oxygen. However, you cannot see nor grab air. Just a couple of minutes without air prompt certain death. Oxygen is the foremost life-giving element for us humans. No oxygen—no life! Little surprise that the first and foremost goal of blood transfusions is to re-establish the oxygen-carrying ability of your blood!

When we discuss the importance of oxygen it is not just about the air quality of the environment. While good air quality does make a huge difference it is the amount of oxygen you are inhaling and processing through your body that is directly responsible for the level of your health. Any lack of oxygen can bring about a large array of issues including diabetes and pre-diabetes related symptoms. We already have seen how disturbances in your acid-alkaline balance directly and rapidly influence your blood pH. These changes, in turn, affect the oxygen-carrying ability of your blood.

Oxygen plays an important role everywhere in your body. Another example of the role of oxygen you have seen when we briefly touched on metabolic acidosis such as in ketoacidosis (p. 81), a kidney condition frequently related to diabetes.

Your thyroid glands too play an important role in the manner in which oxygen is absorbed by your tissues. The function of your thyroid hormones includes two particular actions: One, thyroid hormones influence your metabolic rate by increasing the synthesis of proteins in all your body tissues. Two, your T3 cells, via a fairly simple mechanism, are believed to increase your oxygen assimilation particularly in your kidneys, heart, liver, and muscle tissues.

You may wonder how to best influence and control your oxygen intake and turnover rate. Several approaches work. A combination of all of them is best:

a) Regulate the acid-base balance by eating only healthy, balanced and sufficiently varied low-carbohydrate and—if you are even mildly overweight—low-calorie foods.

b) Drink the right kinds of fluids; and in sufficient quantities (see the *FACT Summary* and the companion volumes, the *DIABETES-Series Little Books,* for additional details). This assists your body in flushing out accumulated toxins and debris, and reduces headaches, brain fog, nausea, and pain.

c) Acquire proper breathing techniques through activities such as Qi Gong, Tai Chi, voice training, or music lessons focused on wind instruments. These techniques greatly tend to improve oxygen circulation through your entire body and brain.

d) Follow an exercise regimen that allows your body to burn off unneeded calories and fat. This will help to prevent toxins from building up and storing in your cells for any length of time.

We will come back to many of these points in greater detail in *Part Three, Diabetes can be Controlled* (p. 243). First, let us understand how your level of oxygen supply influences your state of health or disease and what a lack of oxygen may lead to in your body. Oxygen (O_2), the air you inhale, and carbon dioxide (CO_2), the air you exhale, are not present in equal amounts in your arterial and your venous blood. Instead—assuming that you are a healthy individual consuming a standard diet—you will exhale as CO_2 about eighty percent of the oxygen you inhale. Roughly twenty percent of oxygen, therefore, remains in your body for use in many of its processes.

This "surplus" twenty percent of O_2 is of greatest importance. Via your blood stream it reaches your various body tissues. This oxygen not only keeps your blood balanced, it also nourishes and drives your cells, organs, tissues, nerves, and muscles. As soon as there is less active oxygen available to your system, the proper function of your cells and, eventually also, of your organs is compromised. Dietary fats and carbohydrates directly affect this input-output balance between oxygen intake and carbohydrate output. If you are eating a high-carbohydrate diet your CO_2 output will rise, at worst, to equal your O_2 intake. This does no longer leave enough oxygen for the essential biochemical reactions and the necessary regeneration of your tissue.

Your cell functions consequently strive for a preservation mode. In short order, your metabolism slows down. Nerve endings and cells lack nourishment and impulses. Cells soon start to die off and the vicious cycle is quickly turning into a downhill spiral that affects your levels of energy and wellbeing. Chronic metabolic acidosis, therefore, is the jumping-off point for most of your undesirable signs and symptoms. Once your oxygen levels are below what your body needs it does not take long for your body to enter a state of disease; weight-gain and obesity are but two of the outcomes prompted by lack of oxygen.

If, on the other hand, you are on a high-fat diet you may actually experience an initial drop in your carbohydrate versus oxygen ratio. According to standard medical texts this may avail you of as much as thirty percent oxygen. At first sight this looks favorable. However, your body's workings are based on balance. Your cells are not designed to cope with that great an amount of oxygen. Any of those surplus oxygen molecules are easily captured and converted into less favorable and in fact undesirable compounds.—Once again disease is the logical outcome.

Allow me to remind you of another important function of oxygen in your body: Reduced blood oxygen levels severely impede wound healing and may be a factor contributing to easy bruising and blood clotting problems. We will yet need to talk about the dreaded amputations. Also we will discuss the role of proper blood oxygenation levels in that context in *Complications, The Largely Avoidable "After" Facts* (p. 234).

48. *FACT Summary Lack of Oxygen*

FAVOR	sufficient quantities of clean water, antioxidant-rich and low carbohydrate, low sugar foods.
AVOID	fried, breaded, and otherwise fatty foods, unstable and excess blood sugar loads due to high carbohydrate diet, alcohol, smoking.
CONSULT	your qualified mainstream or natural healthcare professional.
TEST	blood gas and essential mineral levels, blood glucose and other diabetes-related tests.

Your Personal Notes

Symptoms—Date(s) first noticed:

_____

Symptoms—Description:

_____

_____

Consultation Date(s) and with whom:

_____

Tests—Results:

_____

_____

Lifestyle Changes introduced:

_____

_____

Symptom Changes noticed:

_____

_____

Follow-ups:

_____

_____

_____

Gluten-Sensitivity

When dealing with type 1 diabetes patients many health professionals today will check into a possible link with gluten-sensitivity or full-blown celiac disease (CD), also called gluten sensitive enteropathy (GSE). Most celiac patients carry at least one of the human leukocyte antigen (DNA) markers HLA-DQ2, HLA-DQ8 (present in about 43% of the North-American population), or the HLA-B8 marker. Today, HLA-DQ8 is considered a possible genetic link common to a long list of autoimmune diseases and many patients who have been diagnosed with type 1 diabetes. Interestingly, many individuals with Northern European or Mediterranean roots seem to be more prone to developing gluten-sensitivity or diabetes.

The presently available diagnostic methods for gluten-sensitivity (other than screening for your DNA) leave to be desired. The numbers of patients with a confirmed mainstream medicine diagnosis of GSE or CD are still only in the one to two percent range of the population; nowhere close to the rate of potential genetic carriers. Earlier, we have seen that a diagnosis of diabetes may follow eight to fourteen years of symptoms. Celiac disease is another condition where diagnosis on average takes around eleven years.

When we consider the common problem of mineral deficiencies due to absorption issues and the metabolic acidosis brought on by these deficiencies, we can see how much many an individual at risk of diabetes might profit from a gluten-free lifestyle. Since not everybody suffering from gluten-sensitivity is equally sensitive to the three offending proteins (gluten, glutenin, and gliadin) many patients go undetected for years. For instance, nearly half of our North American adult rheumatics have been shown to be gluten-sensitive. Interesting, isn't it? Other conditions that can be possibly linked to a gluten-sensitivity but are not associated with autoimmunity are food allergies, lactose intolerance, constipation, diarrhea and, due to the malabsorption factor, also obesity. Did you count how many of these conditions are potentially reflected in patients at risk of type 2 diabetes?

Here are, in alphabetical order, just a few of the autoimmune conditions that possess potential cross-links with gluten-sensitivity and, maybe, an increased risk of diabetes: Addison's disease (underactive adrenal glands), hypoglycemia, low blood pressure, low body temperature, anemia (iron deficiency), childhood asthma, chronic autoimmune hepatitis, dermatitis herpetiformis, Grave's disease (increased thyroid activity with bulging eyes), lupus, muscle weakness, pernicious anemia (chronic gastrointestinal and

215

neurological disturbances because these patients cannot absorb vitamins and minerals), rheumatism, thyroid toxicosis, ulcerative colitis, and many other conditions.

We have seen that up to now there is no cure for diabetes. Likewise, there is none for gluten-sensitivity or for its full-blown form, celiac disease. But, since the triggers of the physical manifestations are known, there are options: No need to treat when you avoid the cause. The recommendations consequently center on total avoidance of the trigger glutens. For the patient sensitive to gluten a life without complications requires a one-hundred percent strict adherence to a gluten-free lifestyle; even the proverbial one gram contamination factor is a glitch that must be avoided. This requirement is for life. It is simple, and it works!

Naturally, there are no instant cures. It takes time for your immune system and your gastro-intestinal tract to heal. Most newly diagnosed individuals report significant improvements within two weeks of keeping to a gluten-free diet. Those who continue to show symptoms, quite likely, have not yet eliminated all the hidden glutens, or they may be consistently exposed to contamination. The major impediment over and above the hidden gluten in food is this contamination factor. It cannot be stressed enough that it takes as little as one gram of gluten to keep the inflammatory responses in your system active and to stop your gut from healing. Ongoing inflammations are responsible for mineral deficiencies and a chronic metabolic acidosis, which delay any healing process.

While initial improvements may be noted in as little as two weeks of full dietary compliance it may take up to five years for your intestinal system to fully recover. Just remember, a recovered system does not imply that you can once again start assaulting it. Instead, positive results should serve you as prove that your newly acquired lifestyle works and needs to be maintained. But, why is it so difficult to attain and maintain a life-long gluten-free lifestyle? The answer may shock you. At the same time this very same answer might shed some light on why we face such a huge global problem with obesity, diabetes, and diabetes-related complications or underlying factors. The simple answer is: Gluten is addictive!

So much for all those bagels, muffins, white and even whole-wheat breads, pizzas, pasta, and processed foods! Gluten contains opioid-like substances. Yes, you read right, opioids! Dairy products too, contain a small amount of morphine (an opioid) in their lactose component casein. These opioids exert a direct effect on your brain cells where they trigger addiction. Everyone has heard the term "comfort food." As it turns out, carbohydrates are no comfort food to those sensitive to these morphines; for those individuals a large number of the grain carbohydrates are toxic.

Ah, now you understand why you crave pasta, bread, and other of those heavy grain-based and starchy snacks. Yes, you truly are getting a "high" eating those muffins, bagels, pizza, and breaded somethings. Let me be more specific: You are getting at least a "double high." Firstly, the starch converts to sugar and raises your blood sugar levels. That gives you a high or even makes you giddy. Secondly, that fair amount of hidden morphine you ingest unwittingly makes sure that you need to reach for your next starchy snack as soon as your blood sugar high starts dropping. In my natural medicine practice I call this the *"Toxic Trigger Loop"* (see figure 9, p. 126).

In addition, these gluten- or casein-derived opioids affect more than just your cravings control center. It has been known for a while that opioids also interfere with your natural killer cells against cancer. Also—the perhaps most important point overall to remember—these opioids interfere with the hypothalamus-pituitary-adrenal control function of your brain (the HPA axis) by stopping your endocrine glands from producing killer cells. For this reason people suffering from celiac disease and drug-addicts alike show similarly enlarged gastrointestinal lymph nodes. And, like heroin addicts, celiac patients are at an increased risk of developing severe immune system dysfunction, altered spleen and T-cell function, lymphoma, and other forms of cancer. Did you know that diabetics too show higher incidences of several forms of these same cancers?

Due to the presence of these opioids in the gluten grains, gluten-sensitive people, and likewise (at least according to my experience) most diabetics, may develop compulsive eating habits.—Read more on how to counter such tendencies in *Part Three, Battling Carbohydrate Addiction* p. 292.—Like diabetics, individuals sensitive to gluten may experience chronic discomfort, bloating, and physical and mental exhaustion. Thyroid imbalances and low-grade fevers are common too, especially once your lymph system becomes affected and overtaxed.

With the abdomen frequently bloated, stools may tend towards constipation one day and towards diarrhea another. Floating stools are common too. Your abdominal and low back areas are constantly stressed. Do you remember what I said about diabetics and their musculoskeletal lower back instabilities? Just to remind you of its possible value in an early diagnosis of pre-diabetes or diabetes I would like to emphasize that low back pain is yet another issue experienced recurrently by celiac patients and by diabetics alike.

Gluten-sensitive patients also frequently experience low blood pressure, heartburn, shortness of breath, wheezing and stuffiness from mucus defects, iron deficiency anemia, and easy bruising. All these relate to deficiencies in your vitamin and mineral uptake. Here is where we find the perhaps closest match to what a diabetic person experiences. Deficiencies may include the vitamins A, C, D, E, K, and a wide group of the B vitamins. The most frequent mineral deficiencies are those of calcium, copper, iron, magnesium, manganese, selenium, and zinc, along with vanadium and germanium. Does this list not sound vaguely familiar and sufficiently similar to that of a diabetic? In fact, as you shall see in *Part Three, Most Common Supplementing Needs for Diabetics* (p. 300), it is nearly identical except for the additionally missing chromium of diabetics.

One of the actions of the gluten particles makes them look like a particularly good match when we consider them as possible culprits with regards to a risk of diabetes. Grain carbohydrates and perhaps gluten appear to trigger increased insulin production and release. Consequently, particularly those individuals with a tendency towards hyperinsulinism might want to consider such a possible link with gluten-sensitivity.—Remember, it is the job of insulin to move glucose into your cells for the production of energy. If your body is resistant to insulin, or if it produces too much insulin, it has no other choice than converting the extra sugar into fat and storing it in your tissue. This fat, in turn, acidifies your entire system; and there goes the vicious cycle again.

For this process to distress your body, an additional factor and perhaps a specific weak link must exist in your system. We know that the insulin and leptin connection directly affects your endocrine glands, such as the hypothalamus. We have seen that this will lead to thyroid imbalances, which play a pivotal role in both diseases (gluten-sensitivity and diabetes). In the celiac and the diabetic alike, thyroid problems directly relate to many calories and toxins to be stored as fat. Overweight or obese individuals, therefore, should carefully consider thyroid and other endocrine afflictions as an underlying cause. But more so, these individuals are the ones given the greatest opportunity to improve their state of health by simply following a low-carbohydrate and one-hundred percent gluten-free diet. This is a simple recipe and it works!

Historically, celiac disease and diabetes have been linked to weight loss. Today's celiac and diabetic individuals tend to be overweight. While there is no consensus on the actual cause for these changes—other than the endocrine issues mentioned above—natural medicine widely suspects the increase in environmental toxins to be playing an additional and significant role in this switch from weight loss tendencies towards weight gain. Such toxin storage may alter your cells and their function; alterations that we spent quite some time looking at in the chapter on *Thyroid Intoxication* (p. 190).

How large is the issue with gluten? With a world grain harvest of just below 2,000 million metric tons per year (according to 2006 figures) gluten-rich wheat is the grain most consumed worldwide. In the same year, according to the Earth Policy Institute (using 2006 data from the USDA, United States Department of Agriculture), the annual per person consumption of wheat stood at just over 300 kilograms—more than one kilogram of wheat per person every day, six days a week, all year long. That is frightening! We no longer have to ask what happened to a well-balanced lifestyle and health. With or without a gluten-sensitivity factor this excessive consumption of wheat may well be at the root of our growing metabolic health crisis.

49. *FACT Summary Gluten-Sensitivity*

FAVOR	gluten-free, antioxidant-rich and low carbohydrate, low sugar foods, mineral and vitamin supplements as per practitioner recommendation.
AVOID	all known gluten and lactose containing foods.
CONSULT	your qualified mainstream or natural healthcare professional.
TEST	allergy and gluten-sensitivity tests, mineral deficiency levels, blood glucose and other diabetes-related tests.

Your Personal Notes

Symptoms—Date(s) first noticed:

_____

Symptoms—Description:

_____

_____

Consultation Date(s) and with whom:

_____

Tests—Results:

_____

_____

Lifestyle Changes introduced:

_____

_____

Symptom Changes noticed:

_____

_____

Follow-ups:

_____

_____

Summary of Diabetes Risk

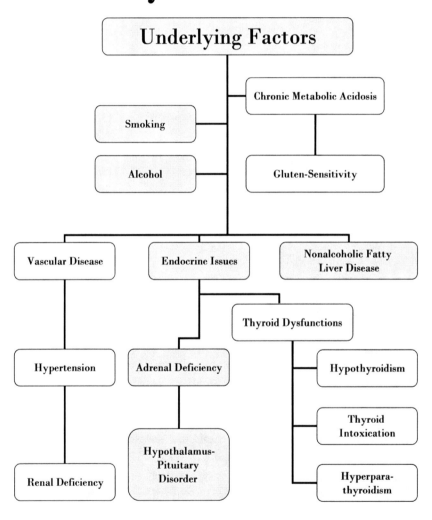

Figure 13 Underlying Conditions - Diabetes Risk Summary

Complications, Your Largely Avoidable "After" Facts

"After Facts" not always are just that, after facts. Mainstream medicine generally views the following conditions as complications of diabetes. Yet, when they surface in a person not yet diagnosed with diabetes, they most frequently treat them as separate and independent conditions. No warnings, no links, nothing! Keep an open mind; if you have a an existing diagnosis of one of these diseases and show any of the previously discussed signs in this book, including the one or the other of beer-belly, obesity, brain-fog, tiredness, sleep issues, and the likes, you might already fall into the high-risk category of developing pre-diabetes or diabetes very shortly—never-mind what your specialist says or doesn't say. Act now and you may stand a chance to avoid diabetes and improve your present issues at the same time!

Heart Disease

In my natural medicine practice I see quite a few patients with cardiovascular disease (CVD) without them having been previously diagnosed with diabetes. Without exception, these heart disease patients show signs of hypertension, elevated blood pressure, and lipid imbalances. At the same time, clear indications are present of the apple-shaped body outline that is so typical of a metabolic imbalance and a pre-diabetic or diabetic disposition. For one or the other reason, unfortunately, these warning signs were considered too insignificant or were missed outright by the medical team of these individuals; likely, because they happened to be on a relative sugar-low at the time their initial blood glucose tests were run.

A correlation between heart disease and diabetes exists and would lead me to assume that a prolonged but unrecognized pre-diabetic condition may long have preceded any heart condition of these individuals. It is common knowledge that erratic and excessive blood sugar values lead to vascular issues; problems that may result in heart disease. It should be imperative, therefore, to check these heart patients for blood sugar levels and patterns on a regular basis and at different times of the day. More than simple glucose testing, all the other factors need to be taken into account also when determining their standing on the path and time-line of a risk for additional metabolic disease.

When a thirty-two year old, hugely overweight and beer-bellied, young man steps into my natural medicine office with all external signs of hypertension and a blood pressure of 155 over 110 and says he wants help to stop smoking I will weep inside for his wife. More than simply support him in his quest to stop smoking I will do my utmost to let such a patient recognize that he is at high risk, not just of heart disease, but also faces a great probability of developing diabetes—if his heart does not kill him first. If you know such a patient or are this type of patient you too must take action. Only immediate and thorough lifestyle changes will do if you want to see your kids grow up. But, these lifestyle changes will effectively prolong your life.

At some point or other, cardiovascular disease patterns correlate with the blood oxygen levels of your body. Blood oxygen levels affect the elasticity of your tissues, including your arteries, and exert a major impact on the health and function of your kidneys. If there are imbalances that are not dealt with early kidney disease may be the unplanned, yet logical consequence. But more about this later; for now let us think back to our chapter dealing with *Metabolic Acidosis* (p. 206).

We found there that unwise food choices and a lack of nutrient absorption nearly always lead to an acidification of your blood. Your body, consequently, retrieves existing calcium and several other essential minerals from your skeleton in order to neutralize the acid-alkaline level of your blood. This dissolved calcium does not indefinitely float around in your blood. Initially, by changing the blood composition it raises your blood pressure; but, eventually, it needs to redeposit someplace. As we have discussed earlier, in some individuals so predisposed, the deposits attach to the walls of your blood vessels facilitating plaque build-up, blood clots, and other vascular factors. This paves the way for a stroke or a diagnosis of heart disease.

Western medicine considers metabolic acidosis an after-effect. Natural medicine sees it as an underlying cause. So, what is the consequence of this inverted association between cause and effect? In short, those of you who already have a history of heart disease stand a real good chance of turning their health around by paying close attention to all the factors involved in the metabolic, pre-diabetic syndrome. By doing so, your body no longer will keep adding insult to injury. Instead, you should be able to reverse your condition, slowly, step by step, by mending what led to your heart issues in the first place—

smoking and alcohol, and unhealthy choices of food and drink. These are largely the same triggers that we recognize as contributing to pre-diabetes and diabetes.

Maybe, some day even our mainstream medical approach will start to reflect this cause or effect connection by placing higher priority on prevention and lifestyle management and less reliance on short term fixes by prescription medications. Such an approach would firsthand reduce the inherent risks and the almost certain side effects associated with any prescription drugs. Many recent, and quite credible heart disease research studies show how further complications can be avoided by medicating early and forcefully. For us natural medicine professionals such an approach is downright irresponsible. Granted, what these studies all have in common is that the patient population surveyed is not expected to make major adjustments to their lifestyle habits and their approach to health.

If these patients were truly being educated as to the cause of their problems, quite likely they would not need to be put simultaneously on a battery of so-called preventative medications, on six, or eight, or more prescription medications (aluminum containing aspirin, blood thinners, cholesterol-lowering drugs, blood pressure reducers, beta blockers, and the list goes on). Mainstream medicine maintains these heart-risk patients in an artificial state of disease by letting them continue to malnourish their bodies on the very same unhealthy fuels (speak destructive foods) that have led them to their downfall. Considering these destructive food intake habits, rightly, prescription drugs will prolong the survival chances of these patients for a little while. Yet, it is quite obvious that none of the prescription drugs will make these individuals any healthier, nor will they spare them a future with additional diabetes; if they live that long.

It is considered a miracle when some of these patients—successfully—take matters into their own hands and strive towards a healthy lifestyle. Against all conventional recommendations, prescription medication—if for relatively short time only—for them may be no more than a transitory and not a life-long approach. To perpetuate illness is not in anyone's interest; to find the level of health that has eluded you is.

In summary, not just diabetes is avoidable. Many forms of heart disease that are connected to metabolic imbalances might turn out to be equally preventable. Like with any illness it is always easier to deal with a disease early, provided you recognize that you might be at risk. Use the suggestions in *Part Three, Diabetes can be Controlled* (p. 243) and in the companion volumes, the *DIABETES-Series Little Books,* and discover the new and healthier you.

50. *FACT Summary Heart Disease*

FAVOR	max. 1-2 teaspoons daily of extra-virgin olive oil or grapeseed oil, antioxidant-rich and low carbohydrate, low sugar and low calorie foods, Mediterranean diet.
AVOID	fried, breaded, and otherwise fatty foods, any oil or fat sources, unstable and excess blood sugar loads, soft drinks, alcohol, smoking.
CONSULT	your qualified mainstream or natural healthcare professional.
TEST	heart related tests, blood glucose and other diabetes-related tests, electrolyte balance, mineral deficiencies.

Your Personal Notes

Symptoms—Date(s) first noticed:

_____

Symptoms—Description:

_____

_____

Consultation Date(s) and with whom:

_____

Tests—Results:

_____

_____

Lifestyle Changes introduced:

_____

_____

Symptom Changes noticed:

_____

_____

Follow-ups:

_____

_____

Kidney Disease

In North America diabetes is the major contributor to kidney disease. A history of ten years or more of diabetes most often ends in a diagnosis of kidney disease; especially if there are concurrent issues with hypertension (blood pressures at 140/90 mmHg or above), possibly retinopathy, and proteinuria (protein loss in the urine). Vascular problems too, such as a stroke, are considered an increased risk for kidney disease—little surprise when we consider that vascular issues are linked to hypertension. Many diabetics end up on kidney dialysis after their kidneys have failed to function properly.

Your kidneys are the most important organ for maintaining your electrolyte and acid-alkaline balance along with your blood pressure and your oxygen levels. Several metabolic imbalances, therefore, can lead to a kidney malfunction. Like blood sugar imbalances, kidney disease frequently is a result of longtime unresolved stress. The higher your stress levels, the more suppressed your kidney function becomes. This may go to the point of your kidneys shutting down.

Every single day your two kidneys need to filter an astounding 1700 liters of blood (1200 ml per minute). In addition, they help your urinary bladder to excrete an average daily amount of one to two liters of urine; up to twenty liters if you are diabetic and do not control your blood sugar levels. Your kidneys also need to filter out toxins that have not been dealt with by your thyroid glands, your liver, lymph, and other organs and systems. If you consider that an individual with uncontrolled diabetes excretes up to twenty liters of urine daily you can easily imagine how overloaded your kidneys may become, especially if blood or urine carry any amount of toxins and other unwanted compounds such as excess and fluctuating sugar levels. Kidney malfunctions result in water retention and edemas. Swollen ankles and feet are clear indicators of your kidneys' shortcomings; as are frequent trips to the bathroom.

Your kidneys also assist in synthesizing the active form of vitamin D, which indirectly aids in your calcium absorption. And, they play an instrumental role in the formation of the hormones aldosterone (responsible for your blood sodium concentration), vasopressin (ADH or antidiuretic hormone, reducing your water loss), and several prostaglandins (lipids extracted from fatty acids by enzymes). The quality of your blood is directly linked to the ability of your kidneys to fulfill their roles.

One of the functions of your blood system is to supply nutrients and oxygen to all your body tissues. Arterial blood rich in oxygen enters your kidneys. After the filtration process the de-oxygenated blood returns to your veins. From there it is carried back to your heart in order to be re-oxygenized in a continuous cycle by means of the function of your lungs. Thus: breathe, breathe, breathe, and breathe again!

Traditional Chinese medicine seems to have gotten it right when its *Five-Element Theory* talks about the functional connection between the *heart* and the *kidneys*, and the *kidneys* and the *lung*. This time we do not even need to substitute any names in order to understand the pictorial language of ancient Chinese medicine. TCM and western medicine use entirely different ways of explaining the connection between particular functions of the heart (movement of blood) and the kidneys (filtering), but here they describe the very same functions and associations.

It appears that your body's inability to regulate its blood sugar levels directly affects your kidneys and their function. As we have seen, your kidneys depend on a regular supply of oxygen-rich blood. High sugar levels found in your blood diminish your blood's ability to carry oxygen to any of your tissues—including your kidneys. Consequently, the blood sugar robs your kidneys of the necessary oxygen supply. It finally all makes sense, doesn't it? Due to the lack of oxygen the various tissues lose their elasticity and lesions are forming in your kidneys (and other tissues such as your blood vessels). These lesions keep your kidneys from filtering out excess proteins and toxins. Since the body cannot handle such toxin levels, in time, kidney dialysis must take on the role of an "artificial kidney." Short of looking at a kidney transplant, dialysis may be your only option if your body reaches these advanced stages.

I am convinced that, once you understand the physiological processes involved in your body's dysfunction, you no longer will lack the necessary motivation to improve your health. You will want to avoid those fluctuating blood sugar levels at any price. Keep in mind that kidney disease, also called diabetic nephropathy, appears to be building slowly over a time period of 10 to 25 years. Kidney disease often remains undetected until it approaches a stage where kidney function becomes seriously compromised. During the years leading up to kidney problems you may encounter several warning signs. Hypertension, blood pressure changes, or lipid metabolism problems are but a few of them.

You also may encounter smaller warning signs that can predict a possible future with kidney disease. For instance, a high percentage of patients on kidney dialysis, like many diabetics, suffer from a phenomenon called restless legs syndrome. As we have seen earlier (p. 144), western medicine does not yet have an acknowledged explanation and cure for restless legs syndrome. Some physicians closer to the natural medicine approach suspect a possible thickening of the veins and, thus, reduced blood circulation. This interpretation may tie in with restricted kidney function. Time will show if something like restless legs syndrome has the potential of becoming a screening tool for early detection of impending kidney damage and a risk of diabetes, as we have mentioned earlier.

In addition, certain mineral imbalances or deficiencies and excesses may serve as indicators. Over the years, several of my patients who potentially are at risk of kidney complications and also complain about restless legs syndrome (day or night time) showed elevated and near toxic levels of manganese deposits in their hair mineral analysis results. Manganese is considered one of your body's essential minerals and, in minimal quantities, it is important for the healthy formation of your bone. This link between manganese, bone formation, and kidney function is interesting. Traditional Chinese medicine too links bone health and kidney function.

Mainstream medicine links manganese to the synthesis of your natural dopamine. This gives it a role in your body's neurological functions. Too little manganese in your body may suppress your glucose tolerance factor. Its levels, therefore, (excess or deficiency) play a direct role as a diabetes risk factor. On the other hand, excess manganese may get in the way of your calcium and magnesium assimilation as well as of your iron absorption. Lower levels of calcium, magnesium, and iron may get you a step closer to chronic metabolic acidosis. To complicate matters, high manganese levels can trigger a whole slew of signs such as rigid facial expression, rigid muscles and tendons, and tremors. According to traditional Chinese medicine such tremors are associated with *liver* function disorders; something we can understand because of our liver's function in the blood detoxification process. The circle closes: too much manganese also may be involved in overstimulating your nerves, such as in certain forms of restless legs syndrome.

Due to the nature of their function, your kidneys respond quickly to even the minutest mineral imbalances. In mainstream medicine many mineral imbalances first are detected when your kidney functions change. For instance, calcifications may form if your electrolyte ratios change; kidney stones are such an outcome. They are made up of minerals drawn earlier from your skeletal structure in order to prevent your blood from turning acidic. These minerals can no longer be assimilated back into your body and need to be flushed out of your system with your urine. As you can well see, there is a fine line between health and disease triggered by imbalances in your essential mineral levels.

In the special form of kidney function changes, called proteinuria, your kidneys fail to properly process proteins. Consequently, western medicine recommends that you largely avoid meat proteins. Meat proteins tend to be smaller and, generally, are better absorbed. However, grains too are rich in proteins and these proteins are of larger size. Along with some other grains, the highest amounts of proteins are found in wheat, barley, and rye. As we have seen in the chapter about *Gluten-Sensitivity* (p. 215) these grain proteins contain one of three forms of gluten and are responsible for the length of time grains can be stored. They also determine the elasticity and stickiness of dough during kneading and processing.

We already know that these grain proteins have been around for a relatively short time only, when we consider the evolution of mankind. And, as we have seen in greater detail in that same chapter about gluten-sensitivity, these proteins very easily cause inflammations in your system. Initially, they trigger an irritation in your gut wall. Subsequently, the proteins leak through your gut into your bloodstream. I know this may sound somewhat farfetched at this time, but could there be a more direct link between these gluten proteins and certain forms of nephropathy (kidney disease), particularly those forms related to issues of hypertension, such as diabetes or stroke? Looking at the interaction of your blood with the various organs and their functions this notion might well warrant some future consideration.

51. *FACT Summary Kidney Disease*

FAVOR	antioxidant-rich and low carbohydrate, low sugar foods, possibly gluten-free diet.
AVOID	unstable and excess blood sugar loads, large amounts of grain proteins, soft drinks, alcohol.
CONSULT	your qualified mainstream or natural healthcare professional.
TEST	kidney tests, electrolyte tests, mineral levels, blood glucose and other diabetes-related tests.

Your Personal Notes

Symptoms—Date(s) first noticed:

_____

Symptoms—Description:

_____

_____

Consultation Date(s) and with whom:

_____

Tests—Results:

_____

_____

Lifestyle Changes introduced:

_____

_____

Symptom Changes noticed:

_____

_____

Follow-ups:

_____

_____

Neuralgia and Neuropathy

In several of the foregoing chapters we have touched on the effect of high blood sugar levels on your state of health and the ability of your body tissues to function properly. Your nervous system may or may not be the first to be affected; yet, if it is affected, it quickly leads to a lot of undesirable complications in a large number of body tissues and organs. Temporary sensations of numbness and tingling—if not caused by spinal misalignments—may be your first indicators of blood sugar imbalances. In fact, being aware of a possible connection with pre-diabetes or diabetes may help you avoid full-blown diabetes by adopting immediate changes to your food habits.

We have repeatedly mentioned that you best act the very moment you realize that you may be facing a problem. Chances are that you already are deep into tissue damage once you experience severe levels of nerve pain. Still, it is never too late to adopt a healthier lifestyle. The worst-case scenario is that you bring to a standstill further deterioration. The best-case scenario allows you to naturally reverse your state of disease by eliminating the constant lifestyle insults to your body. Such improvements, of course, do not happen over night. You might be surprised, though, how much of a difference proper nutrition can make; and how quickly—even in advanced and medicated diabetes and in the management of its many complications.

Because certain biochemical processes and nutritional deficiencies are common in diabetic patients, numbness or nerve tingling over time may develop into severe and crippling shooting pains. This is what we call neuralgia. Therefore, as soon as you experience diabetes-related neuralgia or its chronic and even more severe form, neuropathy, consider asking your natural medicine practitioner for a thorough mineral work-up. By re-establishing their essential mineral balances many diabetic patients suffering from neuropathy have found significant relief.

In most diabetics nerve pain occurs equally on both sides of the body or, at least, alternates between left and right. In contrast, shooting pains due to spinal issues usually are confined to one side of your body. In other words, if you experience real sciatic pain it is probably due to specific spinal misalignments. Knowing the difference can save your healthcare provider a lot of troubleshooting.

Nerves, like any other tissue of your body, need the appropriate nutrients, including the proper levels of your essential minerals and vitamins. Any lack or excess of these essential nutrients may result in your nerves becoming inflamed (neuralgia). Over time, constant inflammation may result in damage to certain nerves (neuropathy). Nerves also need an adequate supply of oxygen in order to function properly. The chapter *Most Common Supplementing Needs for Diabetics* (p. 300) will contain many clues and pointers that can benefit you when if comes to keeping your nervous system healthy.

For a while now, researchers have connected improper nerve function due to inflammation with several chronic conditions. So far, links have been established to asthma and gastrointestinal issues. A special form of neuropathy is a "lazy stomach" (*gastroparesis*). Years of blood sugar damage to one of the major nerves (the vagus nerve) result in the walls of your stomach becoming paralyzed. Consequently, your stomach no longer can churn the food sufficiently and release small portions of it for further digestion to your small intestines. Blood sugar spikes become more frequent. Symptoms of heart burn, nausea, lack of taste after just a few bites, bloating, and abdominal pain, sometimes followed by vomiting, may be related to such damage to your nervous system. More health professionals ought to be aware of this possible link with gastroparesis when they deal with these recurring and supposedly only eating-related symptoms.

While many of these nerve-related diseases may point to a future development of diabetes, persistent numbness and tingling frequently are the direct result of longstanding and possibly undetected diabetes and kidney disease. As such, they need to be taken serious and acted upon without delay. By looking into all the possible causes you may be able to avert worse consequences.

52. *FACT Summary Neuropathy*

FAVOR	antioxidant-rich and low carbohydrate, low sugar foods, regular walks.
AVOID	unstable and excess blood sugar loads, processed foods, soft drinks, alcohol, smoking.
CONSULT	your qualified mainstream or natural healthcare professional.
TEST	neurological workup, blood glucose and other diabetes-related tests.

Your Personal Notes

Symptoms—Date(s) first noticed:

_____

Symptoms—Description:

_____

_____

Consultation Date(s) and with whom:

_____

Tests—Results:

_____

_____

Lifestyle Changes introduced:

_____

_____

Symptom Changes noticed:

_____

_____

Follow-ups:

_____

_____

_____

Amputations

We already know that bad wound healing is a problem for the diabetic patient. Approximately fifteen percent of all diabetics develop foot ulcers. Fluctuating blood sugar levels along with reduced blood oxygen levels greatly delay wound healing. In addition, deficiencies in your essential mineral balance further compound these problems.

Since high blood sugar easily affects your nervous system, loss of sensation in your extremities goes along with progressive diabetes. You may injure yourself anytime you accidentally bang against an object. If you cannot feel properly you may not be aware of an injury. Since there is no pain you may miss a bleeding wound. In time, such wounds become infected and may lead to gangrene. Unfortunately, unless you experience neurological pains early, few diabetic individuals who undergo a partial loss of sensation are aware that their sensory ability is compromised.

Most commonly, ulcers and other undetected injuries affect your legs and feet. If you cannot feel that your shoes are not fitting properly you may be stressing your feet unduly. Corns or blisters often go undetected and commonly lead to open wounds and ulcers. Lack of blood circulation greatly aggravates the situation. Once such injuries become infected it may already be too late. Infections that keep oozing, in time, may even affect your bones by causing a condition called osteomyelitis. Amputations are, although a last resort, often unavoidable at such an advanced stage. Unfortunately, too many longstanding diabetics have to undergo amputations that could have been avoided by earlier and better care and by timely lifestyle modifications.

Prevention is everything! As we have seen, many individuals who suffer from pre-diabetes or already from advanced type 2 diabetes are largely overweight. In this condition it is practically impossible to visually check the underside of your feet or the back of your legs. For this reason, it is highly advisable that you see a properly trained health professional on a regular basis. And again: once a year is not frequently enough if you are at risk!

If you try to take care of these issues early—that is, at a time when you still have full sensation—it may not have to come to the unpleasant consequences necessitating amputation.

53. *FACT Summary Amputations*

FAVOR	specially fitted shoes and insoles, regular check-ups, low-carbohydrate diet.
AVOID	barefoot walking, ill-fitting shoes, pressure points, injuries, blood sugar spikes, mineral deficiencies.
CONSULT	your qualified foot care specialist at least once a month.
TEST	infections, blood glucose and other diabetes-related tests.

Your Personal Notes

Symptoms—Date(s) first noticed:

_____

Symptoms—Description:

_____

_____

Consultation Date(s) and with whom:

_____

Tests—Results:

_____

_____

Lifestyle Changes introduced:

_____

_____

Symptom Changes noticed:

_____

_____

Follow-ups:

_____

_____

Eye Disorders

Longstanding diabetes may lead to several serious eye problems. Diabetes is the most common cause of blindness. Very tiny blood vessels in your body are involved in the proper functioning of your eyes. When they fail to provide adequate blood supply we call this micro-vascular disease, as opposed to heart disease related issues, which we call macro-vascular disease. The longer you have been affected by diabetes the more likely you may be ending up with a form of severe eye disorder. It does not matter if your diabetes has been known to you, or if your diabetes has gone undetected for any length of time. It is assumed that an alarming 85 percent of all people with diabetes will develop one or another form of diabetes-related eye disorder.

By now you should be familiar with the link to your blood sugar levels as a most probable cause. We have looked at the same links when we discussed other complications such as macro-vascular or heart disease. No matter what degree of damage, your ability or inability to control your blood sugar levels is of utmost importance. You stand no fighting chance against serious vision problems without adequate blood sugar control; and, I am not talking about results improved by medication only. Your lifestyle directly influences the years you have to enjoy what sights your eyes can bring you.

Diabetic Retinopathy

Vision problems are common in diabetics and, in most cases, eventually lead to blindness. Complications are to be expected because of the direct effect of unstable or high blood sugar on your various body tissues. Most frequently we notice the so-called diabetic retinopathy going along with the decrease of your natural insulin production. Diabetic retinopathy, therefore, is more common in type 1 diabetes patients; but, in North-America, it is still the leading cause of blindness for individuals suffering from type 2 diabetes.

Your eyes depend on how intact your small blood vessels are. Not unlike the increased bruising that you experience in your muscle tissue, dilated blood vessels may lead to hemorrhaging (a form of bruising) in your eyes. Along with small amounts of blood leaking from these vessels we frequently find the occurrence of edemas (swellings). In addition, lipids (congealed fats) seeping out may impair the function of your eyes and with it your vision; yellowing eyes are a give-away of you experiencing lipid problems.

When dealing with eye disease, just as with any other facet of diabetes-related complications, western medicine approaches your blood sugar control by prescription medication. I cannot repeat enough that, unless you start feeding your body only what provides it with positive nourishment, the downward spiral continues; despite all those medications and the seemingly improved test results.

Retina Detachment

Blurred vision, floaters, or flashes of light might be warning signs of impending retina detachment. These symptoms may appear briskly and fade away over time. But careful, you never should take lightly such outward improvements! Diabetic retina detachment is a result of tiny amounts of blood leaking from the capillaries that supply your eyes. The outcome is that less oxygen becomes available to your eyes. The body self-repairs the damage by reinforcing the leaking blood vessel; but, it thereby blocks your vision and causes blindness.

Retina detachment does not hurt. That is why its early warning signs often go undetected. Not experiencing pain makes it that much more important that you not ignore its early signs listed above. This condition needs to be addressed without delay if you want to retain your sight. For obvious reasons it is best to schedule regular check-ups and to act as soon as you recognize any of the initial warning signs.

Hypertensive Retinopathy

Western medicine discerns diabetic retinopathy from another form of eye disease called hypertensive retinopathy. In hypertensive retinopathy the main trigger is your high blood pressure. If you suffer from hypertension the walls of your fine arterial blood vessels begin to thicken. Hard, yellow lipid deposits may form in your eyes as well. This is of particular concern if you suffer from heart or kidney disease but also if you are pre-diabetic or diabetic. Don't forget: hypertension goes hand in hand with all these conditions.

In summary, the same recommendations we have seen many a time in the earlier chapters with regards to lifestyle changes are valid. Your "to avoid" and your "to do" lists when it comes to preventing vision-threatening eye disorders remain consistent.

54. *FACT Summary Eye Disorders*

FAVOR	active lifestyle, antioxidant-rich and low sugar diet.
AVOID	inactive lifestyle, fried, breaded, and otherwise fatty foods, unstable and excess blood sugar loads, soft drinks, alcohol, smoking.
CONSULT	your qualified ophthalmologist.
TEST	various ophthalmologic tests, blood glucose and other diabetes-related tests.

Your Personal Notes

Symptoms—Date(s) first noticed:

_____

Symptoms—Description:

_____

_____

Consultation Date(s) and with whom:

_____

Tests—Results:

_____

_____

Lifestyle Changes introduced:

_____

_____

Symptom Changes noticed:

_____

_____

Follow-ups:

_____

_____

_____

Summary of Diabetes Complications

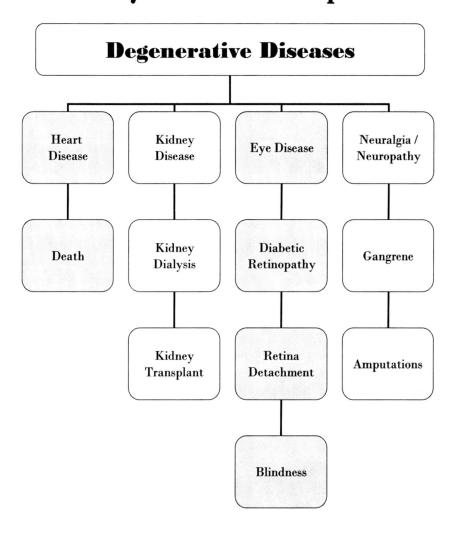

Figure 14 Diabetes Complications Summary

Summary

All serious complications, if not attended to timely, may lead to severe illness and reduced life expectancy. While lifestyle changes at a late point may help delay the unavoidable, lifestyle changes during earlier stages of your symptoms help you avoid many of the dreadful complications altogether. In fact, you entirely have it in your hand to turn your health clock back.

Cells die every fraction of a second and new cells move into their place. This natural renewal process explains why changing your lifestyle can work at any stage of a disease. Obviously, the new cells replacing those that no longer function will directly reflect the level of your nutritional health status at that very point in time. Therefore, if you continue eating the same foods that made you sick, albeit with some minor modifications, you probably will not see much change. At best, you stand to stabilize your present state of health and avoid getting worse too quickly. If, on the other hand, you learn new ways of dealing with your body, eat healthy by avoiding soft drinks, grain carbohydrates, and all the other culprits we have described, and you provide your body with absorbable nutrients in the right amounts and ratios, your new cells will be healthier too.

Needless to say, miracles take time. You can experience minor shifts to the better roughly every three months. However, many toxins and dying cells need to be removed from your tissues at the same time as healthy or healthier cells move into their place. And, naturally, if there is already tissue damage present it will not be that simple. Some tissues do not regenerate that easily; but some do, and that is your window of opportunity.

To some degree the old natural medicine wisdom still holds true that it takes at least as many months to remedy a situation as the problem has been in existence in years. In the case of severe metabolic diseases, however, this may be too short a time frame for a turnaround. Here twelve months may not fix all the damage of twelve years. Think more along the lines of three-month units (the life span of some cells). Most importantly, do not try calculating such an initial date from your first diagnosis by your doctor. Your counting must date back to the time when the actual first biological and biochemical changes in your body took place. In many of today's individuals that point in time could have been even prior to birth.

Once more allow me to give you this most important message of encouragement: cells rebuild! This should be the greatest motivator for you to act—early or not—and to look after your own body at least to the degree that you care for your car. If you keep all this in mind, you will have made your decision to respect your body and to help it get better. The next steps will get easier as soon as you see and feel the first improvements. You may be surprised how quickly you will start feeling better. Let *Part Three, Diabetes can be Controlled* help you with the individual steps towards better health and the avoidance or natural reversal of diabetes!

PART THREE - Diabetes can be Controlled

Keep your thoughts positive,
because your thoughts become your words.
Keep your words positive,
because your words become your behaviors.
Keep your behaviors positive,
because your behaviors become your habits.
Keep your habits positive,
because your habits become your values.
Keep your values positive,
because your values become your destiny.

Mahatma Gandhi

Making Positive Lifestyle Choices

You have no one to blame for the state of your health except yourself. We all are given a set of genetic predisposing factors. That is your (only) canvas, and no more than the canvas upon which you paint with every breath you take, with every meal and every snack you eat or are being fed, with every drink you have, and every action you take or fail to take. In short, your canvas very quickly starts reflecting how you live and nourish yourself.

The economy, the media, and our social environment constantly attempt to influence these very behaviors of yours. Lastly, it is your own choice how and if you decide to play along with this massive convenience food hype. Will you decide for what is good for your body? Or, will you be drawn to destructive habits just because you think that something is "cool?" Repeating vices has never made anyone of us a more valuable person! Remember, you cannot dilute the gas that you put in your car. Similarly, there simply are no short-cuts when it comes to issues of health. If the path of least resistance would work there would be none of our widespread issues with weight control, addiction, and serious illnesses.

If you want to stay off the present or future list of statistics for pre-diabetes and diabetes you must choose sides. The facts are painful but they do not lie. For now, change of lifestyle is the only choice when it comes to controlling diabetes without you heading towards the abyss of almost guaranteed complications.

Fortunately, or unfortunately, we humans do not come with a body warranty like our cars and appliances. You have to take care of yourself and help those around you take care of themselves as well. Most of all, you are responsible for teaching your children habit-forming healthy behaviors. To help them make positive food and lifestyle choices from their earliest years is just one part of this duty as a parent and educator. You are a role model for them. And, sometimes—by them showing you your own shortcomings—your very own children end up serving you as your motivators for change. Thankfully, it is a two-way road.

Yesterday, you chose an unhealthy dead-end road. Today you have been given an opportunity to choose a healthier new path. Time is a factor and so is "technique." Tomorrow may be too late! Allow me to stay with an image I used earlier: When the gas tank gets contaminated with diesel you do not wait until the car breaks down and then decide to change the motor. Instead, you clean out the tank immediately and thoroughly. Lastly, you make sure to never again—by mistake or by neglect—put diesel into your tank. Treating your vehicle in this manner you will have many more years to enjoy it.

When it comes to dealing with health the word is not "little by little." There is no room for compromise. So, do not fall for those that offer you to continue putting garbage into your system if you also take this pill or that supplement. Nor should you be lured by offers of only having to reduce your vices by a little. Change means choosing a new approach and learning to say "no" to what you have recognized as leading you down the wrong avenue. Health means "zero-tolerance" for self-destructive habits. It is you who fills the shopping cart with what your mouth and stomach, or eyes, desire. It is your own hand that pushes the foods you select into your mouth. It is your mouth that opens the door to the chain of events that eventually will keep you alive or make you sick (even kill you). If your engine runs on diesel feed it diesel! If it runs on gas don't mix diesel in for fuel!

You must learn to recognize what works for you and what does not. And once you recognize the positive impact of your initial actions, stick with your approach. You know that you will pay for any of those little "ah, just one piece" moments. So, stay away from them; proudly say, "no!" Because you know that you are doing a good deed for your body by avoiding self-destructive treats. Yes, you must learn to "love yourself!" No matter if you believe that mind and body are one or that mind and body are separate, you will not survive to complete the task you have been assigned (whatever your purpose in this life) without feeding proper and adequate amounts of absorbable nutrients to this one body you have available: yours.

The warning flag of diabetes, or any other serious condition for that matter, is like the "Dead End" sign at the entrance of a road. Would you really have chosen the dead-end road had you noticed that sign? Would you have continued if you had recognized earlier that it was not going to lead anywhere but down into the abyss? For some reason denial, the "oh-it-cannot-happen-to-me factor," is strong. But, once it does happen to you, do you really want to spend the rest of your time keeping busy getting nowhere, continuing your path of systematic self-destruction? Yet, this is exactly what most people do when it comes to their choices for health. They repeatedly and stubbornly keep heading for the dead-end road only to scramble up the embankment to a parallel road in order to avoid drowning in the river. All along, they hope blindly to find another road that may take them to a safe place; all this without them actually having to change their direction. Why is it that we people know full well that any parallel roads lead to the same roadblocks and downhill slides? Yet, we refuse to choose a radically different direction. Inertia may be human, but nothing to brag about.

The good thing is that a clear road is quite visibly outlined and you do not have to fight the undergrowth to get ahead. For the diabetic and the diabetic at risk the path to better health is cleared into a wide and inviting alley. Granted, some parts along the way may not look that inviting. Think of it this way: When you decide to fly to Hawaii or any other destination of lure you willingly put up with the travel delays, long lines at customs, the hassles and perils, and maybe even the nausea and some illness along the way. If you can put up with the ills of travels all for the sake of a beautiful and enjoyable destination, you surely are capable of walking the path to better health. I say: Go for it! Start looking after yourself!

Overcoming Lack of Motivation

Feeling stuck is a common issue for any one in human shoes. Change is never easy. When you finally receive that diagnosis of pre-diabetes or diabetes, remember that there is no need to interpret the diagnosis as a heart-breaking verdict. To the contrary, I would like to hear a deep sigh of relief at the time when your doctor utters the seemingly ominous words "you have diabetes." Finding out that you are pre-diabetic or diabetic, finally, should explain to you why you have experienced these many signs and symptoms and have been feeling tired, unmotivated, even depressed for the past few months or, worse, years.

No question, having to face change sounds daunting. Few people look forward to learning new behaviors. This adds stress and, as you know, stress adds to your cortisol imbalances and to the possibly life-threatening blood sugar roller coaster. How much easier it is at such a time to simply fill the doctor's prescription and to start down the long and slippery road towards the complications of diabetes! Believe me, without changing the triggers that got you to where you are, the scenario I described at the beginning of this chapter will be the unfortunate but entirely predictable progression.

On the other hand, finding the motivation to address change of lifestyle is closely linked to reducing the stress imposed by the diagnosis. Look at it as an opening, as an opportunity to get your life back on track. And yes, do "get a life!" Go for the change; but do not just go it alone. Get your entire family to embark on this new journey along with you. To take a new direction together with your loved ones is much easier than if you are all by yourself. When you include your entire family you become your family's role model for healthy lifestyle choices. The reasoning for an inclusive approach is simple: If you have an issue with your health it is extremely likely that everyone else in your family either already has an issue too or will be developing one in the foreseeable future.

If you are affected by a metabolic disorder it is more than likely that your mate too experiences problems. Not infrequently I see couples where the husband suffers from heart disease or diabetes-related problems while the wife experiences joint pains, osteoarthritis, rheumatoid arthritis, or similar conditions. For both partners inflammatory processes lay at the onset of their respective ills. In one of them the digestive organs are affected most severely, in the other the musculoskeletal system. Both suffer from lack of absorption and an excess of free radicals. Various levels of metabolic acidosis and its related deficient essential mineral levels may affect them both. In their own ways, therefore, both can benefit from proper food, drink, and other lifestyle factor choices.

Your lifestyle, food and exercise choices are part of an effective solution. By including your mate and kids you will spare them aggravation and pain later in their lives. Interestingly, it has been shown that parents frequently fail to recognize that their kids are overweight. Have you noticed how many television shows recently promote healthy food and lifestyle choices? You quite obviously are not alone in this endeavor of looking after yourself in a better way.

Sit down your family and discuss with them how all of you can get involved in getting or keeping yourselves healthy. A group effort makes this entire process more enjoyable and challenging. You will see; the dreaded shift towards a healthy lifestyle may yet turn out to be fun. Even in our *Diabetes Prevention Retreat Model* with its focus on the initial phases of lifestyle changes I like to incorporate this family-inclusive approach.

Reasonable Expectations

How long has it taken you to get to your present state of health? It may not take you this long to turn your life (and health) around, but there are no instant solutions. The natural medicine community frequently uses the one or three months per year guidelines—one to three months of healing period for every year the condition has existed. However, as we have seen, this best-case scenario only has a chance to play out if you no longer and simultaneously are assaulting your body with any of the triggers, destructive foods, and environmental toxins. Your food habit changes must be absolute. Even the smallest exceptions and slip-ups will not allow you to make permanent improvements.

Most people actually report that it is fun to work for the good of their body. Think of it as an exercise in team work: you and your body in conversation! Always remember, "garbage in—garbage out" still holds true! The good news is, the longer you are cooperating with your body the easier it becomes for you to stay on track. The reason for this is simple: As soon as you stop plugging your body full of carbohydrates and other addictive or destructive foods, your body will be able to send nutrients and oxygen to its various tissues. Your rate of inflammation consequently slows down. Most of all, your blood sugar levels stop their roller-coaster behavior. Gradually, you will notice specific or overall improvements. Your mood too will improve. Your brain fog will diminish. Your fatigue will disappear. Your energy levels will increase. Truly, your world will look brighter. Certainly a reason to celebrate!

When I look at the path of several of those patients who came to me with an existing diagnosis of diabetes, I see that those who are not yet on prescription medication on average can make progress very quickly. Prior to being put on medication your body probably has fewer accumulated toxins and tends to be more responsive to your new eating habits. But, even if you are on prescription drugs already, you do have an opportunity to reverse some of your issues, at least in part.

By rigorously watching what is going into your mouth solid changes can be effected in as little as a couple of weeks. Even better results can be achieved if you have a qualified natural medicine practitioner work with you and help you by suggesting specific nutritional supplements, essential minerals or vitamins, and homeopathic or antihomotoxic remedies. Such homeopathic or other remedies should be particularly geared towards your gastrointestinal absorption and your endocrine system function. It is very important that you avoid any undesirable interactions between the various essential minerals or vitamins you supplement with. This means, you may have to space out your supplements throughout your day. Sticking to a timetable may take some getting used to; others have done it, so can you!

Those individuals on medication generally need more time before noticing significant improvements. To be clear: You cannot and must not attempt to stop prescription medications "cold turkey." Such an approach would be irresponsible and could be potentially life threatening. Instead, ask your primary health care provider to help you keep a close eye on your blood sugar, liver, and kidney values while you start adopting healthier food choices. In most cases, your medical doctor will be quite happy to down-adjust your prescription medication once you can prove your consistent dietary compliance. If you are on meds you already should count it as a big success if your general practitioner is no longer upping your doses or putting you on additional prescription medications every few months.

I simply must share this story of one of my patients with you: A diabetic on medication and with several other conditions, this mid-fifty patient went for his regular appointment with his endocrinologist. Over the past months, since he had become a patient of mine, he had kept meticulous daily records. It was quite obvious how his new food regimen was benefitting his blood sugar readings. He explained his recent lifestyle changes and his gentle and gradual reduction of his diabetes medications to the endocrinologist as he showed him his last three months' blood sugar profile. The well-known doctor appeared truly impressed and warmly congratulated the patient for his decisive approach to lifestyle changes. He ended by saying that no further consultations with him were needed as long as my patient was able to keep matters this well balanced. Then the doctor sat down and wrote out a new prescription. When the surprised patient asked what this was for, the specialist answered that it was customary to increase the dosage after this amount of time since the initial diagnosis. Speechless, my patient grabbed his new prescription and left the doctor's office.

This scenario, unfortunately, is not unusual. We must understand that it will take some time until the medical establishment will accept the power of lifestyle changes—even though, for now and according to mainstream medicine, there is no cure for diabetes except for rigorous lifestyle changes. Reasonable expectations, thereby, are as much about what your medical practitioner expects from you as about what you can expect from your medical practitioner. Your path is that of moving forward in baby steps. Still, you must totally stop the assault of feeding your body the wrong foods because any partial or gradual reduction would only perpetuate your internal inflammations. Having said this, you and your health team must not forget to deal with detoxifying your body from all the build-ups that come with prescription medication and unsuitable, processed foods, and drinks.

Be patient and persistent. In time, your body may start once again to respond the way it is designed to. Once you figure out what your main triggers are, stay away from them. Remember, zero tolerance is not just your quickest, but your only way to reach your goal: better health! While we have found that your cells contain a so-called muscle-memory there is no reasoning with your body. There simply is no room for a let-me-have-that-cookie and I will eat-my-greens approach. Get help! Your natural medicine support team can help you get through this process safely and expediently.

The Role of Exercise

We have seen that eating right must be your number one priority. Exercise too has a role to play in returning or creating the healthful you. Let us look at the specific physical actions and functions triggered by exercise:

⇨ Exercise increases your oxygen intake.

⇨ Exercise improves your blood circulation.

⇨ Exercise activates your nerve impulses.

⇨ Exercise contributes to the crucial waste and toxin elimination processes.

And, here is a list of additional benefits of regular, well-designed exercise:

⇨ Exercise promotes weight loss.

⇨ Exercise increases energy.

⇨ Exercise improves sleep patterns.

⇨ Exercise activates brain function.

⇨ Exercise speeds up your digestive processes.

⇨ Exercise makes you "feel good."

Diabetes does not just have physical repercussions; it has a massive mental impact too. Your tool against this is exercise. Exercise helps you increase your coping skills. All these results are pretty well guaranteed. However, your neighbor or mate cannot work out for you, neither can your doctor. It is you who needs to sweat. Your dedication to improving your body's well-being is key, and you must put aside a regular and non-negotiable time-slot for your daily exercise program.

Until you are well into a regular exercise regimen it may appear too daunting to you to even get started. It may help you to understand why this happens. Guilt-feelings do not contribute to stress-reduction. There are several major factors that make it potentially difficult for you to work out on a regular basis:

Firstly, the biochemical processes in your body have slowed down to the point where they cause physiological problems. As you have seen, your body very quickly enters a state of deficiencies (particularly in essential minerals). Electrolyte imbalances are common too. This not only affects your organs, muscles, and nerves, it also directly affects your brain cells. It is, therefore, common for individuals with metabolic imbalances (such as diabetes) to experience brain fog and to feel too tired and unmotivated to exercise.

Secondly, if you are eating sugar-loaded or carbohydrate-rich foods, not only will your body lack the necessary oxygen supply—as we have seen in the previous chapter—it also constantly will find itself in a chronic drug-induced state. In an acidic body the sugar and the carbohydrates turned-to-sugar may cause a high not dissimilar to that of alcohol or drug intoxication. You may become giddy and euphoric, but your stamina will be short-lived. All said and done, it should come as no surprise to you that in such a state you may find it difficult to get serious about a commitment to exercise.

Thirdly, in the chapter about gluten-sensitivity in *Part Two, Predisposing and Underlying Factors* (p. 215) we have discussed how many of the gluten-containing carbohydrates contain minute amounts of opioid-like substances. If leaky gut syndrome is an issue for you offensive gluten proteins may act as possible mood-depressors. These proteins are leaked into your bloodstream and have a toxic effect on many of your tissues. This process results in bloating and a distended gut. It leads to a variety of chronic inflammations that may even affect your nervous centre and your brain. In addition, the blood sugar imbalances the carbohydrates bring with them will doubly affect your mood. It is obvious that you are experiencing fatigue and brain fog. Exercise, once again, may no longer look intriguing in such a state of mind.

No, I am not giving you any of these explanations in order to justify your inactivity. I simply want you to understand why exercise must go hand-in-hand with addressing your underlying physical issues and why It may be difficult for you to feel motivated until your body chemistry is changing by your—albeit grudging—exercising routine and your changes to your food intake.

One word of caution: Do consult with your physician prior to engaging in any physical activity that exceeds your present routine. Exercise is known to directly affect your blood-sugar levels. You may end up dropping your sugar levels too low too quickly. Extra caution is advised, particularly so if you are on prescription medication and experience hypoglycemia (low blood sugar) to start with. Your doctor may need to adjust your medication levels accordingly in order to avoid over-medicating you.

Also, if you suffer from hypertension in general and blood pressures in the range of 150/95 your doctor may advise you to abstain from extreme exercise such as weightlifting, running, or the likes, until your blood pressure levels have reached a more acceptable range. Remember that prescription medications may give you a false security by showing lower readings. Workouts change the way your body responds to medication. You must remain vigilant and open to making adjustments to your prescription medications immediately; but not on your own. Doctors like patients who keep them in the loop.

So, what is the solution to finding the right exercise balance? There are many forms of physical exercise that I routinely recommend to my patients. Largely it is more important how you perform an individual exercise than what form of exercise you choose.

Walking is greatly recommended for pre-diabetics and diabetics alike. The benefit of two daily thirty-minute walks has been amply documented. If you are a dog-owner you are especially lucky. Your exercise regimen fits into your daily routine naturally and without much of an extra mental effort. Your dog's natural needs will force you to get healthy by taking it for its daily walks.

If, however, you already suffer from musculoskeletal issues, especially if there are chronic problems (such as bunions or chronic sciatica) walking may prove difficult for you. To stick to walking as a form of exercise on a regular basis without precipitating further injury may require a careful look at your technique and footwear. Don't hesitate to consult a knowledgeable trainer or fitness coach for an individual exercise plan and to supervise your technique.

There are many other forms of exercise you may want to consider. If walking is not an option for you, or if you are adamant about making more rapid progress and lasting changes, you probably want to look at one of these options:

- ⇨ Qi Gong
- ⇨ Tai Chi
- ⇨ Pilates
- ⇨ Feldenkrais
- ⇨ Alexander Technique
- ⇨ Some forms of Yoga

What these methods all have in common is a gentle and highly awareness-focused approach to your body and mind integration. All of these exercise forms consider the body as an indivisible one and are very apt at quickly bringing you into a physical and mental balance. Any one of these techniques will help you become more aware of your body. Pick the form that appeals to you most and that you anticipate sticking with.

In all of these gentle exercise forms breathing plays a key role. These techniques will teach you how to stop holding your breath (a cause of many further problems and a major trigger of physical stress). You will learn to properly use your diaphragm. You will be amazed how quickly the newly-found connection will help you make surprising progress. The better the perception of your body's internal changes, the easier it will be for you to learn what messages your body tries to communicate to you. This will help you control your blood sugar levels, your hypertension, and your underlying stress levels.

Breathing techniques can be acquired in other ways too. Think of taking up dancing or starting music lessons. If you put your heart and soul into it this can be a fun and cultured way of exercise for any age group. Among many other paybacks, such as stress reduction, playing a musical instrument can actually benefit your blood sugar balance. Experiencing an adrenaline rush is common when you are actively involved in playing music. Your body will take advantage of this, and soon it will speed up your internal metabolic processes. Musicians tend to live longer, happier and healthier lives than the average population.

It could be of even greater and more direct benefit if you start taking voice lessons or learn to play a wind instrument. Both require proper breathing techniques and, very directly, improve your oxygen intake patterns. The exhaling process too becomes more conscious and consequently affects your acid-base balance and helps you to detoxify your system even quicker. Remember, CO_2 is supposed to leave your body to make room for more O_2 to enter it!

No matter what form of exercise you choose and how rigorous or gentle an approach you take, when it comes to drawing benefits for your health, it is all about the frequency of your exercise and about technique, technique, technique. For this reason, it is well worth you getting the best help you can afford right from the beginning. One of Canada's Olympian equestrian riders used to say, "Only perfect practice makes perfect." Practicing wrong techniques is probably the number one cause of more injuries and problems than anything else. Professionals in any field are here to help you achieve your personal goals without detours and damage to your joints and muscles.

Your Personal Notes

My Hang-Ups:

_____

_____

_____

_____

_____

What I can change easily:

_____

_____

_____

What I perceive difficult to change:

_____

_____

_____

What I will look for help with:

_____

_____

_____

_____

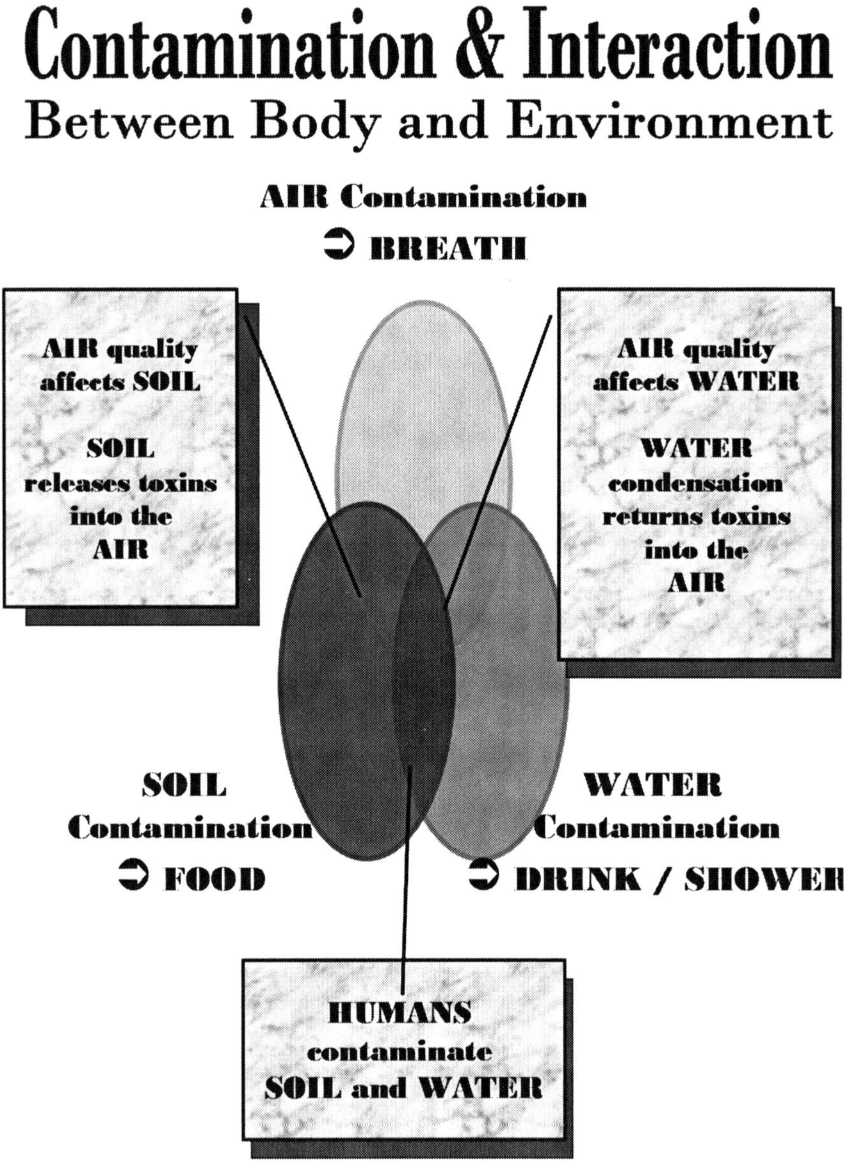

Rivkah Roth DO DNM®

Contamination & Interaction
Between Body and Environment

AIR Contamination
➲ BREATH

AIR quality affects SOIL

SOIL releases toxins into the AIR

AIR quality affects WATER

WATER condensation returns toxins into the AIR

SOIL Contamination
➲ FOOD

WATER Contamination
➲ DRINK / SHOWER

HUMANS contaminate SOIL and WATER

Figure 15 Contamination & Interaction Between Body & Environment

Avoiding Stress of all Forms and Shapes

Stress has become a buzzword. Hyper- or hypo-functioning biochemical processes of your body start biochemical reactions triggered by your emotional or mental stressors. Whenever your body is exposed to stress it not only functions at less than par, it also opens itself up to illness and disease.

Remember that stress always is a primary factor and directly influences your insulin production and your blood sugar levels. In an earlier chapter, *Part Two, Figuring out Your Risk*, we looked at the involvement of your adrenals and other endocrine organs (p. 183). They play a pivotal role. You can work for your endocrine system or act against it, help it work in your body system, or impede its work. You quite easily can control many of the positive or negative triggers responsible for your level of health or illness—and all of that without prescription medications.

In *Part Two, Underlying and Predisposing Factors*, we looked in detail at the metabolic acidosis (p. 206) and the function of oxygen (p. 211) in your blood stream. Let us now address several environmental factors that contribute to your metabolic acidosis and to the high levels of physical and functional, not to forget psychological and mental stress.

Lack of Natural Light and Air Stress

Stress is the wrong light and unclean air. Today's predominantly indoor lifestyle brings with it a whole cluster of additional issues that may compromise your state of health. A lack of natural light directly affects your biochemical balance. It is well known that too little exposure to sunlight causes absorption problems; such as deficient vitamin D levels in people living in colder countries.

Similarly, spending much of your day in artificially lighted indoor environments hampers the energy production ability of your body—not to mention the chemical and electric leakage you are constantly exposed to. Your body needs light, natural light, in order to synthesize many of its hormones. Synthetic hormones deceptively may look as if they help you; but, their side effects are not negligible nor are their actions fully predictable. If you want to be healthy, get healthy by arranging your life in a way that makes it possible for you to spend several hours a day in natural daylight.

You know about all those sun and radiation warnings. Yes, heed them and, by all means, avoid going outdoors during the time of highest radiation. But, think twice before slathering your skin with a slew of easily absorbed chemicals marketed as sun blocks. Become sun-smart and you will reap more benefits.

Absorption of all sorts of toxins through your skin is a growing issue these days. It starts with your make-up and your shavings cream and goes on to the water you take a shower or bath in. Don't forget your laundry detergents and house or office cleaning products. We don't yet know how the absorption rates through your skin are affected differently between natural light exposure and indoor, artificial light exposure. For now, just keep in mind the need for natural light and include these factors in your decision to live a healthier life and to avoid all other factors that might possibly contribute to quickening your risk of diabetes.

Indoor air quality too may contribute to problems. Toxins and radiation levels emitted by the constant artificial light sources along with the recycled air common in today's business environment in all likelihood are much higher than commonly assumed. Add to the hours you spend in such an environment those you spend in your home environment in apartment buildings and other centrally controlled complexes; not to mention your commuting time during which you are exposed to various levels of traffic fumes and smog.

It is easy to see that you are ingesting quite the drug cocktail day-in, day-out. This is not compatible with a healthy lifestyle. In short, you need to come up with your own personalized list and see where and how you can work around these issues in your quest for healthier living conditions.

Environmental Obstructions

Ever increasing numbers of environmental factors are starting to influence your body everywhere. At first glance, some of these obstructions appear to be of natural causes not just of artificial origin. Your natural healthcare professional may advocate a detox regimen and suggest specific supplements. Temporary supplementing of essential minerals, vitamins, and other nutrients may depend largely on where you live. The weather too and the seasons in your area of the globe also play a role. An individual in a fog-covered valley will not be able to access the same amounts of sunlight as someone working on the prairies and, therefore, may have to supplement at different rates and with different nutrients.

You also will not be able to cover your requirements naturally if you work in an indoor office or live in a basement apartment. If you perform shift work your body's chemical balance may be depleted to an even greater degree. Shift work is known to create confusion in your internal clock and puts direct stress on your adrenals and your entire endocrine system. It is for this reason that the simple formulae and recommendations printed on the bottles and supplement containers rarely work. Only a knowledgeable healthcare professional can assess and customize all information specific to your circumstances.

Chemicals and toxins from cleaning agents and beauty products, from your toothpaste to your shavings cream and your underarm deodorant, pose further challenges and are accruing far more quickly than forecast; both, in your environment and in your body. We do not know yet to what extent our car-filled cities change our lives. Nor do we fully understand if and how the shopping bag in which you store your groceries in the fridge changes the composition of your food and, eventually, the mechanisms of your body. However, we do know already that the plastic compounds surrounding us (from the plastic bowl that stores your food to the dashboard of your car) do release into the air certain hormone-altering elements.

Could any of this play a role in the ever-growing incidents of diabetes worldwide? Possibly! Yet, why is the number of diabetics growing even faster in developing countries? Artificial environmental threats may be blamed for many problems. Yet, it is my guess that—when it comes to changing the health of starving nations—there are some additional, more "natural" factors at work. I have long suspected the one natural commodity we call "staff of life:" wheat. Wheat is the one factor that is new to a majority of developing nations. Every year many tons of wheat are being shipped overseas from Canada, the USA, and Russia. Some of this wheat has been in storage for up to six years prior to it being brought to market.

From fertilizers and pesticides in the soil to rat poison and mouse droppings during storage and transport the contamination factor such grain is exposed to is not negligible. Moreover, the milling process of grain largely depletes it of its natural mineral and vitamin content. No problem, says our wonderful food department. It simply recommends that our milled grain be supplemented ("fortified") with nutritive additives derived from in part artificial and in part natural sources. More importantly, in order to improve the storage ability of grain it has been bred for a higher gluten content (the protein determining the storage factor). You already know that gluten-sensitivity may play a role in many conditions from hypothyroidism to diabetes, and that gluten also contains an opioid-like component.

You and I pay the price for such practices, and we have no idea what undesirable effects they have long-term. Who says if there could not be a link between the agricultural and industrial processes involved in the flour production and the surge in diabetes? We have seen it years ago when the government imposed fluoridation of the city water. Many cities today oppose fluoridation after sufficient research has cast a doubt on this practice.

Other Stressors

Often overlooked is the negative and immediate influence of physical, mental or emotional stress on the mineral balance of your body and, thus, your body's homeostasis (internal functional balance).

Thousands of years ago, traditional Chinese medicine has established links between your emotions and the workings of your organs. TCM accepts the emotions of joy, worry, fear, fright, and anger as natural occurrences in your biological system. However, TCM also stipulates that any extremes (too little or too much) of any one of these basic five human emotions will result in a negative or suppressive effect on their related organs (see figure 4, p. 63). Illness, TCM stipulates, is the direct and unavoidable consequence.

In one of our first chapters we looked at the workings of your body's hormone cortisol. Whenever you experience stress, no matter of what origin, the cortisol levels in your body become imbalanced. This cortisol rush in turn depresses your immune system functions as well as the functions of your individual organs. Your body's ability to react becomes hampered.

It is simply quite amazing how often TCM and Western medicine agree on the overall interactions and functions of our body. Disagreements mostly are based on translation problems and on a lack of in-depth understanding of the other system. No matter what angle we choose to look at stress, stress directly can lead to mineral depletion via a temporary or long-term overuse and subsequent burnout of certain of your body's hormones, enzymes or other essential catalysts. Without eliminating such stressful triggers even the best supplements and a balanced food regime will stand little chance of permanently remedying the situation—probably a major reason behind many contradictory research results.

It is for this reason that in my natural medicine practice I, like many other natural medicine practitioners, advocate an integrated approach of internal and external management if I encounter significant mineral imbalances. Namely, external stressors must be brought under control by indirect means such as by stress-relieving techniques (breathing techniques, Tai Chi, and the likes) or by direct means such as offered by lifestyle or stress counseling.

Last but not least, stress also may mean "food stress." Yes, wrong foods will stress your system! Therefore, you want to establish proper eating habits in concert with those measures mentioned above. I tend to get the best and most lasting results by combining these three approaches:

⇨ Indirect and direct stress relieving techniques – exercise, counseling.

⇨ Knowledgeable food and eating habits.

⇨ Emphasis on your internal mineral balance.

Wrong Food Choices Stress

Wrong foods present a form of stress. Wrong food choices affect your system directly by producing less than the essential energy and nutrients for your body's needs. Wrong food choices cause inflammation and chronic metabolic acidosis. We already looked at the impact of carbohydrates on your oxygen versus carbon dioxide mechanism in *Part Two, Chronic Metabolic Acidosis* (p. 206) and will look at additional issues in the following chapters.

Wrong foods overload your system with allergens. These allergens cause inflammatory responses and allow less oxygen-carrying blood to reach your various body parts. This could mean staying away from some seemingly "healthy" foods, such as certain vegetables or fruit. Some of the more common food allergens may include asparagus, okra, pineapple, mango, or strawberries. If you do show signs of sensitivities or allergies towards one of these foods also consider the possibility of your allergic reactions to be related to chemicals or other substances used in the growing process or the preparation of these produce. Many fruits also are coated with a corn-derivative to maintain their freshness. If you are sensitive to corn, that alone may trigger an inflammation in your system.

High on the list of destructive foods are products containing known or suspected carcinogens such as preservatives and a whole slew of other additives such as colorants or artificial flavors. While your average canned and boxed food is supposed to provide you with a more or less trustworthy list of ingredients, assuring possible contents and contamination is more difficult when it comes to fresh produce and open items such as your spices.

Apart from preservatives, artificial flavors, and food coloring, the hidden carbohydrates are the worst offenders when it comes to destructive foods.

261

Unfortunately—in an attempt to improve taste or consistency—starches and sugars along with fats are added everywhere in refined and processed foods from soup bases to salad dressings and designer coffees; you name it. Starch binders even surface in dairy products such as whipping creams, sour cream, and cream cheese. Also, don't forget to check all items for other unwanted ingredients. You might not expect (if at all you buy that sort of lactose-turning-into-sugar containing product) your brand of cottage cheese and other dairy products to list "carbon dioxide" as one of their ingredients! Unfortunately, I know of at least one leading brand that does.

Fats too may be destructive if you ingest either too much, the wrong fats, or too little of the good fats. I probably do not need to repeat that breaded, deep-fried foods, chips, sausages, and fatty meat cuts have no place in a regimen designed to avoid diabetes and other chronic illnesses. Simpler advice is to ask you to stay away from any of the "cream-colored" foods such as those just mentioned. Nutrient-rich foods are colorful; the color "cream" is not one of the positive choices. Most vegetables and fruit fall under the category "colorful." Most processed foods fall under "cream" colored.

Foods rich in sulfur and phosphorus too elevate your acid levels. Although sulfur and phosphorus are natural building blocks of your body, an excess of sulfur or phosphorus renders them toxic. An intake too high in protein-rich foods leads that list. Many of these foods are high in sulfur. Soft drinks and canned foods tend to be high in phosphorus. You will want to cut all soft drinks from your menu plan at all cost—neither drinking water nor drinking tea is stamping you as a "sissy." In fact, in many countries closer to the cradle of the world, drinking anything but tea is considered unmanly.

We have seen that most processed and store-prepared foods are full of harmful preservatives, colors, and other possible cancer causing substances. But, did you realize that even the fresh looking meats in your grocer's counter most likely have been chemically treated to keep their fresh red color? How do you know? If the meat from your ground beef package is bright red on its outside but brownish inside you do know that this is not natural. Therefore, it may pay to find a local butcher who knows where his meat comes from and who does not treat his display cuts with preservatives and other substances.

Did you think that eating healthy means that you can safely help yourself from any public salad bar? Did you know that most of the goodies in the seemingly convenient and fresh salad bar, not to speak of what you buy at your supermarket deli, may have been chemically treated to maintain an air of freshness? This steady presence of additives and chemicals in all your daily foods forces your body to constantly defend itself. In time it burns out your body's own protective mechanisms. This opens the doors to illness.

Before we will look at your most important steps to better food choices let us identify what to avoid. My patients learn the following six simple rules when it comes to foods to steer clear of.

Avoid anything where

1. the ingredient list contains more than four ingredients.

2. sugar, fructose, corn syrup, or any other sweeteners are named as one of the first three ingredients.

3. the product contains starches or binders, including the terms "modified" and "hydrogenated."

4. the carbohydrate count per serving exceeds 6 grams.

5. any of the ingredients are difficult to pronounce.

6. the product contains preservatives, colorants, or artificial flavors.

Labels help, but not if you ignore them! Most of all, reading the label does not refer to the brightly designed, large-lettered package front with all sorts of health endorsements and claims. Reading the label means searching for the fine-print ingredient list and that small white square that displays the calorie, carbohydrate, fat and other analysis. You must make it a habit to read the labels or to inquire with the manufacturer if you want to see positive results when it comes to protecting your health. Reading the glossy and eye-catching package front simply does not do. In fact, these statements may be outright misleading. A package may state "does not contain sugar." But, when you check the ingredient listing, fruit juice or some other sweeteners are pushing the carbohydrate and sugar count through the roof.

Moreover, it is not only about what you eat. As easy as the skin absorbs moisture it too carries into your system any proteins, chemicals, artificial colorants, and preservatives it is exposed to. Among those items that directly affect your system are your daily beauty products such as creams and toothpastes. Yes, you have read right, there too you find all sorts of goodies ("badies") such as sugar and starch that you better avoid; not to mention the number of chemicals they contain. Did you know that by the time the average woman finishes her morning chores she may have exposed her body to well over one hundred chemicals and toxins? Even taking a shower these days you cannot seem to avoid being sprayed with all sorts of chemicals that are absorbed by your skin and inhaled by your lungs. As you have seen, your town water may contain everything from chlorine to the remainders of birth-control pills and prescription medications that have—literally—gone down the drain and are not removed by today's conventional sewage treatment plants.

Why do you want to avoid any of these substances from external chemicals to preservatives to artificial sweeteners and other additives? Remember when we talked about the inflammatory processes in your body? Your body does not recognize these additives as any of its fuel-producing natural elements it was designed to process. It, therefore, mounts an attack on them. Such a defensive attack always involves an inflammation. If you frequently bombard your body with foreign substances your body will—at some point—run out of steam and shut down its fighting response. This gives the cell-altering invaders a free hand. Worse, if you constantly bombard your system with such inflammation-causing substances, your body may get so used to needing to mount an attack on everything that enters it that it no longer differentiates between your own healthy cells and an invader. Such a response over time leads to a so-called autoimmune reaction or disease. Many chronic allergic reactions fit into this category. Over the years, theories tying such autoimmune responses to diabetes and other disorders (such as celiac disease) keep surfacing but have as yet to be conclusively proven.

If you introduce foreign substances or any other toxins to your body on a regular basis, and if your body's health police no longer is able to cope with this onslaught of unnatural substances, these largely toxic particles get lodged in your tissues and cells; your fat cells mostly. In time, and given a favorable environment (in most cases acidosis, a state of excess acidity in the cell environment of your body), these substances effectively alter the function of your cells. This will lead to altered biochemical processes including those involving your acid-alkaline balance and your metabolism. An excess onslaught of acid-producing foods to your system forces your body to neutralize its blood by drawing calcium, magnesium, and phosphorus from your bone and muscle tissue. We call this the process of de-mineralization. While it is the quickest route for your body to rebalance your blood pH, these minerals leached from your skeletal structure make it the fastest way for you to lose your body's essential structural building blocks. This process almost guarantees the start of illness and disease.

Don't feed your body what it does not need—including having seconds when the first serving might have been sufficient! Lack of portion control is a major factor of overeating. Too much food ultimately contributes to obesity because your body burns less food than you ingest. Constantly overeating becomes destructive. Most people never even come close to burning off the daily calories they ingest. The accumulated excess builds up and starts slowing down your metabolism. Consequently, every day your body will burn off and convert into energy a little less. Every day your body will store a little more. Your body no longer can rid itself of its natural waste and soon retains more and more toxins.

To sum up, a destructive food choice is anything that has the potential to negatively alter any of your cells. For a diabetic, pre-diabetic, or overweight individual even simple foods may turn out to be destructive. Such foods include all sugars, carbohydrate-rich compounds, and lactose containing foods. All of them convert into high blood sugar. Please note that the emphasis here is on the word "all." Most of these sugars and carbohydrates are not that obvious. Instead, they are hidden in many refined and processed, plain-colored products. Did we not just talk about avoiding all "cream" colored foods?

The good news is that by changing what you feed your system you can largely reverse your biological clock. Naturally, the longer you have abused your body, the longer it may take for it to recover. A common misunderstanding is that you can experience positive results simply by reducing offensive foods little by little. Unfortunately, this is not the case. Do you remember the example of your car? As long as you top up any one of your required fluid levels with the wrong fluid your car sputters or, worse, you ruin its engine. Your body too has a zero-tolerance policy. You will only be able to attain the required positive changes by completely avoiding all inflammation-causing agents and triggers.

After all, it is easy to generalize these wrong food choices: a bad choice of food is anything that your body does not need. Clearly, your very first task is to avoid and steer clear of any further acidification of your system by making healthy food choices. Let us have a closer look at such choices.

Rivkah Roth DO DNM®

Your Personal Notes

My personal stress factors:

_____

_____

_____

_____

_____

What stresses I can accommodate:

_____

_____

_____

_____

What stresses I would like to eliminate:

_____

_____

_____

_____

What stresses I will need help with:

_____

_____

_____

_____

Understanding Food Choices

At Risk? greatly emphasizes the impact of an acidic environment on your state of health. Nutritional deficiencies or stress may turn your body acidic and lead to a significant deterioration of your organ functions and your entire system. The mostly sugar- and refined carbohydrate-induced damage is rather easy to avoid. Healthy foods are widely available. It takes a bit of a shift of thinking, though.

Firstly, you want to understand that nourishing your body is about providing a balance. If, initially, your body is totally imbalanced this might mean that for some time you need to be even more rigorous in your choices of what you feed it. Think of it as a total overhaul. What food groups you choose matters as much as how much you eat of what. Many rather misleading diet recommendations have been made for people battling with weight issues and with a risk of diabetes (see p. 112). It is obvious that, since any of these recommendations are in place and have been publicly promoted, the numbers of overweight people and those suffering from metabolic diseases are skyrocketing while the numbers of those who are healthy steadily shrink. Something is seriously amiss here!

Allow me to jump ahead and give you a very brief outlook at what the companion volumes of *At Risk?*, the *DIABETES-Series Little Books,* deal with in much greater detail, namely how and what to eat. Smaller, more frequent meals are recommended. We already talked about portion control; this is very important and will be easier after as little as two weeks on a good regimen.

You want to stick to non-inflammatory, non-allergenic foods. That pretty well means "going green" not just for your environment but also for your menu plan. Non-inflammatory foods are antioxidant-rich, green and colorful vegetables. Many of them are classified as alkaline foods. Note that, if you are one of the many individuals who also suffer from chronic gut issues—for instance you experience bloating and loose bowel movements—you may not be doing that well with raw vegetables and fruit. Instead, steam or lightly stir-fry them in a splash of olive or grapeseed oil; your digestion will be grateful for this little bit of extra care.

267

Rivkah Roth DO DNM®

In addition, I recommend the right amount of light proteins (especially for breakfast) and omega-3 rich foods. If you are overweight you also may want to watch your calorie intake apart from sticking to a low-carbohydrate, nearly starch-free diet. Did I mention that individuals on the correct amount of calories for their metabolism—not too much, but also not too little—rarely suffer from metabolic diseases and cravings? You may want to have a natural medicine professional help you establish your personal meal and nutrition plan.

For now, let us have a closer look at how nutritional issues affect you and when and how to supplement before we discuss the three major food groups. Most of all: Be good to yourself! Work for your body, not against it, and learn to take care of yourself and those around you who depend on you.

Malnutrition

If the food you eat does not provide the essential nutrients for your body to work properly this is called malnutrition. Most short- or long-term illnesses are accompanied by periods of malnutrition. Without the proper driving forces in your many bodily mechanisms your daily functions are compromised. In developing countries malnutrition may be the result of starvation, that is to say, of shortage of food or of lack of access to balanced nutrition. In the developed countries, on the other hand, malnutrition most commonly is the result of eating so-called empty calories. In these areas there is plenty of food available, but the wrong nutrients are supplied in excess amounts.

Where malnutrition starts with empty calories these foods include all your processed foods, soft drinks, and other foods that have undergone processing. These foods include anything you buy in a box and most everything that has gone through a grinding, baking, or brewing process. If you carefully read all labels and ingredient lists you will quickly notice that the most common basic foods, such as bread, flour, or milk mention all kinds of vitamin supplements. The answer is simple: milling and heat processing of these foods destroys their natural minerals and vitamins. Subsequently, many minerals and vitamins are added; mostly in a less absorbable or even a synthetic form. As a natural medicine practitioner, I doubt that these supplements are as effortlessly absorbed by the human body as their natural equivalents. It would appear that nature is not easily deceived by crude, manmade look-a-like supplements.

The evidence is quite apparent when we compare scores of urine and hair tissue mineral analysis results from people who use natural supplements and those who do not. For example, many women who have supplemented for years with some obscure forms of calcium still show major calcium deficiencies in their bone density scans; an indicator that some of these supplement forms may not have been recognized by their body and, therefore, have been bypassed.

Naturally, other factors such as, in the case of supplementing with calcium, a lack of sufficient amounts of magnesium or vitamin D_3 may also play a role in creating such a mineral deficit. However, in the end result, it always comes down to either malnutrition, which we define as a lack of access to the essential nutrients, or malabsorption, which we attribute to a dysfunctional intestinal system.

Malabsorption

We call it malabsorption if your intestinal walls are not in a position to properly absorb and process the nutrients provided by your food. Related to the workings of your gut, malabsorption may be a considerable issue for anyone suffering from intestinal disorders, metabolic imbalances, pre-diabetes, and diabetes.

To quickly recap, your gastrointestinal tract is no longer able to work properly when it becomes inflamed. Even beneficial nutrients can no longer be absorbed. This does not only apply to food-derived nutrients but also includes any of the supplements you consume. Crudely formulated: much of the money you spend on your expensive health food store supplements may end up in your toilet instead of in the systems of your body that need such supplements.

Keep in mind that any offensive and inflammatory proteins that are leaked into your bloodstream start a vicious cycle of inflammation and lead to the certain dysfunction of your body's absorption processes. Your skeletal structure suffers as soon as the mineral imbalances affect the ratio between major essential and non-essential minerals. It is forced to give up structural components in order to balance the whole; this is a natural, yet highly disadvantageous process leading to osteoporosis.

In addition, many other factors influence your mineral and vitamin balance and affect your hormones, enzymes and other essential drivers of your body. Let us have a look at some of these processes that may further influence your risk of developing pre-diabetes and diabetes.

Drug-Induced Deficiencies

If you are taking prescription medication some of your mineral deficiencies may become more pronounced. Many of the prescription medications work by suppressing your natural processes. This disables the necessary drivers in your body. Over time your body's own and necessary biochemical reactions slow down.

Having said this, I once again need to stress that under no circumstances must you quit any of your prescription medications after reading these lines. You must work very closely together with your primary healthcare provider in re-establishing your nutritional needs and balances first. Only then—and very gradually—may you be able to phase out some or all of your medications (if and when your hormonal and other balances have become sustainable and reliable). Any unqualified or rash decision to reduce or discontinue prescription medications may bring about further complications or may prove deadly and must be avoided by all means.

Food Source Depletion and Contamination

It is common knowledge that the nutritional value of our vegetables has decreased five-fold over the course of the twenty-five years from 1980 to 2005. In short, today you would need to eat at least five times the number of vegetable servings recommended in the nineteen-eighties in order for your body to receive the required nutrients. At a recommended five daily servings of vegetables and fruit for 1980 that would necessitate twenty or more daily servings today. There is no need to emphasize that this is not likely to happen. What it means, however, is that we all are lacking important nutrients and, therefore, might pass as malnourished.

Whenever you see a label naming "added vitamins and minerals" or a detailed list of added nutrients you can safely assume that these were extruded in the first place. Unfortunately, it is not as easy as re-adding nutrients and minerals towards the end of the manufacturing process. Instead of the unstable natural nutrients more stable nutrients from different sources are added; many of which your body either does not recognize or cannot absorb.

We have touched on this earlier: This day and age, your body also has to cope with an unacceptable level of toxic residues contained in just about everything you eat. These residues stem from pesticides, fertilizers, and treatments designed to extend seed storage life. Vehicle exhaust fumes, airplane vapor trails, and other brilliant inventions of ours too, leave their mark on the fresh food chain from vegetables to fruit to animal source.

You are used to thinking of possible problems with your drinking water. Yet, you often forget that many toxins and chemicals remain in the water even after you filter it for drinking. And then, what about your use of unfiltered water for bathing and for washing your clothes? Don't forget that the water used to water your vegetables and other crops undergoes even less scrutiny. Many unwanted chemicals, therefore, end up on your vegetables and fruit and consequently in your cook pots and your body. In summary, all these stressors from food source depletion to environmental impact very directly affect your health and wellbeing. Knowing where your foods come from, therefore, greatly contributes to a healthier you.

Supplementing Know-How

We have seen that the nutrients we get from our natural foods may be insufficient. But taking nutritional supplements is a hot iron. You are as apt to damage your system as you may benefit it. If you consider supplementing you should discuss this in detail with your knowledgable healthcare provider before you go and spend your money on a bag of this-is-good-for-this and that-is-good-for-that supplements. It is easy to go wrong with vitamins, minerals, or other nutrients. Even natural substances can have side effects if improperly used. The potential dangers are greater if you indiscriminately combine supplements. Some of the most essential nutrients can even be toxic if you take them in excess or in the wrong combination.

Your goal should be to achieve and maintain a careful balance in order to allow your body to work properly; not more and not less. The question is how we define this very fine line. The baseline values you need to strive for may differ depending on your particular individual situation. What is good for you may not be an adequate choice for your partner or your kids.

I do not find the one-a-day multivitamin recommendation helpful. Most multi-products are based on the established natural balances. They simply add a small percentage of everything in exactly these supposedly ideal and predefined proportions. Such an approach may be fine for a healthy body in perfect nutritional balance. But it may be the wrong thing for the body that needs more than a little boost in one particular element and is already too high in another.

I frequently see untenable deficiencies across the board in many individuals who do not supplement. But, I see as many individuals with hugely imbalanced ratios who do supplement without professional guidance. Neither approach is beneficial. Homeostasis (balance) is exactly what has gone askew in a body that is challenged with glucose imbalance or insulin resistance. For such a body it becomes even more important to custom-tailor any supplementing measures. And, as things start working and your symptoms improve or disappear, such supplement plans need to be adjusted on a regular basis.

Your specialized healthcare provider should be able to guide you through the jungle of possibilities and ought to be able to help you develop a workable plan of action. Most importantly, you want to keep in mind your reason for taking supplements. Apart from a lower nutrient content in our food we have seen that, in most cases, the inability of our system to process and absorb nutrients leads to deficiencies. Such deficiencies may persist over any length of time and will result in missing building blocks for your body and its functions. Disease is the predictable outcome. Therefore, you must give your body all it needs in order to work properly and in a balanced manner, but no more. If you have established absorption problems, standard nutrient supplements may do little or nothing for you; you might want to consider homeopathically-based products instead.

Many of your nutritional imbalances that have lead you or are doomed to lead you to illness-shaping essential mineral deficiencies are a direct result of the foods you eat or don't eat. It is easy to remember that there are seven factors, which contribute to proper nutrition. The key is to know how to balance them and includes establishing a proper balance between input and output (such as in physical exercise or absence of exercise levels). Here are your magic seven:

⇨   Proteins

⇨   Fats

⇨   Carbohydrates

⇨   Vitamins

⇨   Minerals

⇨   Fiber

⇨   Water.

The three major food groups, proteins, fats, and carbohydrates all have their specific role to fulfill. Think of them as your car's motor oil, brake oil, and transmission fluid. If you choose right, these foods can supply most of your nutritional needs with regards to vitamins, minerals, and fiber. The better you understand the impact of these three food groups the easier it will be for you to stick to a proper regimen custom-tailored to your body's requirements.

But, there is one more aspect: calories, a measurement of your food energy; call them your car's gasoline octane count. Calories measure the energy a certain food gives off when your body's metabolic conversion mechanism functions properly. Proteins clock in at four kilocalories per gram, and so do carbohydrates. Fats chalk up a whopping nine kilocalories per gram. Let's start with a closer look at your calorie intake.

Enzyme & Coenzyme-Mediated
Vitamins Enable Metabolic Processes

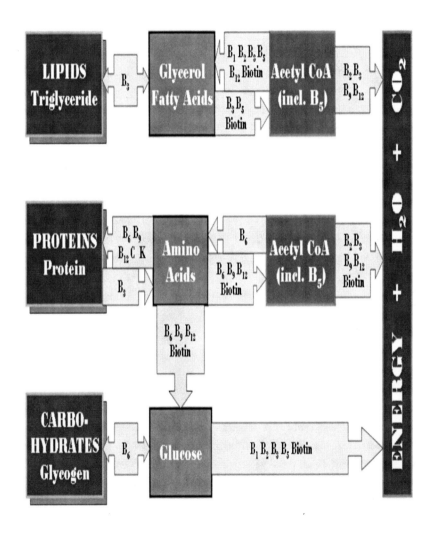

Figure 16 Enzyme & Coenzyme-Mediated Vitamins Enable Metabolic Processes

Developing Healthy Eating Habits

Calorie Intake

These days, many of the calories you ingest are so-called empty calories. They originate from processed foods many of which, during their manufacturing process, have been depleted of their digestible, natural nutrients and essential minerals. These foods, therefore, no longer possess any nutritional value. That is why we call their calories "empty calories." To make up for this the industry likes to add all sorts of seemingly wonderful sounding additives. Such foods are sold as "enhanced," "vitaminized," "enriched," or "fortified." However, to date there is no conclusive research showing that artificial supplementation of junk foods is providing the same benefits as your naturally occurring nutrients. In addition, no one knows yet what the long-term effects will be of all these routinely supplied additives that pass through or accumulate in your body.

The bottom line is: if you are overweight or obese chances are that you are deficient in essential nutrients. No, I am not guessing. A slowing down of your metabolism always is a sign of lacking essential nutrients in proper amounts and ratios. When you eat empty-calorie foods you starve your body even more because such foods lack the essential building blocks. Your body needs those in order to renew its cells. What is the solution? For now, it is important that you rely on calories from foods high in natural, not artificially supplemented nutrients. Apart from very few exceptions healthy foods by design are low-calorie foods. My patients learn the "maximum-four-ingredient rule." I encourage you too to read all labels and to return to the shelf anything that contains more than four ingredients. Read the small print on the back of the label, not the glossy—often misleading—catch phrases on the front of the package!

The first thing you need to work on when you revamp your eating habits is to reduce your calorie intake. For today's more sedentary lifestyle an average of 400 calories per meal for women, and 500 calories per meal for men should be your initial targets; especially while you are losing weight. Nobody says that you need to go hungry by committing to such a lower calorie diet. There are many healthy choices that will satisfy even the biggest hunger if the balance between the foods is right. But, I am jumping ahead; we will come back to this. If you are working out heavily and you are lean you may have to add another hundred calories or so to the above recommendations. But, without the proverbial beer-belly and with lots of lean muscle mass from regular workouts your metabolism is likely active and your risk of developing pre-diabetes or diabetes probably minimal.

The main point to remember is that you eat only as much as what you truly burn off during your workout; not what you wish to burn off, nor what your hunger dictates! With the proper ratios of your protein, fat, and long-acting carbohydrate proportions your hunger and cravings will be a thing of the past within very short time. For most individuals such a time frame amounts to less than two or three weeks. After the initial time period of adjusting, your body should no longer experience the severe nutritional deficiencies and addiction factors. You may be assured that, very soon after achieving better mineral ratios, your hunger pangs and cravings will no longer bother you—unless you relapse to your former eating habits.

This all sounds very simple. But, how do you reduce your calories? Always read the ingredient list on anything you plan to pass through your mouth. Start by checking the "serving size" and compare this with the numbers for the calories and the carbohydrate count (more about latter in the chapter *Carbohydrate Uptake*, p. 289). It might be a very useful exercise for you to have your healthcare professional sum up in writing all the calories you ingest during the course of a day. Then compare this with the amount of exercise you would need to burn up these calories. You may be in for a huge surprise! It is quite common for overweight and obese individuals to ingest a multiple of their daily calorie needs without them being aware of such excesses.

Assuming that you are overweight and that you would continue on the same high-carbohydrate diet that you are used to, you quite likely use up your calorie allowance within your first three to five bites of food. Understandably, this cannot satisfy anyone. Remember that precisely your high-carbohydrate and high-calorie habits got you to experience your present health problems. Therefore, stay off the fuels that have proven wrong for your body!

For starters, if you stay off grain carbohydrates completely, you may not have to reduce your portion size by that much. Unprocessed, fresh foods provide you with a goodly amount of essential nutrients that enhance your digestive processes and help your body absorb what it needs. The major benefit of this? Your cravings soon will disappear. It is simple: from now on eat vegetables only for carbs. But pass on all starchy veggies. It is important to recognize that some of the vegetables are nearly as high in sugar and starches as your grains. Among these vegetables are potatoes, carrots, other root vegetables, and squashes. Legumes too, although high in fiber, are higher in carbohydrates than many of us natural medicine professionals recommend for individuals at risk of pre-diabetes and diabetes. At least in the initial phase an individual who needs to turn the life-clock around and learn to avoid diabetes will want to go easy on them too.

You should remove all starchy foods completely from your diet until you have reached your proper weight and blood sugar values. By that time you quite likely will feel so much better, and will have lost your craving and taste for starchy foods. No longer will you experience any desire to reintroduce them. But, if for whatever reason, you do occasionally reintroduce some of them into your menu plan you must be very watchful of portion size. In most cases, one or two regular size tablespoons of these vegetables per meal are more than enough. Anything more will put you back on your blood-sugar and cravings rollercoaster and will counteract any of your weight control measures.

Here are some of the worst empty calorie providers; those you want to eliminate first. Note that I did mention "eliminate!" I did not say reduce. Soft drinks are out, completely! Apart from coffee they are some of the worst causes of metabolic acidosis. One twelve ounce glass of pop contains in excess of 150 calories and close to 40 grams of carbohydrates. This is already 30% more than your daily allowance of carbohydrates for a successful diabetes avoidance program. Soft drinks may contain 11 to 17 teaspoons of sugar per can and nothing else than making you crave another one. North-Americans consume a frightening 52(!) teaspoons of sugar per day much of which from soft drinks. Yet, studies show that women who consume one or more cans of soda on a daily basis stand an 85 percent increased risk of developing diabetes compared to those skipping on soft drinks.

Alcoholic beverages count also. Their carbohydrate and their calorie counts are disproportionally high; lots of calories, little or no nutrient value. A 12 ounce glass of beer easily adds 150 calories along with at least 13 grams of carbohydrates. Also, don't forget that—if you are one of the people who experience bloating and fatigue—beer is out of the question since you may be sensitive to the gluten contained in the malt (barley). Compare the above values with those of a cup of brewed tea (obviously without sugar or milk) at less than two calories and no more than half a gram of carbohydrates! What a boon; what are you waiting for: switch to tea!

Wine and other alcoholic beverages too are high in calories (seven kilocalories per gram!) and tend to maintain your body in its safe-it-for-later mode; exactly what you do not need! A glass of red wine has been touted for its high antioxidant benefits. In some people wine tends to lower your blood sugar, temporarily at least. This could become dangerous, especially, if combined with blood sugar-lowering medications. When you look to lose weight and need to stick to highly nutrient, enzyme- and mineral-rich foods even that one glass of wine is detrimental. If you wish to remain true to your calorie and carbohydrate regimen—as you should—this one glass alone will put you over the top without your body even coming close to receiving its essential nutrients.

What about that supposedly healthy glass of milk? One glass of whole milk rakes up approximately 150 calories and over 11 grams of carbohydrates; 1% low-fat milk counts in at 100 calories and at an even slightly higher carbohydrate count of just below 12 grams. For the individual at risk of pre-diabetes and diabetes the higher carbohydrate count of the low-fat version is unacceptable. However, using the example of one glass of milk, this would equal more than a quarter of your caloric intake per meal and uses up your entire carbohydrate allowance for a lunch or dinner meal. Wouldn't you rather spread out your enjoyment over a whole meal of vegetables and meat packed with flavor and nutrition for the same 12 grams of carbohydrates or less?

Did you know that most of your commercially available over-the-counter and prescription cold medicines also contain caffeine and sugar? Therefore, they too ought to be included in your calorie and carbohydrate counts; a good reason to put them high onto your "to avoid" list. Don't forget to discuss such medications with your specialized healthcare professional before embarking on them. And, last but not least, do not forget that any of these offenders increase the acidity level of your body (see *Chronic Metabolic Acidosis*, p. 206).

Rivkah Roth DO DNM®

Your Personal Notes

My personal issues with calories:

_____

_____

_____

_____

_____

What calories I can accommodate:

_____

_____

_____

What calories I would like to eliminate:

_____

_____

_____

What calories I will need help with:

_____

_____

_____

_____

Protein Intake

Of all the three major food groups the value and impact of proteins has become the most publicly disputed over the past few decades. We have gone from "proteins are bad" to "proteins are key," and back again. The truth probably lays somewhere in the middle. First of all, I strongly believe that we cannot simply lump up all proteins into the same category. Both, source and size of the protein portion matter. We also must not forget the particular health issues of the individual that consumes these food groups. Some people simply do better on proteins than others.

Let us look at the function and action of proteins in some greater detail: Except for water, your body consists of more proteins than of carbohydrates or fats (unless you are hugely overweight). Your body converts nutritional proteins into one of twenty amino acids. These amino acids make up many of the proteins in your body and are programmed for specific functions. Proteins are needed as tissue building blocks by anything from your brain to your muscle tissue, your organs, and even your skin, hair, and nails. Hormones regulate your metabolism; and, they too can only be formed if the right proteins are available. With their link to hormone production, protein deficiency appears to play a key role in the development of pre-diabetes and diabetes.

Your enzymes are another form of proteins. They are needed for your digestive system to work properly and for any cell regeneration to take place. Enzymes present quite a direct link to diabetes. Without proper enzyme function your insulin release will be impaired and may result in uncontrolled blood sugar values. It is for this reason that natural medicine considers changes to your blood sugar a result, not the cause of diabetes. This is another one of those important points that you may want to double-underline!

While protein deficiency is a problem, did you know that your body converts proteins eaten in excess to sugar? Eating unreasonable amounts of proteins on a daily basis forces your body to produce an excess of lactic acid. Not a good thing; we have seen earlier what chronic levels of metabolic acidosis can do to your nutritional state and your blood sugar! Ingesting excessive quantities of meat proteins, however, on average lead to cardiovascular problems before they affect your sugar balance. On the other hand, in my natural medicine practice, I have found that most people who are into high-carbohydrate diets have totally neglected their protein intake. Here is the difference between neglecting protein intake and binging out on proteins:

⇨ A lack of nutritional protein intake deprives your body of its necessary building blocks.

⇨ Any excess of nutritional proteins forces your body into storing them.

The short answer is: no excess in anything. The question is how to define "excess." If you are like most people, you consider your present habits as "normal." That may be correct if you are entirely healthy and at your ideal weight. However, most individuals believe that they need bigger portions because they are big people. Unfortunately, this is far from the truth. The only justifications for eating bigger portions are intense daily workouts or heavy physical labor on a daily basis. And, talking exercise, your 30-minute walk three times a week does not count as a license for eating larger meals; neither does your Yoga or Tai Chi session.

When it comes to proteins there are several different forms of protein; they all work differently and all are needed for your body to function properly. Let us look at the foods that provide a form of protein:

⇨ Grains

⇨ Legumes

⇨ Nuts

⇨ Fish

⇨ Eggs

⇨ Meats.

First, there are your whole grain proteins: Whole grain proteins are heavily recommended by mainstream medicine because of the additional essential minerals they supposedly provide. Never mind that processing and storage largely deplete them of many of these beneficial nutrients. Remember, what we said about the commercial habit of enriching foods with synthetic or different natural forms of some of the vitamins and minerals destroyed during the manufacturing process? Probably the chief reason for whole grains to become so heavily recommended is that most research is based on the comparison of a whole grain versus a processed grain diet, and not a whole grain versus a no-grain diet.

Even if the whole grains you are eating are unaltered, the problem with grain proteins is this: if your gut does not properly process the grains, you get all the carbohydrates, but not the proteins nor their heavily touted essential minerals. In addition, these grain proteins may be difficult to digest and can cause swollen bowels. Complaints of bloating, flatulence, leaky gut syndrome, and eventually a whole slew of gastrointestinal conditions are becoming more and more common. The bottom line is: grain proteins (no matter if whole grain or not) are apt to cause inflammations in many individuals. If that is you—and you will know if you experience one of the above symptoms—stay away from grain proteins, whole grain or not!

Legumes too contain a fair amount of proteins. Their carbohydrates are longer acting. For this reason dieticians recommend them for people with diabetes. In my natural medicine practice I have seen that legumes too may cause many problems; including blood sugar spikes. Therefore, you should carefully assess how legumes affect you before making them an integrative part of your diet. Also, if you are sensitive to gluten, you carefully have to watch for contamination. Legumes frequently are processed and packaged on equipment used to process wheat. You, therefore, may experience bloating and other gluten-related discomforts with one brand while you can safely eat legumes from another.

Nuts are a great source of proteins and make for a wonderful snack. A word of caution though, I recommend raw, untreated nuts. Roasted nuts are heavy on the kinds of fats that you do not want to burden your system with. All nuts contain natural oils. Heating these oils during the roasting process turns them rancid quickly. This makes your body acidic; not something you want to promote if your metabolism already is affected. Salted nuts are another no-no because they mess with your electrolyte balance and force your body to retain water. This will overburden your kidneys, and possibly lead to hypertension and even heart issues.

The rule of maximum one small handful of plain nuts a day is a good one, especially if you are overweight. Suffice it to say that the trail mix idea for a snack does not work for anyone who carries extra weight and is at risk of pre-diabetes or diabetes. As its name implies, trail mix with its dried fruit and roasted nuts belongs on the trail; not from the office to your house but on an exhausting all-day march and climb across the Alps or Rocky Mountains. Only there do you need the extra energy from the concentrated sugars, fats, and proteins along with the salt to help you retain what little water you have access to.

Fish proteins are some of the best source of protein because they also provide you with essential fatty acids (more about this in the companion volumes, the *DIABETES-Series Little Books*). The problem with fish is their potential levels of heavy metal toxins, such as mercury. There are ways around this that your natural medicine professional can help you with; for instance with homeopathic remedies to help you clear unwanted toxins. The benefits of fish are simply too great to have your body miss out on them entirely. The oilier fish such as salmon and mackerel provide the highest amount of Omega-3s. On the other hand, I strongly recommend that you stay away from eating scavengers. This, at least, reduces some of the toxin accumulation effect in your body.

Lighter meats such as chicken and turkey may even provide you with a few nice choices of proteins for breakfast. Watch out for prior antibiotic treatments of feed and birds. Any birds not raised on feed free of antibiotics might add to your toxic load of arsenic and other undesired substances. Also, many people are allergic to a natural amino acid in turkey called tryptophane, which they may want to avoid. On the other hand, many overweight individuals—particularly those at risk of diabetes—appear to lack sufficient amounts of natural tryptophane and might benefit from putting turkey on their menu plan more often. Learn to listen to your body. Feeling any added pressure on your bladder and experiencing a more frequent need to look for the closest washroom may indicate an allergy or other problem with your food. Your kidneys will try to eliminate the hidden toxins such as mercury, arsenic, and the like. If you keep a food diary it will be quite easy to make these connections, to experiment with eliminating certain foods, or to look for other, purer sources.

Similar reservations as with poultry meats go for eggs. When you buy eggs make sure that the carton states something to the effect that the chickens have been raised free of antibiotics and medication-containing feed. Arsenic and other toxins added to antibiotics and supplements are not what you want your body to ingest. The bad reputation that eggs have received due to the fat content of the yolk (about five grams of fat in a medium-size egg of fifty grams) is rather unjustified. The fat is unsaturated fat and, therefore, not something you should worry about. You will see that it is not fat that makes you fat; it is starch that makes you fat, raises your blood sugar, and leads to insulin resistance. And, when it comes to the cholesterol in the egg yolk, these natural cholesterols are mostly of the HDL kind, the "good" cholesterol.

Overall, eggs are a great source of protein and choline, an essential nutrient and important component of your cell membranes and neurotransmitters. Many people tout eating raw eggs. However, the protein contained in raw egg whites is only about fifty percent digestible, whereas that of cooked egg whites is more than ninety percent bioavailable. Therefore, cook your eggs—not just to avoid salmonella poisoning, but simply to get better nutrient absorption. Also, many people who are allergic to eggs are actually allergic to the egg white. Yolks may still work for them.

Some of the leaner beef cuts make for a wonderful source of protein. Just remember, the portion size ought to be nothing in excess of the palm of your hand! This rule should remain in effect no matter what meat or fish source of protein you choose. The high-cholesterol scare with beef comes mostly with the plate-size steaks so popular in many restaurants in North-America. They really drive up your body's acid levels and burden your kidneys. They also may result in arterial build-ups due to cholesterol deposits and due to your blood's need to flush calcium from your bones in an attempt to maintain its slightly alkaline pH balance. So, stick to your guns, eat portions no larger or thicker than the palm of your hand or a 9 oz. steak.

Lamb too is a great choice and, if properly prepared, can be very enjoyable to eat. However, traditional Chinese medicine does consider it one of the more "hot" meats and discourages people with a tendency towards cardiac events from regular consumption of lamb.

Some of the wild meats are becoming fashionable, particularly in Europe. Venison, buffalo, moose, pheasant, goose, or duck are other options—as long as these animals did not snack on freshly sprayed wheat crops or drink water from creeks or ponds that carry industrial run-off.

Natural medicine frequently frowns on eating pork. Pork is commonly advertised as a "lean meat." Did you know that pigs are omnivores? Therefore, there is a greater likelihood of you ingesting concentrated toxins by eating pork than by eating any other meat. The possible toxicity of pork is a particularly interesting topic when we look at the traditional Chinese medicine food cure system. As much as Chinese cuisine loves pork, their traditional medicine system considers pork "toxic." Did the ancient Chinese know something we are just finding out? Thus, forget your breakfast bacon and your ham. Salmon trout, salmon, or maybe even a piece of chicken breast work just as well for breakfast and without the oxidizing fats and nitrate additives of ham or bacon.

Let me end this short overview of meat protein sources by warning you about your deli meats. Today, the large majority of processed meats and sausages contain preservatives, nitrates, and recently also wheat gluten to assist in better storage, consistency, and taste. As you have seen, all of these are big factors in raising your body's acid and lipid levels. You don't have to be gluten-sensitive, therefore, to benefit from avoiding them at all cost. Sausages and deli meats may trigger inflammatory processes in everybody. Skip them!

You may wonder why I have not mentioned dairy products for their value as a source of proteins. Most individuals at risk of pre-diabetes and diabetes are subject to chronic inflammatory processes. Their bodies tend to be acidic. Most dairy products would make such an underlying condition even worse except for a few high-fat, low-carb plain yoghurts. Dairy, therefore, is rarely a positive choice of food; at least not in the initial stages of diabetes avoidance. In addition, we have seen the unfavorable carbohydrate count from most dairy products. There are exceptions; but I will talk more about this hot topic in my companion volumes, the *DIABETES-Series Little Books*. For now, remember that dairy products contain too much sugar (lactose ups your carbohydrate count) particularly in any of their low-fat versions and, to make matters worse, contain many additives in excess of my maximum four-ingredient rule.

Your Personal Notes

My personal issues with proteins:

_____

_____

_____

_____

_____

What proteins I can accommodate:

_____

_____

_____

What proteins I would like to eliminate:

_____

_____

_____

What proteins I will need help with:

_____

_____

_____

Rivkah Roth DO DNM®

Fat Consumption

Fats are as much in dispute as carbohydrates; maybe even more so. Like the building blocks of most of your body tissues the basic components of fats are carbon, hydrogen, and oxygen. Their ratios in the fats you consume also define the category of fat or oil that you are dealing with. As you will see, it is up to you to stick to the good fats only. Fats are high in calories. This makes most healthcare providers suggest that you stick to a low-fat diet. While I entirely agree with the need to stay away from transfats and any fried foods because they turn your body acidic, I have three major concerns about this "lean" approach that mainstream medicine postulates:

⇨ When you eat the right fats they do not directly turn into fatty body tissue.

⇨ When you don't eat the right fats your body lacks the basis for processing your fat-soluble nutrients such as your vitamins A, D, E, and K.

⇨ When there is an excess of glucose in your system your body stores such surplus sugar as fat.

In summary, we already know that sugar and carbohydrates produce the most glucose and glycogen in your system. Therefore, to put it in clear text: Not all fats make you fat; but all excess sugars and carbohydrates do!

Your body needs fats (good fats!) for a number of essential processes. Among them are your nerve conductivity and your brain function. Every cell in your body needs a certain amount of fatty acids in order to rebuild new cells. Just keep in mind that fat is useful only in amounts that your body can convert. Any accumulated excess will be destructive. Excess, or the wrong fat, is one of your strongest contributors to chronic metabolic acidosis and, therefore, to kidney disease and all your micro-vascular (e.g. eye problems) and macro-vascular problems (e.g. cardiovascular disease).

Think of it this way: You don't want the fat in your kitchen pantry to go rancid. When it comes to butter, oil, cheese, and other fat-containing foods you only buy what little amounts you need, and you keep replenishing it regularly. It is the same with your body. If your body receives more fat than it can turn into energy or, if it is being fed the wrong fats, it has no other option than storing the surplus in your body tissue. This affects anything from your

286

waistline or thighs and buttocks to your arteries and your actual organ tissues. Not a very pleasant thought, is it!

Naturally, the wrong fats—especially those having undergone a process of hydrogenation—are detrimental to your health and must be avoided. During their production cycle unsaturated fats undergo a process called hydrogenation during which they become exposed to heat and light. The resulting fats contain transfatty acids and are some of the worst for your system. I, therefore, recommend that you avoid all products containing these highly oxidized fats because they will very quickly lead you towards a state of chronic metabolic acidosis. Although the trend is away from transfats in chain restaurants, many processed and restaurant foods still are among the worst offenders.

Having said this—instead of going on a fad fat-free diet—learn to use the right fats for the right reason and you will be able to make a huge difference in your body's ability to function properly. With suitable management it will not be long until you will see your essential mineral levels adjust. Consequently, your energy levels will pick up, your sleep will improve and, overall, you will feel in much better health.

As you have seen, your body can turn your excess carbohydrates and sugars into fat to store them. At the same time, there are also several fats that your body cannot produce itself but needs to access from the outside in order to function properly. These are called "essential fatty acids" or EFAs. They must be supplied to your body as part of your daily diet in the form of Omega-3 and Omega-6 fatty acids. It is very important to remember that too much Omega-6 can suppress your ability to absorb the necessary Omega-3s. For this reason, I generally recommend in my natural medicine practice to avoid supplements that combine the two in the same formula and, instead, use them individually.

One of the functions of your essential fatty acids is to regulate the oxygen transport throughout your body. EFAs also are important for your cell structure, your immune system, your hormone production and, last but not least, they are instrumental for your body's blood clotting mechanism. The latter is a function that frequently seems to be compromised in those with a tendency towards diabetes and diabetes-related complications such as cardiovascular disease.

Fish such as salmon, mackerel, sardines, and others provide many of your essential fatty acids—including the coveted Omega-3s. A multitude of research papers has alternatively recommended or disavowed fish as a good source of protein and healthy fats. The concern about high heavy-metal toxin levels is well founded and leads me to recommend to my patients to stay away from those kinds of fish higher up in the food chain. Most of these, such as shark, swordfish, even tuna scavenge on smaller fish and, therefore, condense the

Rivkah Roth DO DNM®

toxins. Still, the nutritional benefits and their unique ability to supply essential fatty acids are so great that you do not want to miss out on fish.

In summary, we differentiate between animal- and vegetable-source fats. Fats are grouped into three categories: saturated fats, (mono)unsaturated fats, and polyunsaturated fats. Most animal fats belong to the first category, vegetable fats and fish to the second, and many seeds and nut oils to the third. Since there are a gazillion of books out there offering education about the fat categories I will constrain myself here to a few positive suggestions.

I advise my patients to avoid canola oil, peanut oil, soybean and similar oils because these crops tend to get exposed to heavy pesticide use. Instead, my preference is for cold-pressed extra virgin olive oil. Each brand has its own taste and flavor. You may want to check around until you find an olive oil that works well for your palate. I prefer olive oil for most cold applications, drizzling over steamed vegetables, or cooking at lower temperatures. When it comes to high temperature cooking with oil (such as browning meat) my choice is grapeseed oil. Its smoking point in excess of 250 degrees Celsius (485 degrees Fahrenheit) is higher than needed for most purposes. Grapeseed oil is also one of the highest antioxidants nature has to offer. Its taste is very fine and gentle, and it blends well with just about anything. You must give it a try!

Sesame seed oil has not been well established in western cooking. Yet, for centuries, it has been used as a traditional Chinese food cure to help reduce high blood pressure. Used in moderation—at the rate of about one tablespoon per day—you may want to drizzle a little sesame seed oil on your steamed or stir-fried vegetables, on salad, and fish. For additional suggestions on how and where to use sesame seed oil check out the food ideas in my companion books, the *DIABETES-Series Little Books*.

Used in moderate quantities the following also provide you with acceptable fats: avocados, nuts, and seeds (raw, not roasted, and definitely not salted), flax seed oil, pumpkin seed oil, walnut oil, fatty vegetables such as the occasional squash.—You should, however, remember to watch the sugar, speak carbohydrate level, of the squash vegetable group and eat it in moderation only.

Your Personal Notes

My personal issues with fats:

_____

_____

_____

_____

_____

What fats I can accommodate:

_____

_____

_____

What fats I would like to eliminate:

_____

_____

_____

What fats I will need help with:

_____

_____

_____

Carbohydrate Uptake

No matter if you are underweight, at standard weight, overweight, or outright obese, your primary focus must be centered on avoiding blood sugar spikes at all cost. Any blood sugar high over-engages the free radicals in your body and makes it difficult for you to escape the chain of damage caused to your system in vicious cycles. Anytime your blood sugar readings surpass 7.0 mmol/L (USA 126 mg/dl) cell damage may be initiated. Therefore, pay due diligence; it is all about avoiding the sugar roller coaster!

Your body does not think and count in days, months, or even years. It records offenses immediately and responds instantly. The stronger your defensive system is the less you notice the changes; the further down the road towards tissue destruction you have inched the quicker or more sudden the changes become. Awareness plays a huge role here. Unfortunetely, along with cell damage, your perception may be impaired as well. You can play to this tune and try to cover up the damage with prescription medicines or, slowly step-by-step, you can start turning your biological clock around by eliminating and avoiding all the offending factors. The choice is yours! Radical changes of lifestyle still offer the best and only lasting protection and hope for improved health.

Worldwide, diabetic specialist dieticians still recommend a fair share of carbohydrates for each meal. Special diabetes meal plans add up to 220 plus grams of daily carbohydrates (an offense to your body, compared to our recommended 30 grams per day!). Recommendations of 52 grams of carbohydrates for breakfast, 75 grams of carbohydrates for lunch, and 65 grams or more of carbs for dinner—with an additional allowance of two snacks packing another 15 grams of carbohydrates each—are not uncommon but are shocking to many natural medicine professionals. Assuming that such an approach would work, more newly diagnosed diabetics should be able to get their blood sugar values under control. I don't need to stress that this is not the case. It is time for a thorough reassessment of the public recommendations for those individuals who suffer from pre-diabetes or diabetes, or find themselves at risk thereof.

This is not the only complaint that I have with the mainstream dietary approach. If the nutrients contained in that substantial amount of whole grains recommended by these same dieticians truly would be absorbed, fewer diabetics should be noted with significant zinc, chromium, vanadium, and other essential mineral deficiencies. In addition, the common nutritional recommendations do not appear to result in a significant elimination of the nutritional problems. Sadly, we see more and more people following their physician's nutritional guidelines; and yet, they need progressively stronger prescription medications. Something is greatly amiss with this approach!

What is it that we do differently in our natural medicine practice? In patients of all weight categories I have seen blood sugar levels stabilize when they reduce or totally cut out their grain carbohydrates. Whole grains concededly contain more essential minerals and nutrients than processed grains—although, even that is doubtful with today's processing approaches, as we have seen. However, their carbohydrate count is no lower than that of your refined grains used in most processed foods. And, remember, if you cannot absorb the minerals because of intestinal issues even whole grains do not benefit you.

We mentioned it before: the most important step is to eliminate the glucose roller coaster and to keep to proper oxygen intake versus carbon dioxide output levels (see chapter *Lack of Oxygen*, p. 211). The most efficient way to achieve this is to stay altogether off anything that puts the roller coaster in motion, i.e. off grain carbohydrates—any and all grain carbohydrates! Your psyche plays a large role in how successful you will be in this step. First and foremost, you want to adjust your way of thinking. Linguistically the word "reduce" subconsciously is understood (interpreted, manipulated, whatever term you like to call this phenomenon) by your mind as "so long as I eat one-and-a-half grains less than before my diagnosis of diabetes I will get the disease under control." Okay, I am a bit sarcastic here. But honestly, this is how your mind does respond to the carbohydrate addiction factor. Maybe you want to go back and reread the chapter in *Part Two* about *Gluten-Sensitivity* (p. 215), where we discussed the gluten-equals-morphine aspect of grain.

The thought of reducing one factor in your daily habits rarely works. Even one drop of diesel in the gas tank will still spoil your entire trip. Your mind must undergo a total shift before you can experience any success with adjusting your food intake; and, believe me, it can be quite an exhilaratingly positive experience! When you come off a standard breakfast of 58 gram carbohydrate cereal with milk and orange juice, or a 600 calorie bagel and cream cheese that boasts 60 grams of carbohydrates, any amount of reduction will end up no lower than at best in the twenty gram range of carbohydrates per meal. Such a supposed reduction simply will not bring any results, remains unacceptably high, and still ends up triggering a sugar high.—Look at it this way: When a river has gone over its banks and flooded your neighborhood up to the first floor, you still call it a flood when the waters recede to the level of flooding your basement. You only revoke the flood status once the river is properly contained within its river bed. Why should it be any different with your health and your sugar levels?

Remember that on anything more than maximum 30 grams total per day of grain carbohydrates, you miss any opportunity to overcome your cravings or your blood sugar roller coaster. No one comes off drugs or alcohol while staying on them! Why should this suddenly be different when it comes to food? Your seatbelt on the carbohydrate merry-go-round can only be unlocked once you start with a zero-gram grain carbohydrate balance. If you start from a zero-gram basis even six grams of grain carbs soon will look and taste like luxury. One word of caution: as we have seen earlier, if you are the type that experiences bloating, remember that you may be sensitive to gluten and that your only option is to stay off all gluten grains no matter what.

More and more professionals successfully advocate the rule of 1/5th of grain carbohydrates for breakfast and 2/5th each for lunch and dinner for a maximum of 30 grams of carbohydrates per day. I do not see the need for my patients to count their non-starchy vegetable carbs as part of this 1/5th-2/5th-2/5th pattern. But, I have them apply the rule to either grains or starchy vegetables such as squash, parsnip, carrots, corn, sweet potatoes, and all legumes. Throughout all this, greens are pretty well free choice. Many of these non-starchy vegetables have high anti-oxidative qualities and greatly assist in keeping your inflammatory processes in check. You do not want to limit those.

Unlike those healthcare practitioners who recommend fruit for their wonderful anti-oxidative qualities, I restrict most fruit, except for some berries here and there and fruit such as pomegranates or dried goji berries. Due to the high sugar values in fruit even their good qualities do not compensate for the destructive overall impact they have on your blood sugar. The "apple a day keeps the doctor away" simply is not true for individuals at risk of metabolic syndrome, pre-diabetes, or diabetes.

Battling Carbohydrate Addiction

Food can be addictive! It is well known and documented that we tend to crave those foods that we are allergic to. Food allergies and sensitivities are on the rise all over the world. Have you ever eaten a standard American breakfast and felt the need to stop at the donut shop a couple of hours later? Have you ever experienced hunger pangs within 20 minutes to 2 hours after a pizza or a pasta meal? Do you ever feel like you need to go for a nap after a meal or even after a simple sandwich? Do you suffer from either diarrhea or constipation?

The answer to all questions is that you may suffer from addiction to a protein contained in many of the grain carbohydrates that you are ingesting. What concerns us in the context of diabetes is its underlying addiction forming mechanism. The most offensive three gluten proteins are called gluten, glutenin, and gliadin. These are found largely in wheat, barley, rye and, in North America due to the contamination factor, also in oats. Other sources for gluten are spelt, triticale, and kamut.

From prescription medications to creams, the glue strip on your envelopes, to lipstick and toothpastes, from malt in cereals and beer to soy sauce, the list of gluten content in processed foods is long. So what is it that makes gluten-containing carbohydrates so addictive?

In search of an answer we must consider several patterns:

1. The grain connection
2. The gastric connection
3. The mental addiction factor.

Let us look at each one of these three components in greater detail before we consider some of their effects, namely how the macro-mineral and the trace mineral balances are affected by gluten in people sensitive to it.

Rivkah Roth DO DNM®

Your Personal Notes

My personal issues with carbohydrates:

_____

_____

_____

_____

_____

_____

What carbohydrates I can accommodate:

_____

_____

_____

_____

What carbohydrates I would like to eliminate:

_____

_____

_____

_____

What carbohydrates I will need help with:

_____

_____

_____

_____

Carbohydrate Addiction
Your Vicious Cycle

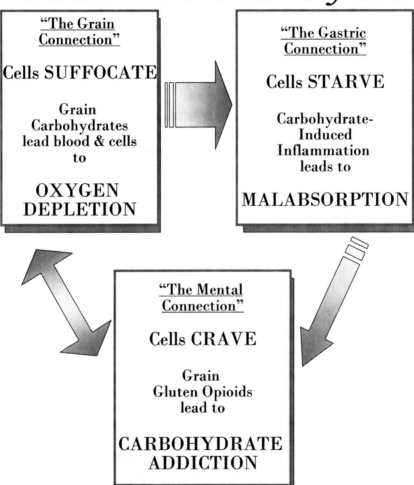

"The Grain Connection"

Cells SUFFOCATE

Grain Carbohydrates lead blood & cells to

OXYGEN DEPLETION

"The Gastric Connection"

Cells STARVE

Carbohydrate-Induced Inflammation leads to

MALABSORPTION

"The Mental Connection"

Cells CRAVE

Grain Gluten Opioids lead to

CARBOHYDRATE ADDICTION

Figure 17 The Vicious Cycle of Carbohydrate Addiction

The Grain Carbohydrate Connection

As you have seen, most grain carbohydrates contain a series of proteins called gluten. Gluten is the binding factor and, for this very reason, plays a major role in all baked goods and is routinely included in a large majority of processed foods. The gluten content also influences the storage ability of the grains. Considering that, for instance in Canada's grain silos in Manitoba, grain is stored for up to six years before it comes to market a higher gluten content in grain becomes a major asset for its market value.

Grain carbohydrates also act in a way that deprives your body of the necessary oxygen reserves. You have learned earlier in this book how a high-carbohydrate diet may have you exhale an amount of carbon dioxide equal to that of your oxygen intake. This leaves your body short of the roughly twenty percent oxygen surplus from every breath that it needs to nourish your various tissues. Allow me to use a somewhat drastic but real picture of what grain carbohydrates do to your body:

⇨ **Excess Grain Carbohydrates Suffocate your Cells!**

The Gastric Carbohydrate Connection

When, earlier, we looked at the leaky gut syndrome, you have seen how grain is apt to prompt the absence of certain enzymes (proteins) and essential minerals and how this interferes with your digestion. The constant bloating and the presence of gas easily lead to a distension of your gut and to a constant level of inflammation.

You have seen how your intestinal cell walls become perforated and allow undigested food molecules into your bloodstream where they cause further inflammation. At the same time, the normal function of your gut no longer works properly. Many of the valuable essential nutrients and minerals are being lost. Your body's power plant goes on strike. To stay with our somewhat harsh picture:

⇨ **Reduced Gastrointestinal Health Starves your Cells!**

The Mental Carbohydrate Addiction Pattern

Earlier in this book, I have shown you that some grain proteins contain a small amount of morphine. Is it conceivable that in people of a specific genetic make-up even these relatively small amounts of grain- and casein-derived opioids lead to a massive addiction factor? While more research into this aspect of carbohydrate-induced addiction is needed, we can safely assume that—in conjunction with today's accumulated toxin levels from heavy metals and a variety of plastic compounds—any addiction factor is more likely to become exacerbated.

It is worse for today's kids because, already prior to birth, they have experienced this carbohydrate rush in their mothers' womb. It is uncanny how many mothers-to-be over the past few years have mentioned to me how—during their pregnancy—they mostly lived or wanted to live on pasta, breads, and other "comfort foods." They all claim that vegetables and all "the healthy stuff" made them feel nauseous. There is quite a simple explanation to such a bout of nausea. With good and healthy foods your body starts an immediate and natural detoxifying action. As the toxins leave the fat cells where they were stored and reenter your active system nausea is but one of the signs you can expect to experience. Shouldn't we truly clean our bodies before allowing them to nurture a new life? Wouldn't that be the first step towards height-weight proportional, healthy, and addiction-free kids, teenagers, and young adults?

This mental addiction factor of carbohydrates appears to be the third nail in the coffin of your body:

⇨ **Your Body is Out of Control!**

Mineral Deficiencies

As we have seen, your food choices directly affect your state of health. Food does not simply pass through your body unprocessed. All foods and drinks—in fact, everything that goes through your mouth including your over-the-counter and prescription drugs—prompt certain functional reactions and changes. If what you eat is not what your body needs, acute or chronic problems are sure to follow. Inflammations and mineral deficiencies are a predictable and certain result whenever you consume the same unsuitable foods or drinks repeatedly.

According to the United Nations Food and Agriculture Organization this globe of ours presently counts 854 million of undernourished people, 820 million of which in developing countries. I suspect this number to climb the more the wealthier nations promote to many of these traditional non-farming areas the supposed benefits of modern high-yield grain farming. From an evolutionary standpoint, these populations have not had the time to adapt to carbohydrate digestion. In these areas the initial attempt of "elimination" of world hunger may yet turn out to be the start of unimagined levels of immune system deficiencies and of a rise in gastrointestinal and endocrine diseases, such as diabetes.

However, the problem of malnutrition is much greater than simply that of lack of food. Malnutrition exists very close to "home." Unfortunately, there are no statistics available as to the number of people who experience malnutrition due to malabsorption and mineral deficiencies—other than a lack in the three or four of the minerals that the above named organization suggests as defining mineral deficiency. A very large percentage of low-income people in the industrial countries live largely of processed grain-carbohydrates. The majority of these people can be classified as malnourished. Unlike the peoples who starve from hunger—not by their own choice—these homegrown cases of malnourished people indulge in destructive lifestyle choices—by their own volition. These individuals actively starve their bodies by giving in to destructive food choices; the diner next door makes things all too easy! As a result, their bodies lack the ability to properly absorb any nutrients. Rare? Not so! If I claim that at least fifty percent of all North-American individuals (one in two) already suffer from nutrient deficiencies I am probably being extremely conservative.

In my personal opinion malnutrition and malabsorption are the very clear and obvious causes of our hugely disproportionate increase of pandemic illnesses and diseases such as pre-diabetes and diabetes. Other gastrointestinal conditions too, such as irritable bowel syndrome, Crohn's disease, and a wide array of immune system disorders, including asthma and allergies, may be linked to mineral imbalances and deficiencies due to malnutrition or malabsorption. "Malnourished and overfed," we have previously called this condition so prevalent in most diabetics and those at risk of diabetes.

Cravings go hand-in-hand with malnutrition. If you experience cravings for sweets, fats, salts, and even cold drinks, you should first and foremost consider them as an indication of malnutrition or malabsorption. Mainstream medicine rarely considers cravings as a significant indicator of any physical illness. In fact, it is common for doctors to stamp patients as simply "depressed," "weak," "undisciplined," or "mentally unstable," if they are not able to resist their cravings.

From a natural medicine point of view it is rather obvious that you should look to correct the causes rather than simply try to resist and ignore your cravings. The bottom line is that your body is trying to tell you that it misses something. But beware: A craving for sugar does not mean that your body needs sugar! In fact, it is known that we often crave what we are allergic to and should avoid. Every craving is connected with very specific mineral deficiencies. When these deficiencies are corrected most of your cravings disappear and you may find that some of your organ functions improve too.

Let us look a little closer at what you can do to overcome a state of malnutrition. Yes, it is important that you avoid sweets and sugars in any form because they directly and most strongly affect your mineral balance. You also need to limit your excessive salt intake and the habit of chilling your drinks. But, more importantly, you need to eliminate the underlying cause of your cravings, namely the disproportionately high intake of grain carbohydrates and maybe wrong fats. Only, when you no longer feed the wrong stuff to your body, does supplementing with essential minerals, vitamins, and other nutrients become effective. May I suggest that you learn the preceding sentence by heart! How easy it is to forget this connection, particularly when your undernourished brain cells are having your thoughts spin in circles!

When it comes to absorption problems you may need supplements even if you eat the best quality of vegetables. Just keep in mind that all capsules, tablets, and pills that go through your gastrointestinal tract maybe useless if you show even the slightest indication of a compromised digestive system and the inflammations going along with it. If bloating and other digestive issues are part of your pattern you always can rely on one of the many traditional and modern forms of homeopathy. Anti-homotoxic and homeopathic remedies and preparations allow absorption of vaccine-like minute forms of plant and mineral matter through the mucous tissue of your mouth. These homeopathic formulas, therefore, can be effective where your standard capsules and pills are not. The key is to find a trustworthy professional who is trained in these forms of homeopathy or homotoxicology and has a deep knowledge of human biochemistry and organ function requirements.

In summary, you need to:

⇨ Work out a low-calorie, high-antioxidant, balanced meal plan.

⇨ Avoid grain carbohydrates.

⇨ Stick to low quantities of the good fats; this includes a fairly high ratio of Omega-3 essential fatty acids and avoidance of too much Omega-6.

⇨ Eat a colorful array of vegetables and go easy on those that are high in starches and sugars such as squash, corn, or the root vegetables—including carrots.

⇨ Don't neglect your meat proteins; but stick to a portion size not in excess of the size of your palm, and include fish as part of your diet.

⇨ Drink sufficient amounts of clear spring water in addition to organic green or white, antioxidant-rich teas, or unflavored rooibos tea.

⇨ In order to avoid interactions, overdosing, side effects, or ratio imbalances, let a knowledgeable healthcare practitioner help you work out and adjust an individualized plan of nutritional and essential mineral and vitamin supplements.

Most Common Supplementing Needs for Diabetics

Due to the gastrointestinal malabsorption factor and the reduced enzyme function common in most pre-diabetic and diabetic patients supplementing should not be taken lightly. In natural medicine practices all over the world the one-a-day pill approach is frowned upon. Most all-in-one supplements are based on the supposed ideal ratios of a healthy person. Someone with a pre-existing health condition and certain deficiencies or absorption problems, however, may require entirely different ratios. Such ratios must be monitored on at least a biweekly basis, and amounts or ratios must be constantly re-adjusted depending on your progress.

For those of us who in depth have studied the actions and interactions of essential minerals, vitamins, and other nutrients, it is a known fact that many of these substances counteract or reinforce each other if they are ingested simultaneously. Let me give you an example:

We all know that zinc deficiency is common among most diabetics; so are calcium and magnesium deficiencies; along with a slew of other nutrient imbalances. However, your calcium absorption may be obstructed for instance by high doses of magnesium that provide more than the target ratio of 2 to 1 calcium to magnesium. If you take zinc at the same time, or high amounts of fiber, they too have the ability to block your calcium absorption. To top it all off, your boron levels may be exceedingly low, thereby depressing your estrogen production and triggering further bone loss and calcium leaching from the hormone side of the triggers.

Why then would you want to waste your money and effort by taking calcium at the same time as you take zinc or magnesium in excess of your individual and momentary target ratio? Would it not make more sense to start with the factors that trigger calcium loss? That way you can work out the ratios and amounts in the exact way your body requires them (provided that you simultaneously balance your nutrition).

Daily foods too may interfere with the absorption of your nutrients. In fact, most of these foods also cause a state of chronic metabolic acidosis. The most common offenders that increase your bone breakdown and the rate of your calcium excretion are:

⇨ Alcohol

⇨ Caffeine

⇨ Excess Protein

⇨ Sodium

⇨ Phosphates

⇨ Sugar

⇨ Aluminum-containing antacids.

To put an additional spin on this: Many nutritional elements in your body are working according to a natural body rhythm; we call it "bio-rhythm" or "circadian clock." While we need to learn much more about this internal clock of ours, we already know quite a bit when it comes to certain enzymes and hormones; this understanding includes the workings of adrenalin, cortisol, melatonin, seratonin, and many, many others. Therefore, the time of day may matter when it comes to taking supplements. In my practice, I usually prefer individualized time tables to the everything-at-once method and I would like to urge you to discuss a similar approach with your responsible healthcare provider.

Your body will be able to give you quite a detailed feedback if you spread out your medication and supplements according to an individualized time and dosage schedule. You will know what works and what makes you feel queasy. In time, you will even learn to truly fine-tune your supplementing efforts and be able to cut cost by avoiding counterproductive nutrient combinations or excesses.

I have mentioned before that, in patients with a compromised gastrointestinal system, I have had better success with homeopathic and antihomotoxic remedies. These are easily absorbed by the mucous tissue of your mouth and do not get lost in a possibly compromised digestive process. Just remember, supplementing is very important and, since it is a very delicate subject, it should always be attempted only in careful communication with your knowledgeable and dedicated healthcare professional.

Also, do take serious my earlier warning: The greatest mineral imbalances I have experienced in my natural medicine practice, I saw in individuals who consumed hefty amounts of what I call "this-is-good-for-this and that-is-good-for-that supplements" that they had bought over-the-counter from their local health food store. These individuals were proud of "looking after themselves." But, for lack of qualified professional guidance, they may have wasted significant sums of money. Worse, they actively moved their bodies into a state of dys-regulation and homeostatic imbalance that resulted from unnatural ratios, excesses, and deficiencies. All their good intent opened them up to future disease.

Nature's minerals have long been identified as the essential building blocks for health. In the sixteenth century the Swiss physician Paracelsus already set himself apart from the alchemists of his times. His primary goal was to find out about the medicinal properties of plants and minerals. No longer did he strive to produce gold from substances of lesser value like it was the aim of his contemporaries. Paracelsus believed in the harmony and interrelatedness between microcosm, man, macrocosm, and nature. He stated that certain mineral balances needed to be present in the human body and, in fact, he concluded that various minerals could cause or cure specific illnesses.

Still today, we find strong opposition from mainstream medicine to this view about the importance of minerals to our body and health. Would it not seem appropriate to start acknowledging that, as much as everything else in nature, our human bodies too are the results of biochemical processes? And, even more so, is it not time to accept that these very biochemical processes ultimately depend on the presence of a respectable list of minerals in precise amounts and ratios in our body?

All living organisms are made up of four major building blocks, namely the chemical elements carbon, hydrogen, nitrogen, and oxygen. It has been long acknowledged that we humans too—and yes, this includes our bodies and functions—are made up of these same molecules. In addition to these four elements—and in order for all its processes and functions to work properly— our body needs a number of additional nutrients in varying quantities and ratios.

Without going too much into detail, let me list for you some of these major and essential nutrients and catalysts. Most of all, your body needs calcium, magnesium, phosphorus, potassium, sodium, and sulfur. In addition, your body requires a fair amount of iodine and several so-called trace minerals. Some of these trace minerals are chromium, cobalt, copper, fluorine, iron, manganese, molybdenum, selenium, and zinc. Several other minerals that now are being considered as essential are boron, molybdenum, nickel, silicon, and vanadium. Even minute amounts of arsenic appear to be essential. However, the threshold before many of these substances turn toxic is extremely low and, in today's environment, that limit is easily exceeded.

Paracelsus seems to have gotten it right when he emphasized the importance of the balance or—as we would call it—ratio among the various minerals. It is for this precise reason that many experienced natural medicine professionals today too caution against the widespread practice of consuming indiscriminate amounts of nutritional supplements. Let us look at where else we encounter minerals and why the environmental conditions providing them must be taken into consideration in any individual supplement regimen.

Where you live strongly influences your mineral levels, presence and absence, excesses or deficiencies of individual elements. Soil and air are as much a source of toxins as they are a resource for the minerals that end up in your environment and your food chain (see figure 15, p. 256). The soil surrounding you, to a large extent, codetermines what the outdoor air quality is like around you. In return, any airborne particles—such as those dispersed by acid rain— contaminate the soil. Even the indoor air, recycled by air-conditioned buildings, does affect you; unfortunately, not always positively.

More than soil and air, the water you drink and shower in is of greatest importance. During your shower, your skin directly absorbs moisture and, along with it, many chemicals carried in your water. When you inhale the moist air droplets your lungs easily absorb any foreign substances. Town water is treated with chlorine and, sometimes, other not so favorable components. Chlorine kills all bacteria, good or bad. For a sensitive body even the presence of minute levels of chlorine may have a negative accumulative impact on mucous tissue and immune system. Furthermore, treated water commonly lacks in many essential minerals. In addition, it often carries potential toxins that block or cancel out whatever good minerals it might contain. Filters and water softeners add to raising your hidden toxin levels. Silver, carbon and other minerals they use as antibacterials, over time, may accumulate in toxic levels in your body. And, lastly, rarely do filtering units replace any of the good and essential minerals in an absorbable form.

The food you eat makes perhaps the greatest difference, as we have seen. Healthy living does not consist of eating meat from animals raised and slaughtered in mass production; animals fattened on polluted grains that were supplemented with antibiotics, which contain toxic elements such as aluminum or arsenic. Even eating vegetables may not prove that much safer. Vegetables dowsed with chemicals or grown near major highways, a sewage plant, an industrial area, a transformer station, or an overland power line, probably lack as many nutrients of one kind as they provide toxic levels of another. And, if those same vegetables have been trucked any distance to your supermarket they will have been exposed to a hefty dose of exhaust fumes and, quite probably, will have been irradiated, a process that recently has become popular and further reduces their vitamin and nutrition value.

Are you surprised at me mentioning power lines? There are big discussions going on regarding the impact of their proximity on your health. In Europe we buried the power lines a long time ago. Not that burying them eliminates all problems! I am not the only one convinced that the static fields emitted by high power lines influence the molecular structure in all living cells within their range. Just consider for a moment the fact that all cells in your body carry an electric charge and that your heart function largely depends on the interaction of such positive and negative charges.

Once you understand this constant interaction between positively and negatively charged ions in your body, it appears not just possible but rather plausible that there will be an interaction between living cells and their surrounding, external power fields. Even all your electrical equipment, computers, TVs, kitchen gadgets, and more, build up a constant field and interaction with your body's own biochemical mechanisms. Electrical leakage in your home or office environment has been known to pose problems for people's health. We will further discuss some of these interactions when we talk about the roles of sodium and potassium in your cells and for your overall metabolism (see figure 18, p. 315). The electrolyte activity in your system is the greatest determinant of health or illness. For these and many more reasons, I believe that the possibly negative impact on living organisms—from plants to animals and humans—of electric leakage from any source should never be discounted.

The higher up the food chain we go, the more complex the potential for mineral deficiencies becomes. Deficient or toxic pastures will not suddenly turn into nutrient-rich hay for the cows that produce your milk or end up as steaks on your plate. Apart from their exposure to airborne particles remember also what we said about the additives and medications routinely fed to these animals. It stands to reason that they would not need supplementing if the natural ingredients that make up their feed had their mineral balances and ratios intact. But, without supplementing these animals do not remain healthy. Therefore, know where you buy your food and how it was treated and raised!

Eating less than optimal foods over time will cause mineral deficiencies in you. And, as we have seen, such imbalances cause functional and eventually organic problems. How can you find out what your body lacks? Blood tests—to some limited degree—show you what is circulating through your body. Urine tests show you what your body excretes. Mainstream medicine does not use any tests to show you what is actually being deposited inside the cells of your body—short of taking a liver biopsy; but who wants to go through that procedure!

Prior to anything being deposited in your cells it passes through your body's interstitial fluid, the fluid that surrounds all your cells. Since every organ cell or function displays its own ideal ratio and flow of electron exchanges innovative approaches to diagnosis are being developed. New and wonderful diagnostic tools such as the *Electro Interstitial Scanner*, or *Somatograph*, are slowly finding their way into our medical practices and hospitals. With the help of such tools early recognition and, therefore, prevention of many illnesses should no longer be an impossible quest.

Other methods are already more widely available. But, their application is largely restricted to finding out what minerals and toxins there are present. One of the areas in your body with the quickest change-over of cells is the hair at the back of your head, just above the nape of your neck. These days, several well-established and well-respected laboratories do specialize in the analysis of hair tissue samples. Few mainstream doctors use these tests. You, therefore, may want to ask around for a specially trained natural medicine professional who offers hair tissue mineral analysis testing and who is experienced in the interpretation of the results.

The hair tissue mineral breakdown may give the experienced practitioner an insight into the past couple of months of biochemical changes in your body. In fact, I find that quite frequently the hair tissue mineral analysis picks up on changes and looming problems long before either urine or blood analysis give any indication of disease. Using such early indicator methods gives you time to correct the imbalances and helps you prevent serious disease. I don't need to stress that avoiding disease is always preferable to healing disease. At the same time, I do recognize that these tests are only useful if the person who interprets them for you is knowledgeable and properly trained. Such a professional needs to possess a deep understanding of the biochemical processes in your body and should be able to suggest ways for you to strengthen your body's make-up without causing additional imbalances. It is imperative not to fall into the trap of simply supplementing those factors that show up as deficient on the result print-out.

Let me illustrate this by using once again the example of zinc, one of the most important minerals in your body. In diabetics and in people at risk of diabetes zinc levels are commonly low. If a zinc deficiency persists for any length of time, many of the toxins—such as aluminum, cadmium, and a few others—will accumulate in your body rather easily and any time you are exposed to them; not a good idea! If, on the other hand, you indiscriminately supplement zinc you may feel better for a little while. But, in short order, you may be crashing even worse. What happened? Excess zinc rarely causes much harm directly; however, it will reduce other of your essential mineral levels to dangerously harmful lows such as for instance copper. Copper, in turn, will affect your iron levels; and iron will negatively affect your blood's oxygen-carrying ability. Because of the interaction between many of your body's minerals a vicious cycle establishes itself this easily.

What can you do about this? Your first step is to develop good eating habits by avoiding foods and drinks that deplete your body's mineral composition. Secondly, have a well-qualified natural medicine physician help you map out a strategy to slowly, but lastingly, rebuild your body's mineral balance. For now, I would like to help you understand a bit more about some of the most important individual building blocks of your body and how they affect your various diabetes-related conditions and the overall level of your health.

Macro- and Micro-Mineral Supplements

Calcium (Ca)

Calcium makes up roughly two percent of your total body weight, and 98% of it is found in your bones. Most of the calcium is absorbed in the first part of your small intestines, the areas of the duodenum and jejunum. Less than ten percent of calcium is absorbed by your large intestines. Interestingly, it is the duodenum and part of the jejunum section of the small intestines that are bypassed in gastric bypass surgery. Up to 95 percent of the individuals who undergo this radical surgical measure are considered free of diabetes after the procedure. However, similar to celiac patients whose absorption is compromised, these patients then have to cope with significant mineral deficiencies and the danger of bone loss. It may yet turn out to be highly noteworthy that precisely these same duodenum and jejunum sections are affected most by gluten damage. Could it be that gluten and the ensuing inflammations, after all, do play a role in the development of obesity and subsequent diabetes?

If calcium is being absorbed by your small intestines it plays an important role in your enzyme activity, in the release of your neurotransmitters, in your muscle contraction, the regulation of your heartbeat, and the blood clotting within your arteries. Very low calcium levels may trigger muscle spasms and leg cramps; particularly at night, since that is the time when your body needs the most calcium. All these symptoms are problems both celiac patients and diabetics complain about.

For calcium to be absorbed sufficient amounts of vitamin D must be present. Exposure to sunlight synthesizes vitamin D in your body. At times, it is a toss-up between staying out of the sun for fear of radiation damage and getting enough sun for your body to manufacture its own vitamin D. But, the further north you live the less natural vitamin D you may get, especially during the winter months.

Vitamin D is not the only vitamin that influences calcium absorption. During my nutrition studies we used to repeat the following catchphrase: "vitamin K keeps calcium in the bones and out of the arteries." This is the reason for many natural medicine professionals to consider moderate supplementing with vitamin K, a vitamin that is important for the reversal of bone loss and for effective prevention of plaque build-up in your arteries. Luckily, your body makes a lot of its own vitamin K in your small intestines before storing it in your pancreas. But, if you experience bloating and other gut problems, your intestines may not be able to make enough vitamin K. You can help: kale and other leafy greens are great natural sources of vitamin K.

Calcium has an extensive job profile. Without appropriate absorption of calcium, iron cannot pass through the cell walls of your body tissues. This, more often than not, results in a lack of strength and, in time, may cause anemic tendencies. Therefore, consider the possibility of chronic underlying calcium absorption problems if you have been a candidate for repeat, but ineffective, vitamin B_{12} and iron shots. In such a case, only by solving the issue surrounding your calcium absorption deficit will you solve your chronic iron deficiency! This relationship between calcium and a lack of iron is something I see frequently in patients with gastrointestinal problems—as well as in those suffering from celiac disease and gluten-sensitivity. For many diabetics calcium deficiency is an often neglected but important factor.

Low calcium levels also may contribute to high blood pressure, osteoporosis, and colon cancer. Calcium supplements seem to reduce blood pressure in many hypertensive patients. However, allow me a word of caution: this may work for patients who are salt-sensitive; that is, whose blood pressure can be lowered by reduced salt intake. The few who are salt-resistant (their blood pressure rises after salt deprivation) may find no improvement or might even get worse by taking calcium supplements. You may find the probable cause for how your body handles its sodium balance in the pH values of your body tissues and blood. The acid-alkaline balance in your blood (your pH value) must always remain constant. If your body detects an imbalance, it causes calcium to be drawn from your bones and teeth in order to reestablish the equilibrium of acid and alkaline values.

Once dissolved into your bloodstream, calcium does not float around in your blood indefinitely. Eventually, the calcium drawn from your skeletal structures must be re-deposited in other body tissues. This leads to plaque build-up, or arthritis, rheumatisms, fibromyalgia, and the like; all are causes for many complications. Nevertheless, enough new and absorbable calcium must be made available to your body in order to replace the calcium leached earlier from your skeletal structures. Have you ever had a bone-density test that indicated decreased bone-density in an area that appeared fine last time, but you found improvements where the last test showed deficiencies? There is a fair chance that the reason for these apparent inconsistencies is that your bone-density issues are directly related to mild to moderate chronic metabolic acidosis (see *Chronic Metabolic Acidosis*, p. 206).

Calcium cannot act alone. We have seen the primary role of vitamin D. Apart from vitamin D, calcium also needs magnesium, which—by prompting the thyroid gland into producing calcitonin—aids in depositing calcium where it belongs, namely in your bones and teeth. Since magnesium is known also to work against unwanted calcium in your cells its role for the pre-diabetic and diabetic patient is significant, and we will discuss this in greater detail in the following chapter.

If you know—for instance from the results of a hair tissue mineral analysis—that your body is leaching calcium and magnesium (Ca and Mg will be showing high in the HTMA) you must supplement sufficient amounts of magnesium. Your normal supplement ratio of a well-balanced body is 2:1 calcium to magnesium. Depending on your situation, your natural healthcare professional for therapeutic purposes may want to choose the otherwise uncommon ratios of 1:1 or 1:2 calcium to magnesium for a short initial treatment phase. Once your calcium to magnesium ratio is properly balanced, the common 2:1 calcium to magnesium proportion will be the ratio to be considered for all of your further supplement needs.

For reasons of absorbability, I prefer the form of calcium citrate and magnesium citrate with the addition of vitamin D_3. There are many other and cheaper forms of calcium available. However, absorbability is an issue. Citrate seems to work best. Some words of caution: watch out for significant levels of lead toxicity in your calcium supplements. As with all supplements it pays to buy supplements from a trusted source and not to use less absorbable forms.

If you see calcium praised as an additive to antacids don't fall for it; antacids do not contain absorbable forms of calcium. In addition, many brands of antacids contain aluminum, which is known to block your calcium absorption and is toxic after all. Did you know that NSAIDs, aspirin, and several other drugs reduce your magnesium and, to some degree also, your calcium absorption? If you are on any of these remedies you may require additional calcium and magnesium supplements. Make sure you discuss your supplement regimen in detail with a medical professional who is knowledgeable in these biochemical processes.

In the context of speaking about over-the-counter and prescription medications it has always baffled me that toxic substances—such as aluminum, arsenic, mercury, to name but a few—are a consistent component of many prescription medications, vaccines, and of commercial animal feeds. The argument is that in the concentrations provided these substances are not toxic. We know that these toxins get stored in the human body. Has nobody ever calculated the accumulative impact of a simultaneous consumption of these substances in the form of medication, cosmetic products, cleaners, environment, and food? And, what about their impact on today's ever growing problem with bone loss leading to conditions such as osteoporosis?

Do you recall our discussion of other essential minerals such as boron (p. 92)? A boron deficiency can hugely speed up your bone loss. If excess testosterones or deficient estrogens are part of your picture you may want to supplement boron temporarily and under the supervision of your healthcare professional. This may solve some of your calcium deficiency problems along with several other endocrine issues.

Let us look at the natural food sources and deterrents for calcium. Including caffeine, coffee contains thirty acids that are instrumental in coffee's diuretic property. This diuretic effect of coffee doubles the normal rate of calcium loss. As we saw earlier—by raising the acidity levels in your blood—this is but one of the switches that prompt your parathyroid gland to mobilize calcium from your bones. It does this in order to maintain a stable blood pH value. In short, if you don't want to experience bone loss, stay away from that regular cup of coffee a day!

Some of your best natural sources of calcium are: carob flour (watch for its sugar levels!), almonds, parsley, Brazil nuts, and watercress. Seaweeds too, such as dulse or kelp, are ideal sources for calcium. They contain up to five times more calcium than all the other sources, but you have to watch out for the presence of pollutants and toxins. In general, green leafy vegetables are perhaps your best source of absorbable calcium from plant origin. These include kale, broccoli, collard, mustard greens, and many others. Other vegetables, such as turnips, provide good nutritional values too and are better than dairy products. Getting calcium from greens helps you avoid the problematic lactose (sugar!) connection that you would have to factor in if you needed to rely on milk products for your calcium. This is a major reason for us not to buy into the "drink milk" scheme.

Last but not least, if you suspect any thyroid imbalances you should discuss your choices with your trusted healthcare practitioner. Only the professional who is knowledgeable in these biochemical processes will be able to help you determine what the underlying causes of your calcium deficiency are. This is particularly important when it comes to the function of your thyroids. Depending on your thyroid condition (hypothyroid versus hyperthyroid) it is particularly important for your healthcare provider to figure out if seaweeds and other plants are an acceptable source of calcium for you. They contain quite significant amounts of iodine and you just might have to stay away from all natural iodine containing foods if you are hyperthyroid.

Magnesium (Mg)

Your bones contain 60% of the magnesium in your body. You find about 26% in your muscles and the remainder in other soft tissues such as your brain, your heart, liver, kidneys, and your body fluids. Magnesium is required in more than 300 enzyme driven reactions. These include your energy production (ATP), protein formation, and the cellular replication. Magnesium activates the so-called sodium-potassium pump by moving sodium out of the cells and potassium into your cells. This means that deficient magnesium levels may lead to lower potassium levels inside your cells, to water retention, and to cell function disturbances.

Once you understand the major functions of magnesium, it no longer should surprise you that magnesium frequently is low in diabetics. Most importantly, magnesium is involved in the secretion and action of your insulin. It may be for this reason that it is also said to prevent complications such as heart disease, and retinopathy. Chronic diarrhea, malabsorption syndromes, and pancreatitis, all may cause low levels of magnesium. Note that all of these are inflammatory diseases. Magnesium deficiency may lead to heart disease, high blood pressure, nerve conduction problems, muscle cramps, insomnia, and fatigue. Too much magnesium can block calcium from entering smooth muscle and heart muscle cells and, it may lower your blood pressure excessively.

High calcium intake, alcohol use, and liver or kidney disease may interfere with your magnesium absorption. Antibiotics, too, may lower your magnesium assimilation; so does surgery. Contraceptives and diuretics, along with several digitalis-based heart drugs and insulin injections tend to dissolve magnesium from your bones and tissues. I suspect this may be related to either the drugs causing a more acidic environment, or the oxygen-carrying ability of your blood being negatively influenced by these same drugs.

When it comes to supplementing with magnesium you need to remember a few basic guidelines: The higher your calcium intake, including dairy products—and, particularly, if these are fortified with vitamin D—the less your body will be able to absorb magnesium! On the other hand, vitamin B_6 assists magnesium in many enzyme and cellular functions and, therefore, may be an important addition to your supplement regimen. Commonly recommended for diabetics is a daily intake of 300 to 500 milligrams of magnesium together with a minimum 50 milligrams of vitamin B_6 to help move the magnesium into your cells. You see, it is all about balance; and, since your body's mineral ratios are not like mine, multi-vitamin supplements rarely make sense.

Rivkah Roth DO DNM®

A majority of your commercially available supplements contain calcium, magnesium, and a whole slew of other vitamins and minerals all in one "handy" product. Keeping in mind all the interactions between the minerals, I strongly advise that you take your calcium-magnesium-vitamin D_3 supplement separately and at different times of the day from any of the other mineral supplements. The only exception to this one-a-day type practice may be if you take the other substances in homeopathic form, in which case their absorption via mucous tissue should not be compromised to the same extent.

Many new patients of mine tell of being used to taking their vitamins and minerals all at once (usually in the morning). These patients quite often turn out to be the ones whose hair tissue mineral analysis shows the highest imbalances and toxin levels. I would not be surprised if the reason for this is that such indiscriminate popping of supplements presents a major shock to the body's system. The kidneys simply cannot keep up filtering out the overload. This contributes to the excess nutrients being stored in your fat tissues. The problem is that, with all the repeat onslaught, your body never gets around to dealing with these stored components. They become an inaccessible burden to your system and, eventually, may reach toxic levels and affect other synergistic or antagonistic minerals.

Because of certain and potentially severe interactions you absolutely must consult your primary care physician before attempting to supplement with magnesium if you suffer from kidney or heart disease. Only after you have received the go-ahead from your physician—along with specific dosage recommendations—should you commence on a magnesium supplement regimen if you suffer from any of these conditions.

The best natural sources for magnesium are kelp, dulse, wheat bran, wheat germ (if you are not suffering from intestinal malabsorption issues due to gluten-sensitivity, celiac disease, or similar conditions), almonds, cashews, buckwheat, Brazil nuts, hazelnuts, and peanuts. Make sure that the nuts are untreated and raw, not roasted. During the roasting process the natural oils in nuts turn rancid; and eating rancid nuts will quickly acidify your system—thereby canceling out any of their health benefits.

Potassium (K)

Potassium is the most important of our three dietary electrolytes, potassium, sodium, and chloride. The body's electrolytes conduct an electrical charge whenever they are suspended in fluid. Electrolytes are found in pairs. For instance, a potassium molecule or a sodium molecule with a positive electrical charge will pair up with a negatively charged chloride molecule. Potassium co-regulates your acid-alkaline balance, your water balance and function, your muscle and nerve cell function, your heart, kidney, and adrenal functions. Most importantly—for the pre-diabetic or the diabetic individual—potassium helps in the conversion process of blood sugar into glycogen and, thereafter, in its storage in your liver and muscle cells.

Potassium itself is not stored in your body. Instead, it needs to be supplied daily through your food intake. When you sweat excessively—for whatever reason (exercise, stress)—you lose potassium. Other factors that may cause loss of potassium are over-the-counter drugs such as aspirin, laxatives, diuretics, and several prescription drugs. Your potassium levels may be low if you experience urine leakage the moment you sneeze, cough, or laugh. Potassium deficiency affects your sphincter muscle's ability to contract and, generally, may be corrected easily by taking homeopathic, sublingual potassium.

These problems with low potassium levels frequently improve as soon as you pay more attention to your dietary potassium intake. Potassium deficiencies may be involved too if you experience muscular weakness, overall fatigue, and brain fog. If your potassium intake is low, but your sodium intake is high, your blood pressure rises. This situation with high blood pressure is common among many diabetics with a tendency towards kidney disease and cardiovascular events. This high-blood pressure and potassium deficiency link presents an interesting situation that I want you to consider more carefully: As you have seen, low potassium levels partnered with high sodium levels—over time—may lead to kidney and heart disease. However, if you suffer from kidney disease mainstream medicine guidelines demand that you must carefully follow your physician's orders and that you may have to limit your potassium intake. This includes nutritional potassium from potatoes or bananas.

According to mainstream medicine guidelines, supplementing potassium is also contraindicated if you are on any digitalis-based heart prescription medications or any enzyme-inhibiting blood pressure medications. Why? By eating healthier without simultaneously down-regulating these heart and kidney drugs you could very well end up overmedicating yourself. Your doctor, therefore, must be willing to coordinate a switchover with you. Remember, prescription medication is based on the premise that you will not change your food intake habits—even if those habits are known to have caused your problems. Once you are on any of these prescription medications it is extremely difficult to revamp your functional health status unless your prescribing physician is aware that you intend to change your lifestyle and dietary habits.

So much for low potassium levels! High potassium levels, on the other hand, are more commonly related to bacterial forms of cystitis and other bladder and kidney related problems. In all these latter cases you should immediately consult with your primary healthcare provider. Natural medicine approaches that supplement chromium, magnesium, manganese, sulfur, and niacin may help counteract a potassium excess in some urinary tract infections. But, again, that is for your healthcare professional to suggest.

Barring any information or recommendations provided in the previous paragraphs, it is generally suggested that your potassium to sodium intake ratio is that of two units of potassium to every one unit of sodium. Those of you at risk of pre-diabetes or diabetes must be aware of many weight loss formulas that contain excess levels of potassium. Such high potassium doses may, initially, help you lose weight from extra water in your body, but not by curbing your fat storage. In fact, this may backfire; particularly, if your body tends to veer towards the side of low blood sugar (hypoglycemia). Any extra potassium from those weight loss formulas is likely to reduce your sodium further. Yet, you need a certain level of sodium as an insulin antagonist.

At the same time, these high levels of potassium commonly provided in weight loss formulas reduce your chromium and manganese levels long-term. This starts a vicious cycle of undesirable diabetes-enabling biochemical imbalances and deficiencies. For this reason, I tend to caution all my patients and suggest they stay away from these sorts of weight loss formulas.

Your best natural potassium food sources are: avocados, potatoes, cooked lima beans, peas, several vegetables, fresh tomatoes, bananas, and nuts. You know what people say about craving nuts? One is a craving for the salt (sodium); the other is that, for instance, Brazil nuts contain up to 1000 times more potassium than sodium. Still, this is no license for binge-eating. A small handful of nuts a day is fine; everything else may tip the scale with excess fats. Flounder, salmon, haddock, and white chicken meat are also quite high in potassium but, at the same time, they contain a fair amount of sodium. You may have to go easy on them if your sodium is high already.

Sodium-Potassium Interactions

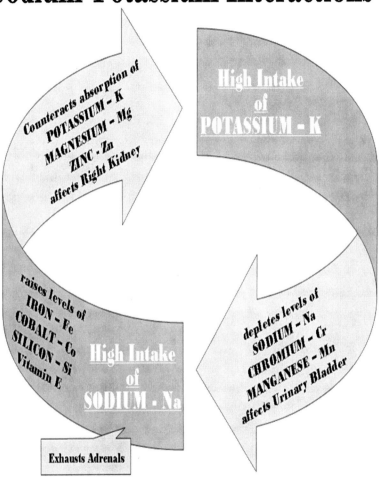

Figure 18 Interactions between Sodium, Potassium, and Phosphorus

Sodium (Na)

Never mind its bad reputation, sodium has an important role to fulfill in your body. Hormones produced by your pituitary gland and your adrenals control your sodium balance. Sodium levels determine the volume of fluids outside your cells while potassium levels, as we have seen, determine the fluid levels inside your cells. The sodium-potassium interaction determines the osmotic pressure in your body (what helps certain fluids move across your cell walls). It takes small amounts only of sodium to help regulate your acid-alkaline balance.

For anyone at risk of pre-diabetes and diabetes it is most important to know that sodium also acts as an insulin blocker. The higher the sodium level in your body the less your insulin is able to perform its function, namely to move glucose into your cells where it can be burnt and produce energy. As we shall see your adrenals and other endocrine hormones control your sodium balance. Stress—any kind of stress—depresses your adrenals and affects their function. Everything in our intricately fashioned body is interrelated. Therefore, keep in mind that salt cravings, not surprisingly, are more common in individuals who have metabolic issues. Heart disease and the risk of pre-diabetes and diabetes rarely lag far behind.

From among the electrolytes, sodium is the most common culprit in today's population. Salt for dietary consumption usually comes in the form of sodium chloride. Today, many households also use commercial water softeners based on salt. Did you realize that your body absorbs more than its daily requirements of salt alone by showering or bathing in such treated water? Yet, you also add salt to your foods or buy processed meals that are chuck-full of salt. No wonder then that so many people suffer from hypertension.

High salt intake, over time, affects your adrenals most strongly. Your adrenals easily become overworked and exhausted. Adrenal exhaustion depresses your aldosterone levels, one of the hormones produced by your adrenals. Aldosterone plays an important role in the interaction between sodium and potassium in your kidneys. The more sodium your system is exposed to the more aldosterone your adrenals need to secrete in order to cope with this onslaught of salt. This leads to increased sodium and water retention in your tissues and to an increase in blood volume. More blood needing to be pumped through your blood vessels results in hypertension, a condition that becomes even more precarious if your blood vessels have lost their elasticity or show plaque build-up.

Let us look at some numbers: Many vegetables and fruit contain large amounts of potassium and very little sodium, which makes them truly your food choices for good health. Yet, only five percent of the sodium in most people's diet comes from natural and unadulterated food sources. This amount alone would be enough to cover most of your requirements. Unfortunately—on average and on a daily basis—you also ingest from prepared foods close to twenty times more sodium than your body needs in order to function properly. A majority of this excess comes from commercially prepared foods and through the cooking process, which always concentrates the sodium. Lastly, a small amount from spices adds up to your 95% sodium overdose.

This is like using twenty people for a task that one person can perfect alone. You would not do such a thing at work or in business. So, why are you forcing your own body to work in this manner? Just as the extra people will only end up getting in the way and possibly will undo the good work the one does, so it is with the natural processes in your body. All that excess sodium gets in the way of many other processes. Oh, and I have not even included in this calculation the above mentioned sodium flood from externally absorbed sources such as water conditioners and water softeners.

Sodium interferes with your potassium levels. Moreover, it also keeps down your magnesium, zinc, vitamin B_2, folate, and long-term vitamin B_6 levels. From a natural medicine perspective, there is a clear link between excess sodium consumption or absorption and pre-diabetic or diabetic predispositions and conditions. The influence of sodium is significant: Sodium can raise your iron, cobalt, silicon, vitamin E, vitamin B_1, vitamin B_{12}, and short-term also your vitamin B_6 levels. Have you ever wondered why many cardiac patients are warned to stay away from vitamin E? Guess what, the reason is that, in many individuals heading towards hypertension and even a cardiac event, sodium has boosted these nutrients to toxic or near-toxic levels. Additional vitamin E supplements, therefore, would prove disastrous.

Here are your first steps towards healthier salt intake habits: Stay away from commercially prepared foods (this includes most canned foods). Use your table salt to clean your kitchen sink and iron skillets. Buy true "Sea Salt" or "Himalayan Rock Salt" for all your salt needs instead. These salts contain many additional essential minerals—not just sodium chloride. They also do not contain the same byproducts such as toxic aluminum remnants from processing as does your table salt.

Phosphorus (P)

High phosphorus levels are not unusual in anyone drinking one or more soft drinks a day. There is a direct link between phosphorus and calcium: adequate levels of vitamin D determine their absorption. High phosphorus levels have been linked to bone loss by their ability to reduce your calcium absorption. High phosphorus levels also lead you a giant step closer to chronic metabolic acidosis and other illnesses such as fibromyalgia.

In traditional Chinese medicine we make a difference between the functions of your two kidneys. Interestingly enough, our old western medical textbooks too teach such a difference. In a healthy human being the right kidney appears to predominantly regulate your sodium, while the left kidney is responsible for your phosphorus and protein mechanisms. These old theories teach us that, if the right kidney is compromised, your sodium levels are high and you may need additional magnesium, potassium, zinc, folate, and vitamin B_2. If your left kidney is affected, this theory stipulates that your phosphorus levels are too high. In this case you should consider supplementing calcium, zinc, and vitamin B_5 (also called pantothenic acid). And lastly, if you suffer from bladder complications, your potassium levels, as we have seen in one of the previous chapter, may be high. In this case your body needs additional chromium, magnesium, manganese, possibly sulfur, and other B vitamins such as B_3, also called niacin (see figure 18, p. 315).

I am mentioning these details because many individuals heading in the direction of diabetes might be pinpointed earlier as being at risk if they were identified by one or the other of these above-mentioned complications. However, once again, I would like to caution you. You cannot and must not simply run to the next health food store and pick up any of these nutrients in supplement form. Using the wrong ones or in the wrong dose, form, or combination may cause grave consequences. In many instances, even your natural medicine savvy healthcare professional may resort to the use of homeopathic substances in order to avoid unpleasant side effects.

High phosphorus sources to be avoided are all soft drinks. Good phosphorus sources are—if eaten in moderation—red meats, eggs, and some dairy products. Fish, seeds, and nuts too are sources of phosphorus, but are more likely to provide you with no more than the adequate levels needed for an already balanced diet.

Zinc (Zn)

In the introductory paragraph of this section about minerals I mentioned Paracelsus. In 1526, he introduced the name "zinc" for this mineral in allusion to its sharp and pointy form and the German word *Zinke* for the points of a fork. Zinc is a powerful antioxidant and immune system booster. It contributes to more than 200 imperative enzyme reactions in your body. There is no RNA or DNA synthesis without zinc, and it assists in the transport of vitamin A from your liver. Zinc plays an important role in the proper functioning of your hormones. Thymus, growth, and sex hormones all rely on zinc. It is one of the most important nutrients for those at risk of pre-diabetes or diabetes. Its presence or absence directly affects your insulin production.

In a healthy adult you should find roughly 260 mg of zinc allocated throughout your entire system at all times. About 65 percent of the zinc present in your body is stored in your muscles and in your white and red blood cells. The sites with the greatest zinc concentrations are your pancreas, liver, kidney, prostate, retina, bone, and skin. Is it not interesting that in our natural medicine practice complaints relating to these organs are some of the most common! Zinc deficiency is widespread. Neither your muscles nor your brain cells function properly if your zinc levels are deficient. No wonder that many individuals at risk of pre-diabetes and diabetes report brain fog and memory loss; and show highly deficient levels of zinc!

Stress has a tremendous impact on your zinc levels. During stressful events your body may excrete up to eight milligrams of zinc in your urine; the more constant your stress the greater your loss of zinc. Are you still surprised that zinc deficiency is so widespread in today's rat-race population? It does not always take this kind of outside stress though to change your zinc levels. Zinc appears to be a key component of life in general. Did you know that zinc is an important component of human sperm? Every ejaculate contains 7mg of zinc; a great start for the new life to be created, but a big temporary loss for the male producing it!

Remember, how we mentioned that erectile dysfunctions might be alerting you to a problem with impending diabetes? While there has not yet been any research available that proves such a connection beyond any doubt, I personally believe that in certain types of men—particularly if they tend towards hypertension or hypothyroid and overweight conditions—the depression of zinc levels might well provide an explanation to growing problems with loss of libido. Where are the oysters? If the zinc deficit is not replenished quickly enough your entire organism will be affected. And, as you have seen, your pancreas and its production of insulin may be the first to pay the price.

You also lose zinc in your sweat. Zinc affects your sense of taste and smell. Its presence or absence may influence your appetite, your mood, your learning ability, your body odor, your joint and muscle health, your vision, and your fertility. Without the proper zinc levels your serum testosterone levels will become imbalanced because zinc plays a regulating role via the enzyme aromatase, which determines how much testosterone is being converted into excess estrogen. I routinely caution my patients that alcohol intake will reduce their zinc levels and will increase their estrogen levels; certainly not a desired effect in male individuals!

Zinc deficiency affects women too. Did you ever suffer from night sweats that improve after your gynecologist prescribes a progesterone cream? New patients are frequently surprised when I voice disagreements with such an approach. Progesterone raises your potassium and zinc levels. It is quite likely that paying attention to your zinc or potassium intake will help you more than any progesterone preparation; most of all, without its many side effects.

The bulk of naturally occurring zinc routinely is removed during the refining process of flour. Many of the additives used in processed foods too have a direct impact on zinc. EDTA (*ethylenediaminetetraacetic acid*), for instance, is a widely used chelating agent that is not removed during wastewater treatment and has been found to cause reproductive and growth probems. It is customarily added to commercial foods for its ability to bind to and eliminate unwanted metal contamination. While this may help reduce the toxic load of lead and other undesirable minerals from foods such as legumes it, unfortunately, also eliminates sought-after metal minerals such as zinc, copper, and iron.

You should be careful, however; there is such a thing as too much zinc. In larger doses than needed, zinc may cause inflammations such as in your prostate. Left-sided cancers of the ovaries and testes quite commonly are said to be showing a link with high zinc levels. Taking too much zinc also may cause hair loss, possibly gastrointestinal issues, and a whole lot of other problems by affecting its ratio with other minerals and vitamins. Therefore, remember that supplements should only be taken under the close supervision of a knowledgeable healthcare provider!

Zinc is a very sensitive mineral. It competes for absorption with copper and with iron. For this reason many natural medicine professionals recommend supplementing zinc to copper at a 14 to 1 ratio. Zinc absorption can also be blocked if you take it together with calcium and diets high in fiber, phytates (*innositol*), or chelating agents (see above). Many nutritionists recommend a high fiber diet for diabetics. With few exceptions I thoroughly disagree with this approach. Chelating agents such as phytate or phytic acid occur in plant seeds as the primary storage form of phosphorus. Unlike ruminant animals, humans cannot digest it because humans are missing the necessary enzyme. When you consume high fiber diets other and essential nutrients attach to the fiber and are flushed out of your system. This particularly affects your calcium, magnesium, iron, and zinc levels, but also your glucose tolerance factor chromium. Fiber, therefore, is helpful wherever we have an excess of minerals or toxins to get rid of. But, most individuals at risk of pre-diabetes or diabetes already suffer from deficient levels of minerals and do not want to compound their underlying problem.

For similar reasons, I do not like multi-vitamins. Instead I use homeopathic forms of zinc or have my patients take it in smaller doses and away from calcium and fiber. Zinc tends to be absorbed better this way, and any danger of larger doses that could lead to toxic levels is greatly reduced. In addition to its interaction with calcium, your various levels of zinc may be reflected by its interactions with iron, phosphorus, sodium, selenium, nickel, tin, copper, and the vitamins A, B_1, and C, along with niacin, niacinamide, folic acid, lecithin, and choline.

Zinc is naturally available in oysters, eggs, soybeans, wheat germ, pumpkin and other seeds, nuts, milk, and yeast. Lamb meat, beef, chicken, and herring are also reported to be high in absorbable zinc. For many of my patients preparing a Middle Eastern tahini (sesame paste) has become a big hit when it comes to supplementing with zinc. Check out tahini serving suggestions in my companion volumes *DIABETES-Series Little Books*.

Chromium (Cr)

Discovered in France the year the French Revolution spread throughout Europe (1797), chromium's role in blood sugar regulation was not established until the middle of the twentieth century. These days, chromium is largely used in the metal industry to produce alloys and paints. It is toxic in this industrial (hexavalent) form and may cause allergies even on contact. Because of its industrial use, toxic chromium may be found as one of the worst and most common environmental pollutants in your soil and groundwater.

In its less toxic, so-called trivalent form, chromium is an essential trace mineral for the human body. Yet, while sufficient chromium is essential for the human body, even in this form any chromium excess might lead to cell damage.

321

One of the actions of chromium is that of a glucose tolerance factor (GTF). Chromium works in conjunction with your insulin and assists in moving glucose into your cells. If your chromium levels are low, most likely your blood sugar is high—it is this simple. Chromium also plays a role in the protein transport and helps in the breakdown of your glycogen and lipids. Remember those transferrin numbers in your blood tests? Chromium is using transferrin in order to get to your liver from where it can be distributed to your blood and tissues. Low transferrin levels may—in a roundabout way—indicate low chromium levels.

Arduous exercise may lower your chromium too quickly. Chromium deficiencies may result in fatty deposits in your arteries, high blood cholesterol and triglyceride values, infertility and, lastly, reduced life expectancy. As we have seen in the chapter about zinc, chromium deficiencies are especially common in individuals on high fiber and phytate diets. But also, eating refined commercial foods and simple sugars are major contributors to low chromium levels. High sugar intake easily depletes chromium.

We have spent quite some time discussing carbohydrate addiction and cravings. Supplementing minute doses of chromium picolinate has been shown to reduce carbohydrate cravings. My personal take on this is that chromium supplements are able to reduce high copper levels, commonly associated with food cravings. It is interesting to know that, when you start supplementing chromium in cases where copper is high, the chromium will go up only after your copper—and also your potassium—have come down to normal levels. Magnesium, on the other hand, can be helped by chromium probably precisely by eliminating its antagonist potassium.

Many weight loss formulas contain chromium because of its glucose tolerance factor. Disregarding the ratios and balances in your system may cause far greater problems than benefits. Don't fall for advertisements touting high chromium supplements for the reversal of diabetes. It is not that simple. Bringing up your chromium values by working on its antagonists shows far greater promise and needs to be done under the close supervision of a health professional knowledgeable in these matters. Because of the fine line between deficiency and excess I prefer to use homeopathic forms of chromium for many of my patients. This allows me to adjust the balance with the other essential minerals without jeopardizing ratios and other mineral levels to the same extent. Especially elderly patients and the very young people appear to be highly sensitive to chromium supplements. The safe homeopathic route, therefore, is always preferable in those cases in the long run.

Natural sources of chromium include brewer's yeast, liver, beef, chicken, eggs, and dairy. Fish and seafood too contain a fair amount of chromium, as long as they are not too high in copper. While keeping in mind their potassium levels, also think of bananas, green peppers, and whole-grain products. Moreover, beer contains chromium; but, beer is simply too high in calories and carbohydrates to be considered an option. Moreover, beer should be avoided by anyone at risk of pre-diabetes or diabetes. Also check your drinking water; it too may provide you with more than enough chromium—hopefully, not of the toxic kind!

Copper (Cu)

Copper has been known for probably at least ten thousand years. The manufacture of bronze from copper and tin was instrumental in naming the time period from 3500 BC to 1100 BC the Bronze Age. Today, you are still exposed to large amounts of copper through the use of copper water pipes, copper roofs, and many other applications. Copper is important for more than a dozen enzyme reactions throughout your body. In a healthy adult, 80 mg to 120 mg of copper are stored; mostly in the liver. Copper co-determines how iron is integrated in your red blood cells and, therefore, indirectly determines the oxygen-carrying ability of your blood.

If your copper levels are too high, your needs for vitamin C grow. When copper is high along with high zinc—and you, therefore, cannot reduce it by increasing your zinc level—natural medicine practitioners frequently recommend large doses of vitamin C or ascorbic acid to bring down your near toxic copper levels. Another important aspect is that aluminum has the ability to keep your copper levels artificially high. As we have seen earlier, it too can be found in anything from your town drinking water to your prescription medications. You may want to be extremely cautious especially if you live in a newer home: it takes at least five years for your copper pipes to build up enough coating with hard calcium to reduce copper leakage into your water. I reluctantly recommend to my patients to let the water run until all the standing water has been drained from the pipes. This is costly though to the environment and to your purse.

Infections and pregnancies too may raise your copper levels. So do birth control pills or hormone replacement therapy due to their ability to raise your estrogen levels. This may directly affect your blood sugar levels as well as the oxygen-carrying ability of your blood. And, have you asked your gynecologist what your IUD is made from? Copper IUDs are still common. Worn internally, naturally, they raise your body's copper levels. Remember the need for extra vitamin C! The right amount of copper is imperative.

If copper is already low, supplementing zinc might damage your copper levels even further. However, once your body has arrived at proper copper levels and is starting to store it, zinc will no longer lessen it. Copper deficiency may be connected to elevated cholesterol, cardiovascular problems, and a large number of musculoskeletal issues. Low copper levels not only have been linked to joint problems but also depress your good HDL cholesterol and raise your LDL cholesterol levels—possibly prompting arterial and heart conditions. In addition, low copper should be suspected in many gastrointestinal problems, such as leaky gut syndrome and gluten-sensitivity. Low calcium and low potassium, frequently, go along with low copper levels.

Because of the side effects often associated with copper supplements (nausea) I always suggest alternative ways to bring up your copper levels. Homeopathic approaches work extremely well and are rather safe. As simple as it sounds, copper bracelets too appear to be an easy way to bring up moderately deficient copper levels.

Many of the foods rich in copper appear to be addictive; so, therefore, go easy on these: cocoa, chocolate, coffee, cola (common cause of toxic levels), and tea all contain high levels of copper. Black tea, in fact, is even higher in copper than coffee and seems to have some other benefits. Seafood, shellfish, liver, mushrooms, soybeans, wheat germ, seeds, and nuts too contain a fair bit of copper, as do your tap water and draft beer due to copper leakage of the water pipes.

Vanadium (V)

Industrial use of vanadium is common in the production of surgical steel and in many anti-corrosives. The airplane industry too uses vanadium. Vanadium is needed in minute quantities only in your body. It is an interesting mineral and appears to imitate insulin. Vanadium seems to play a role in your blood sugar and lipid metabolism. It also appears to affect your skeletal growth and reproduction. A vanadium deficiency is linked to many of the symptoms and conditions displayed by those individuals at risk of pre-diabetes and diabetes.

You should know that calcium, potassium, sodium, iodine, sulfur, rutin, and sugar may work against vanadium. Zinc on the other hand, may help maintain your vanadium levels. However, vanadium may work against chromium if it is paired with selenium. For this reason, I never recommend supplementing with vanadium but, instead, have my patients rely on dietary sources for the small amounts the body needs.

Fish, dill, olives, black pepper, and some of the unprocessed vegetable oils appear to provide the highest vanadium levels and rarely make supplementing necessary. The water coming from Mount Fuji is said to be particularly high in vanadium also. Anyone want to travel to Japan?

Molybdenum (Mo)

In industrial use molybdenum is part of many heat- and corrosion-resistant alloys and electronic transistors. It is used to remove organic sulfurs in the course of petroleum production. Mammograms use x-ray tubes containing molybdenum too. When it comes to the human body, molybdenum is one of the essential trace elements. It helps in the conversion of carbohydrates, fats, and nitrogen. It plays a key role in detoxifying sulfites and alcohol. Frequently, molybdenum is found to be deficient in patients who suffer from chronic or recurrent allergies.

Molybdenum deficiencies are more frequent among those at risk of pre-diabetes or diabetes and those with Crohn's disease. Low molybdenum and, sometimes, also vanadium levels quite frequently point to degenerative problems of your spine. Maybe, in this context, we find another explanation for the prevalence of back problems in individuals heading towards diabetes (see p. 164).

Furthermore, molybdenum is intimately linked with your copper metabolism. In fact, it may not be easy to distinguish between copper deficiency and molybdenum toxicity. There seems to be a regulating interaction between molybdenum and vanadium on one hand and copper and chromium on the other. If copper is higher than chromium, molybdenum in most cases will be lower than vanadium. Get your healthcare professional to help you figure out where you fit in this equation.

Molybdenum may reduce intestinal iron and copper absorption. It acts as a copper antagonist and, in this role, competes with sulfur. This ability to contain excessive copper levels may have something to do with the rumored ability of molybdenum as an anti-carcinogenic. As with many of these trace minerals, high levels can have severe negative implications. This presents some problems; especially, if copper is low to start with or, if both, copper and molybdenum, are

Rivkah Roth DO DNM®

low. Such a relationship between the minerals clearly illustrates how important it is to work with a healthcare professional who is extremely well versed and knowledgeable in these matters of mineral interactions.

Natural sources of molybdenum are non-modified grains, beans, sorghum, soybeans and lentils. Organ meats too, often, contain molybdenum. However, I do not recommended eating organ meats because of their high count of toxic substances. On a similar note: If you grow your own vegetables and ever have seen onion greens with bleached out tips this is quite possibly due to a molybdenum deficiency of your soil.

Manganese (Mn)

Manganese levels in diabetics have been noted to be less than fifty percent of those in healthy individuals. It is important to know that manganese may block the absorption of zinc, copper, and iron and, therefore, plays a major role in maintaining your entire trace mineral balance.

Manganese deficiency may result in glucose intolerance, hypoglycemia, and a reduced lipid metabolism—along with high cholesterol values. A lack in manganese is reflected in decreased pancreatic cell function. Other manganese deficiency-related problems may include ovarian cysts in women, blindness, or a propensity towards joint dislocations—all potential warning signs of a possible risk of diabetes.

Excessive manganese levels, on the other hand, may block iron absorption and need to be addressed in order to correct an underlying anemia. Excessive manganese levels may also be found in hypothyroid conditions, colitis, urinary incontinence or frequent urination, and water retention. Among natural medicine professionals it, furthermore, is well-known that excess manganese is frequently connected with nerve inflammation, low back pain, menses problems, and endometriosis. If you look back over our list of potential concurrences with a risk of pre-diabetes you find that we previously discussed all of these conditions.

Natural sources of manganese are nuts and seeds, whole grains, spinach and other leafy greens, dried fruit, and black tea. Unfortunately, many of these foods may have been exposed to unacceptable levels of fertilizers, fungicides, and exhaust fumes (fuel additives), and may contain high levels of toxins.

Germanium (Ge)

Although germanium is needed in your body in minute quantities only, it plays an important role in your immune system and improves the oxygenation of your tissues. A lack of germanium often seems to go hand in hand with circulation problems, heart or eye disorders and, most obviously, metabolic acidosis.

All simple sugars and carbohydrates depress germanium levels. For this reason, it appears to be vital for those at risk of pre-diabetes and diabetes to keep a close eye on germanium levels. However, as mentioned many a time, it is important not to over-supplement since kidney or liver damage might be the undesirable consequence.

Natural sources of germanium are garlic, onion, ginseng, aloe vera, comfrey, shiitake mushrooms, watercress, and the spice sumac. Sushi too provides high levels of germanium.

Nickel (Ni)

Your body's requirements for nickel are small but significant. Nickel is part of your body's nucleic acid and protein structure. It too provides an important enzyme action for the breakdown of glucose. Nickel affects the iron and zinc metabolism and, if it is present in excessive levels, may interfere with the Krebs Cycle (energy production), and with your DNA and RNA production.

Nickel deficiency relates to impaired glucose metabolism, hyperglycemia, and high blood cholesterol. These are all issues that directly affect you if you are at risk of diabetes. Low nickel levels, on the other hand, may result in reduced stomach acid levels, iron-deficiency anemia, and general malabsorption issues. All of these are issues diabetics or individuals at risk of diabetes frequently are confronted with.

Lower adrenal and thyroid function—along with the resulting hormone imbalances—may stem from nickel deficiency and may be a reason for fatigue. Sinus congestion too has been linked to low nickel levels. Extreme deficiencies are common in cases of liver cirrhosis and kidney failure.

Natural foods containing nickel are nuts, legumes, lentils, and soy beans.

Tin (Sn)

Tin is mostly involved in the oxidation process. In addition, it supports your adrenals. Low tin along with low vitamin C and maybe also vitamin B_1

levels appears to be found whenever there is reduced adrenal function and left-sided cardiac insufficiency. It, therefore, relates to diabetes only in a round-about, but important, way via its adrenal and cardiac influence. It is a more widely acknowledged culprit when it comes to asthma and breathing problems or cancer.

Toxic levels of tin may accumulate in your body from the use of tin cans, tin foil, food additives, solder used in water pipes, some of the fluoride toothpastes, and from air pollution adhering to foods.

Natural sources of tin are asparagus, broccoli, spinach, cabbage, Brussel sprouts, dulse and other seaweeds and, of course, all canned foods.

Iodine (I)

Iodine is mostly involved in your body's hormone production due to the role it plays in the function of your thyroids. Iodine is also important for your cell respiration. Your thyroid function is involved in conditions such as hypothyroidism, obesity, lowered vitality, water retention, and an overall lowered basal metabolic rate. Since these conditions are common in many individuals at risk of diabetes iodine deficiency should always be considered as a possible underlying cause.

Please note that iodine supplements should only be considered under the careful and continued guidance of an experienced health professional since some individuals must strictly avoid any sources of iodine.

Natural food sources of iodine are plentiful: sea salt, iodized salt (watch out for unwanted aluminum content), seafood, kelp, garlic, onions, lettuce, spinach, squash, mushrooms, whole wheat (if you are not sensitive to gluten), and cheddar cheese.

Lithium (Li)

Lithium appears to play no more than a secondary role when it comes to diabetes. The reason I mention it here is that many diabetics and individuals at risk of diabetes show low to very low lithium levels in their hair tissue mineral analysis results. Lithium may act as an iodine, magnesium, or chromium antagonist and, therefore, may need to be considered when looking at your total mineral balance.

Lithium acts as a modulator of your essential fatty acids. It also plays a role in the phosphorus to sodium balance (always an issue with those who drink one or more soft drinks a day). Gastrointestinal disorders, bloating, low stomach acid, and heart burn frequently do go along with lithium deficiencies. Moderate toxicity and lithium excess, on the other hand, may prompt hypothyroidism, obesity, fatigue, edema, or diarrhea; all again conditions that we have looked at in the context of an increased risk of pre-diabetes and diabetes.

Have your natural medicine professional help you make the distinction between too much and not enough and avoid a possibly disastrous wrong approach. In many cases it is preferable to rely on the support of the natural sources. Magnesium, and chromium help reduce excess lithium levels, while manganese, silicon, sodium and cobalt, along with vitamin D assist in its absorption.

Natural sources of lithium are mineral waters, seaweed, and sugar cane. Please do not interpret this as me advocating you drinking rum for this purpose; it would be the surest ticket to an unwanted blood sugar high. Water that has not been demineralized is a perfect alternative. One of the mineral waters we used to drink in my native European country was particularly praised for its natural lithium levels.

Rivkah Roth DO DNM®

Mineral Interaction Diamond
Essential & Other Minerals

Toxic Minerals

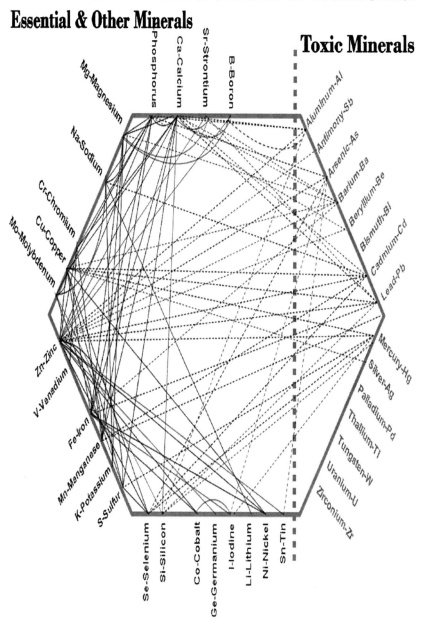

Figure 19 Mineral Interaction Diamond

PART FOUR - Support Structures

For Further Studies

*Your living is determined
not so much by what life brings to you
as by the attitude you bring to life;*

*not so much by what happens to you
as by the way your mind looks
at what happens.*

Kahlil Gibran

Natural Medicine—a Viable Approach

Not everyone is familiar with the concept and approach of natural medicine. Natural medicine presents a different philosophy from that of mainstream medicine. Your natural medicine professional will focus strongly on early detection and prevention of any condition, while a mainstream medicine physician basically must wait until you are sick before assessing and treating you. Earlier, I called this the "health care" versus the "sick care" approach.

A natural medicine doctor has many different tools in his or her toolbox. Some of the modalities are of strictly diagnostic value, such as tongue and pulse diagnoses (borrowed from traditional Chinese medicine), hair mineral analysis or other noninvasive tests such as muscle testing, even iridology. Other modalities are used for treatment and include a variety of herbal treatments, homeopathy, homotoxicology, trace mineral therapy, nutrition, and many hands-on modalities.

Throughout *At Risk?* I have mentioned several differences between how natural medicine approaches a certain issue and how mainstream, allopathic medicine might react. Allow me to summarize a few of the most obvious and important of these points:

⇨ Patient versus Disease: Natural medicine looks at any condition within the whole make-up of the patient; mainstream medicine treats an isolated disease. This is commonly summarized as: Natural medicine treats the patient—mainstream medicine treats the disease.

⇨ Cause versus Symptom: When it comes to treating a condition, natural medicine will want to find and treat the cause; mainstream medicine mostly addresses the obvious symptoms.

⇨ Support versus Suppression: Treatment in the case of natural medicine means supporting your body in its attempt to heal itself—slowly and systematically. Mainstream medicine often suppresses a disease in order to quickly remove the most obvious symptoms, pain and inflammation.

⇨ Chronic versus Acute: Because of its ability to work with your body and bring about improvements slowly, natural medicine is particularly suitable for the treatment of chronic, ongoing conditions. Mainstream medicine is excellent at handling acute situations and all cases where surgery is required.

⇨ Prevention versus Sick Care: Preventive care is easy for natural medicine since it critically looks at early and subtle changes in your systems and functions. Mainstream medicine relies mostly on blood and urine tests for diagnosis. These show changes only once you are quite seriously ill.

⇨ Lifestyle Change versus Prescription Medication: Where possible, natural medicine advocates lifestyle changes that include nutrition and exercise. Mainstream medicine in most cases starts immediately with synthetic prescription drugs—some for life.

During my work with individual patients I have noticed how difficult it is for an individual with pre-diabetes or diabetes to cope with the need of making changes in their lifestyle and their approach to food. Change is particularly difficult if you are newly diagnosed and decide to remain in your regular environment during your adjustment phase. Natural medicine is especially suited to help you reinvent yourself. It will support your decision towards making a shift in your thinking and will help you take responsibility for the health and well-being of your body.

Why is it that natural medicine may hold a promise for change where mainstream medicine almost always will guarantee "more of the same?" A natural medicine approach looks at your body as alive and evolving. It does not isolate one organ or one physiological process. Natural medicine modalities support your body's functions and mechanisms where mainstream medicine mostly suppresses anything that does not fit the pattern. In summary, the main difference is that natural medicine works "with" you, not "on" you.

Whichever natural medicine support system you choose, in the end you, the patient, is the only one able to change your life—and health. Your dedication towards healing, therefore, starts with a greater involvement and commitment that goes well past popping prescription medications one to three times daily. Your health professional can guide you but cannot entirely do the work for you. Your full and total commitment to helping your own body is a strong prerequisite. Never forget that your body is alive and, like any live matter, you can either keep it healthy or destroy it—cell by cell—by the way you nourish or neglect it. Diabetes is no laughing matter after all and, certainly, no reason to boast with defiance!

Physical invincibility does not exist. Patients who are in denial usually are the ones addicted to carbohydrates. They are finding the healing process most taxing. Unfortunately, their non-compliance is proverbial among the ranks of their healthcare givers. Thus, remember: To continue the same lifestyle that has brought you to the edge of the abyss and to simply pop some pills and stick yourself daily with needles may sound simple enough in the beginning. But, as you have seen, only a proactive shift in your attitude and habits will actually show promise of real improvements and may bring about long-term avoidance of further complications and, at best, a reversal process. This requires a good understanding of your situation and a solid support system.

Many different approaches might help you. A natural medicine doctor, or a naturopath, may use several modalities depending on his or her training and expertise. In my own clinic I favor nutritional and lifestyle recommendations along with a combination of antihomotoxic remedies, an individualized supplement plan, and a specific work-out regimen that includes teaching my patients how to deal with their daily stress triggers. I have found it particularly beneficial to spend a goodly amount of time instilling food shopping habits and meal preparation along with a deeper understanding of the nutritional processes involved in maintaining an acid-free, healthy body. And, last but not least, I have found it very important—in fact necessary—to get a patient's entire family involved in this process.

The Ten Pillars of Natural Diabetes Avoidance

The ten main pillars of a successful diabetes avoidance model are:

1. Health assessment (review of your test results and present state of health).

2. Risk assessment (in-depth family history and individual risk analysis).

3. Goal setting (establishing short- and long-term goals and how to successfully work them into your daily routine).

4. Medical supervision (control of daily vitals and progress monitoring).

5. Mental support system and coaching (group and individual support).

6. Nutritional support (learning about food choices and individual supplement needs).

7. Practical support (learning how to work with your individual issues and how to prepare your own meals).

8. Physical regimen (developing a viable daily exercise routine).

9. Stress reduction (developing personal routines such as creating a safe space, meditation, or writing).

10. Process evaluation (periodic reassessments and redirection).

Your Mental Support System

Learning how to cope mentally with your new situation is of utmost importance. Your body is already amply strained on a physical level. Any specific medical diagnosis on top of this is apt to add so much stress that it may evaporate whatever little strength your adrenal system still possesses to draw on.

Counseling and coaching support is designed to fulfill a variety of roles, namely to:

⇨ Help you understand what factors contribute to your health crisis.

⇨ Motivate you to consider positive changes.

⇨ Help you to effect the necessary changes.

⇨ Help you to rearrange your environment.

⇨ Help your family and friends to understand the "new you."

Most of all, counseling must help you overcome your specific addiction factor or factors:

⇨ Carbohydrate addiction

⇨ Mental resistance to change

⇨ Perceived physical blockages

⇨ Other "I need" stances that may become counterproductive to your recovery.

As part of your daily routine, your natural medicine professional may suggest meditation classes and certain other group activities such as Tai Chi or

Qi Gong classes. These activities will help you improve your breathing technique, something you might never have learned or might have lost—either through stress or through bad eating habits.

Then there is your approach to life and, specifically, to your body. Mindfulness and awareness are some of the major qualities you will learn when you work with a natural medicine team. In fact, you will probably learn why any mindless routine from repetitive movements in an uninspiring exercise routine to an unadventurous outlook on food may be counterproductive. After all, an effective natural medicine support will be designed to empower you and to motivate and enable you to take charge of your own life and health long after you leave such a support program.

Before concluding this first volume dedicated to the early risk recognition of pre-diabetes and diabetes allow me to introduce you to several of the more common natural medicine treatment options and modalities used in diabetes avoidance.

Nutrition

Sometimes GPs refer their newly diagnosed diabetes patients to a specialized dietician. According to my experience such counseling sessions, more often than not, are limited to advise on how to use glucose meters, how important it is to stick to your meal times and medicine schedule, and to take a twenty minute walk three times a week. I have yet to see the individuals who attend these sessions and follow this information significantly improve their blood glucose levels, lose weight, or reverse their condition.

Unfortunately, the nationally established diabetes model simply does not work for everyone; nor is it stringent or specific enough to help make a real difference in those who attend its sessions. Most of these mainstream diabetes programs work on the unspoken assumption that you will not change your daily habits. This take is quite understandable when we consider that mainstream medicine still widely views an illness as the beginning of a problem and not, as we natural medicine professionals look at it, as its culmination.

Mainstream medicine and natural medicine, both, acknowledge the power of lifestyle changes for coping with diabetes. Yet, the two approaches differ quite substantially in how you should go about it. In an earlier chapter (p. 112) we have discussed how misleading diet recommendations can be counterproductive. An intimate understanding of the chain of biochemical processes in the body is paramount. Most natural medicine professionals understand that food is the beginning and the end of any diabetes avoidance, prevention, or reversal tactic.

Many of these professionals are well prepared and trained to help you find your balance from where illness and health start: your food intake.

Food is medicine, or food is poison. Every morsel of food, every ounce of liquid that goes into your body affects how that internal system of yours works. If the foods you eat are full of chemicals, contain empty calories, and addictive carbohydrates—not to speak of the fats added to make them tastier—then your body pays the price. There are no exceptions! Equally as important is what your body does not get; namely, the nutrition consisting of the right amounts and ratios of essential and non-essential minerals, vitamins, and other factors needed to form enzymes, hormones, and the drivers for your body's functions.

It is simple, bad foods destroy cells; lack of good foods hampers healthy cell development. Neither one is preferable. The only solution is to stop eating bad foods and to start eating foods that provide absorbable nutrients and positive building blocks to your body. Better health is an almost guaranteed outcome of proper eating! This is where a specialized natural medicine professional can help.

I used to wonder why most diabetics and those at risk prefer cream colored foods and show little interest in the wonderful array of colorful plants and herbs we have so widely available. At some point, I understood that it actually might be the other way around. People who love and consume a wide variety of colorful foods rarely develop diabetes or heart attacks, kidney failure, and other of these nasty conditions.

It is easy to discuss a certain approach to food with a patient or even to prepare an individualized meal plan. However, the healthcare professional does not live with you; the pitfalls are many, so are the numbers of possible slip-ups. The hard work is your work not that of your healthcare professional. Unfortunately, the trick is precisely how you put in action what you have recognized to be necessary adjustments of your lifestyle. You never get out of your toxic trigger loop as long as you have the little "oh, just this once" and the "it's only this one little piece" moments. Don't believe any of the well-meaning suggestions that you start by eating just a little less, or by eating one healthy food for every destructive food.

This is why it is so important that you get the right team lined up to support you in your quest for better health. We have taken a step in this direction here at the *Natural Medicine Centre*. Instead of simply holding one-on-one in house consultations for patients who live locally, we offer online-based services for individuals and groups with regular follow-ups and question and answer sessions. This approach allows us to reach wider geographical areas and work with a larger group of people keen about looking at their possible risk of pre-diabetes and diabetes and willing to work on avoiding it. Many natural medicine professionals are offering this kind of service and help nowadays.

Food and nutrition is a wide topic and is much more involved and detailed than can be done justice to in the framework of this book. For greater insights look to the companion volumes of *At Risk?*, the *DIABETES-Series Little Books*. You will find more detailed information about specific essential nutrients and supplements along with a simple format of basic food preparation tips for anything from breakfast to dinner, and snacks, or drinks.

Phytotherapy

Phytotherapy (*phyto* is Greek for plant) is a form of herbal medicine. It describes the use of whole plants—fresh or dried. Remedies are prepared in liquid form as teas, potions and compresses. They also may be ground-up and prescribed in the form of powders, capsules, or tablets. Drinking a soothing cup of linden tea is a form of phytotherapy; so are compresses of chamomile for a burning eye, or gargles of a sage infusion for a sore throat and for gum problems.

Phytotherapy is probably as old as mankind itself. It is the oldest and most proven form of doctoring. The medicine traditions of many of the indigenous peoples are speaking for themselves. Some of these traditions have merit; others appear dubious or are outright harmful. In these latter cases the believer-patient mindset probably contributes to any possible healing effect—more than do the potions that are prescribed.

In Europe phytotherapy, or botanical or biological medicine as it is also called, has been popular since before the times of Paracelsus (1493-1541). European medical tradition is a strange mix of deeply rooted botanical knowledge that prompted the development of its many plant- and mineral-based approaches and of straight-out herbal pagan magic. This overlap, unfortunately, lead to the medieval witch hunts and caused the demise of many true and gifted healers. Many plant-based modalities found their roots in this European tradition; among them are homeopathy, homotoxicology, and many other lesser known healing forms using herbal remedies. Among these lesser known forms is *spagyrik*. It uses a very pure form of highly filtered plant mother tinctures and only minute amounts of alcohol.

Especially in the European Alpine realm, plant medicine is immensely popular. Still today, many of my study colleagues in Switzerland who now are practicing mainstream medical doctors use herbal medicine approaches before they resort to prescribing synthetic remedies. Let us not forget that modern pharmacology has started from botanical medicine. For example, aconite and digitalis are toxic plants. Yet, they were used in the production of some of the first effective prescription drugs for heart disease. Even today, in its search for new breakthroughs in medicine, the pharmaceutical industry is keen on getting its hands on previously unknown herbs and plants that have a longstanding tradition in indigenous cultures. This interest of the pharmaceutical industry helps in decoding the active constituents of these plants. Unfortunately, it also bears the danger of isolated ingredients being synthetically manufactured or being used out of context.

We know the problem with isolated herbal substances from traditional Chinese medicine where it has long been acknowledged that the action of one and the same plant part can be modified according to its pairing with other complementary or counteracting substances. This very basic knowledge is rarely incorporated in western pharmacology and, unfortunately, is frequently also neglected in the production of many natural supplements and vitamin compounds. Such indiscriminate combinations and extrusions may explain unexpected side-effects or a lack of efficacy of many products.

Plant-based remedies can be strong and, in the wrong application, potentially damaging. It, therefore, stands to reason that you use such approaches only under the strict guidance of a knowledgeable natural medicine professional and avoid self-administering of any plant remedies, supplements, vitamin compounds, and other nutrients.

Homeopathy

Out of the tradition of botanical medicine a branch of natural medicine was developed in the 18th century by Samuel Hahnemann (1755-1843) in the German Alpine realm. Unlike phytotherapy, which uses whole plant parts, homeopathy further processes the so-called mother tincture made from roots, leaves, flowers, or other specific plant or mineral parts. Homeopathy uses a process of ultimate dilution, called potentization, in conjunction with what it calls succussion, a low-amplitude, fast-impact shaking method. Depending on the degree of dilution or potentization few or no molecules of the initial substance are left in the resulting remedy.

It is this dilution process and the potential lack of actual molecules in its remedies that has drawn the greatest criticism from mainstream medicine. Strange then, that Swiss and German medical doctors still like to treat with homeopathic remedies before they will prescribe side-effect producing pharmaceutical drugs! Critics of homeopathy tend that there can be no effect on the organism if there is no actual molecule present. Yet, mainstream medicine for many decades quite successfully has been using a very similar approach to that of homeopathy with its technique of vaccines. Vaccines use minute amounts of live or dead pathogenic organism in order to activate your body's defense mechanism. The difference in approach here is minimal except that homeopathic remedies do not contain mercury and other harmful carriers. They also do no longer contain the actual molecules of potentially harmful bacteria or other components that might be able to cause side-effects and long-term negative consequences as do many of our vaccines. This is what renders homeopathic remedies so ultimately safe.

The following is how I like to explain to my patients how and why homeopathic remedies work in the body: A molecule consists of a chemical grid with its lock and key components attached to certain receptor sites. During the homeopathic dilution process of potentization the active substances are diluted out and the chemical grids remain behind. We reach this state whenever we dilute the mother tincture past 23 times ($x10^{23}$, called *Avogadro's number*). This chemical grid then, true to the Law of Similes—according to which "like heals alike" (*similia similibus curentur*)—offers open attachment sites to pathogens in your body. These resemble the original substance that the remedy was made of. In their rush to spread through your body the pathogens attach to anything that seems suitable and "alike." In fact, attaching to the "empty grid" of the homeopathic remedy may render them harmless. Your body's killer cells can attack them there, and the pathogens can be flushed out of your system.

In classical homeopathy we have available over four thousand remedies. More remedies are added every year as new plants and substances are discovered in previously inaccessible areas of the globe. Historically, case descriptions and other empirically gained data were used in order to assemble the healing profile of a particular homeopathic remedy. Today, many studies are performed on homeopathic remedies. Europe is leading in the production of these remedies and must follow strict government guidelines in their production. For this reason most credible research on homeopathic remedies also comes from Europe.

I find homeopathic remedies particularly effective in all cases where there exists a mental component to the disease or where there is any form of gastrointestinal malabsorption present. Since the homeopathic globules (tiny coated pills) are absorbed directly by the mucous tissue of your mouth they bypass your intestines and achieve a more direct effect. By using this approach your intestinal tract has a chance to heal before once again being asked to absorb any nutrient, mineral, or vitamin supplements given in liquid, pill, or capsule form.

Overall, homeopathy is a very safe approach to healing. Still, the wrong remedy at the wrong time can have quite an unpleasant outcome. As I have mentioned many times during the course of this book, it is very important that you work together with a healthcare professional who is properly trained and experienced in the use of the modality you intend to draw on; homeopathy, in this case.

Homotoxicology

At the beginning of the twentieth century the German medical doctor and homeopath Dr. Hans-Heinrich Reckeweg (1877-1944) developed a more integrated approach to homeopathy. He recognized that the industrial revolution not only brought with it an increasingly multifaceted lifestyle, but that diseases and illnesses too started to present a more complex picture. As a result, Dr. Reckeweg developed a concept that helped him formulate a line of compound homeopathic remedies that where built on the synergistic action between several remedies or potencies—much as we discussed this synergism in the context of the herbal remedies used in traditional Chinese medicine. Dr. Reckeweg called these new remedies "antihomotoxic remedies," using a Latin term that implies their ability to counteract toxins in man. He considered these remedies a bridge between homeopathy and western medicine because they allowed prescribing according to the disease patterns. This approach sufficiently differs from the time-honored, but narrowly defined approach of classical homeopathy that mostly treats according to the patient's constitutional patterns.

One of Dr. Reckeweg's greatest achievements is the formulation of his "Six-Phase Table." We briefly looked at it in the first chapter *Diabetes Avoidance is Key* (p. 19). His chart or table presents a medical classification of the progression and reversal of illnesses and conditions. Dr. Reckeweg, for the first time in the history of medicine, clearly formulated and described the pathways along which illnesses proceed or heal. The process, which he named Homotoxicosis, may be described as follows:

When a pathogen enters the body it causes a reflex reaction designed to expel it (diarrhea, vomiting, cough, tears, etc.). This is Phase 1; he called it the "Excretion Phase."

If your body fails to get rid of the offender in this initial phase the disturbance will move deeper into your system and cause an infection or inflammation in specific areas (any condition ending in -itis). He called this Phase 2, the "Inflammation Phase."

Suppose you suppress such an inflammation—as it is done routinely in mainstream allopathic medicine—the pathogen may become dormant. As a result, more chronic problems tend to follow at a later time. For now it remains hidden away in the interstitial fluid, the fluid surrounding all your cells. Dr. Reckeweg called this Phase 3, "Deposition Phase." We know that your lymph pathways and your interstitial fluid is where your T3 and T4 immune system cells are springing into action. As a result, your lymph, your body's cleaning pathways, go into overload.

Any disease and condition up to this third stage may be reversed quite easily. Dr. Reckeweg was clear to explain—in good homeopathic tradition—that, in order to find lasting healing, an illness needs to be guided back step by step in the reverse direction through all its stages. In other words: Once a pathogen has reached your cell fluid, the healing process may have to pass through another stage of inflammation (Phase 2) before the body has the opportunity to get rid of the pathogen (Phase 1). Homeopathy refers to such a possible initial deterioration as a "healing crises."

If a healing crisis should happen to you at any stage of taking homeopathic remedies consult your natural medicine provider for direction. Don't be surprised, though, if you make your practitioner smile and happy—never mind that you feel under the weather. Homeopathy usually considers a reaction as a positive sign indicating that this vicariation process (reversal of the disease) has been successfully initiated. Still, since this shows that you have entered a different phase of your disease your practitioner may decide to change the potency of your remedy or even the remedy itself. As I frequently pointed out, healing requires team work; team work between you and your body and team work between you and your trusted healthcare professional.

Let us continue with the next three phases of disease development according to Dr. Reckeweg's "Six-Phase Table." If a pathogen is not bound and repelled through any one of the first three stages it can find its way into your cells. Dr. Reckeweg called this Phase 4, the "Impregnation Phase." It is getting much harder now to find effective ways to get rid of the invader. Phase 4 is where glucose intolerance, malabsorption issues, autoimmune deficiencies, irritable bowel disease, ulcerative colitis, Crohn's disease, and many other—often hard to diagnose—conditions are categorized. All too often, these problems are not properly diagnosed because laboratory tests, commonly used by mainstream medicine, in this phase rarely are indicative or conclusive.

If the vicariation (reversal) process is unsuccessful at Phase 4, the pathogenic development will proceed to Phase 5, the "Degeneration Phase." The presence of the invader inside your cells starts interfering with your normal cell functions and processes. As a result, your health noticeably degenerates. Finally, at this stage, your laboratory tests start picking up that you have a problem. The diagnosis of diabetes too falls into this phase.

What happens next? If it has not done so earlier, natural medicine quickly jumps into action and attempts to pull your body back to Phase 4, then Phase 3, and onwards in the process of vicariation. Mainstream medicine, on the other hand, by using drugs in most cases suppresses the disease rather than helping your body, step by step to get back to its original function. With some luck those prescription medications may stabilize the disease at this level. But, remember, changes in your cells keep taking place. Therefore, it is likely that the disease process is starting to affect other organs and functions too, eyes, kidneys, heart. You get the picture; we call these the complications of diabetes.

If the disease factor is allowed to linger in this Phase 5, further deterioration is possible. This depends largely on the state of your immune system. There are two possible outcomes in what Dr. Reckeweg called Phase 6, the "Dedifferentiation Phase" or the "Neoplasm Phase." One, the damage in your cells continues to the point where the cell function impairs or shuts down one or several organs. Two, the pathogenic cells start taking over, develop a plan of their own, lead to cancer and—if not detected early enough—metastasize, that is, spread through your body to other structures.

This disease model of Dr. Reckeweg quite directly illustrates most of the issues that we face with today's healthcare system and its inability to recognize potential problems early and to prevent disease. If a patient has to reach Phase 5 before positive laboratory tests have the warning lights in our mainstream medical offices go on, no wonder that early diagnoses are rare and that the cost of healthcare is skyrocketing. Should it not be the other way around? Would you not expect that the more sophisticated modern medicine becomes the less the cost of healing disease, the earlier the detection of illnesses, and the more effective the treatment should be?

On the other hand, Dr. Reckeweg's understanding and method of homotoxicology as a system of the natural disease progression, along with our ability to coach the healing process back through all the stages of vicariation, may be the very explanation for many so-called unexplained remissions in a variety of diseases. By whatever approach—and, mostly by removing all their specific disease-causing factors—individuals who are able to get their disease to reverse have followed the path of reverse toxicosis. It can be done! This is healing, true healing. Conversely, prescription medications rarely heal. Granted, they may stop a disease; but that is our inability to reverse the disease process and to eliminate continued aggravation.

Stopping an illness is not equal to healing the patient from the disease. It is time for all of us to recognize this correlation. And, it is for precisely this reason that in my natural medicine practice and in my diabetes avoidance programs I base our approach towards control and possibly reversal of diabetes on a combination of biochemical knowledge and this system of homotoxicology.

Beginner's 6-Phase Table According to Dr. Reckeweg
Using Limited Examples of Illnesses

	Humoral Phases		Matrix Phases		Cellular Phases	
PHASES	Phase 1	Phase 2	Phase 3	Phase 4	Phase 5	Phase 6
			Deposition	Cell Impregnation	Cell Degeneration	Neoplasm Dedifferentiation
YOUR ORGANS & TISSUES	Electrolyte Imbalance	Acute Infections	Immune System Deficiencies	Chronic Illnesses	Immune Deficiencies	Cancers
	Diarrhea	Acute Pancreatitis		Chronic Pancreatitis		Organ Failure
	Bloating Indigestion	Lipid Metabolism Problems	Obesity	Metabolic Syndrome	DIABETES	Diabetes Complications
	Inter-Cellular	Inter-Cellular	Interstitial Fluid	Interstitial Fluid	Intra-Cellular	Intra-Cellular

BIOLOGICAL DIVIDE

Figure 20 Beginner's 6-Phase Table according to Dr. Reckeweg

Acupuncture and TCM

Acupuncture and traditional Chinese medicine have long promoted health and well-being. Diabetes was known already in ancient China. Many rather successful treatment modules for a variety of diabetes-related conditions have been handed down and, since, have been further refined. The TCM approach does not focus on your diabetes alone. It is geared towards eliminating the underlying causes that lead to your health problems and symptoms. In many cases such a root cause is identified as an imbalance between basic energy patterns or function disturbances. "Too much yin, not enough yang" or "mixed upper heat with lower cold" and so on, might be what your acupuncture practitioner mumbles to you. Don't let yourself get alienated by these seemingly outlandish and strange pictorial approaches.

While the language and approach to diagnosis seem to be so different from that of western medicine I have found that, in actual effect, most TCM expressions find parallels in our western medicine approach. Using the above examples we would probably use terms such as adrenal exhaustion, aldosterone imbalance, or we might look at hypoactive versus hyperactive thyroids. When we consider medical frameworks from cultures unfamiliar to us it is all about keeping an open mind and finding the parallels that validate them. Remember, we have one body with one functionality, no matter what name the different traditions and modalities call them by.

Acupuncture and Chinese herbal medicine approaches might be well worth your while to explore and are frequently offered by natural medicine practitioners. At best, they help you directly improve your condition; at worst, an acupuncture treatment can be relaxing and energizing. Keep in mind, though, that any particular healing modality is simply as good as the understanding, expertise, and experience of the person who practices it. This is particularly true in those areas of the globe where acupuncture and TCM are not yet regulated. Therefore, check out carefully what aspect of your health issue it is that a particular practitioner plans to work on with you and why. Checking references is not always good enough. You must feel comfortable too with any treatment you are subjecting yourself to. And, you do want to be able to communicate openly and clearly with the practitioner you trust with your illness and health.

Never forget, it is your body and you always have the right to speak up and make decisions; that goes for natural medicine as much as it holds true for mainstream, allopathic medicine. Be an informed patient and you will find in

Rivkah Roth DO DNM®

your medical professional a true doctor and healer. Your doctor will be even more willing and effective in working with you if you present yourself as an active participant and not simply as an enduring, passively accepting "patient."

Conclusion and Final Recommendations

⇨ Your body is one indivisible whole and you want to treat it as such.

⇨ Your risk of diabetes may not be like your friend's or neighbor's diabetes.

⇨ Rule out and preventatively treat underlying causes, imbalances, inflammations, and conditions.

⇨ Stick to a low-carbohydrate (possibly gluten-free), antioxidant-rich, and—most certainly if you are overweight—also low-calorie diet.

⇨ Avoid anything promoting an acidic pH that may lead to chronic metabolic acidosis (including grain carbohydrates, processed foods, soft drinks, fat, alcohol, or smoking and many of the prescription medications).

⇨ Follow a progressive and well planned, daily exercise regimen.

⇨ Avoid stress and other triggers, or effectively learn to deal with them.

⇨ Never forget that the path towards better health may mean teamwork.

⇨ Choose your support team wisely and share all your treatments and approaches with any of its members.

⇨ Develop a close partnership with a knowledgeable healthcare professional or a medical team that is prepared to treat *you*, their patient XY, and not simply one or the other of your diseases.

⇨ If there is a need for a specialist for the one or the other condition—should your internal workings have gone greatly out of balance—keep in mind the effect of such approaches on any of your other body systems.

⇨ Know that diabetes avoidance rests chiefly in your own hands. You pull the strings; even to the intensity with which your healthcare professional and medical team assist you in achieving your goals.

⇨ Always remain positive and proactive. The renewal of your cells is your opportunity to effect change and healing, increment by increment.

⇨ You can avoid the negative effects of diabetes and—to a greater or smaller degree—you can reverse your biological clock and return to better health!

⇨ There is no better day to start taking care of yourself than today.

⇨ Take responsibility for your own health, and surprise yourself with the "New You."

Bibliography

Books for Further Studies

Arem, R. *The Thyroid Solution.* New York, N.Y.: Ballantine Books, 1999.

Balch, J.F., and Balch, P. *Prescription for Nutritional Healing.* Garden City, N.Y.: Avery Publishing Group, 1993.

Balch, P.A. *Prescription for Herbal Healing.* New York, N.Y.: Avery, 2002.

A Barefoot Doctor's Manual. New York, N.Y.: Crown Publishers, 1985.

Beers, M.H. (ed.), et al. *The Merck Manual of Diagnosis and Therapy.* Whitehouse Station, N.J.: Merck & Co. Inc., 1999.

Bensky, D., et al. *Materia Medica.* Seattle, WA: Eastland Press, 1993.

Bensky, D., et al. *Chinese Herbal Medicine Formulas and Strategies.* Seattle, WA: Eastland Press, 1990.

Bernstein. R.K. *The Diabetes Diet.* New York, N.Y.: Little Brown and Company, 2005.

Bernstein, R.K. *Dr. Bernsteins Diabetic Solution.* New York, N.Y.: Little Brown and Company, 2007.

Beukes, V. *Killer Foods of the Twentieth Century.* Johannesburg, South Africa: Perskor, 1974.

Bianchi, I. *The Principles of Homotoxicology.* Baden-Baden, Germany: Aurelia Publishers Ltd., 1989.

Bianchi, I. *Homeopathic Homotoxicological Repertory.* Baden-Baden, Germany: Aurelia Publishers Ltd., 1995.

Bieler, H.M. *Food is Your Best Medicine.* London, U.K.: Neville Spearman, 1968.

Braly, J., and Hoggan, R., *Dangerous Grains: Why Gluten Cereal Grains may be Hazardous to your Health.* New York, N.Y.: Avery Publishing Group, 2002.

Brownstein, A. M.D., *Healing Back Pain Naturally.* New York, N.Y.: Pocket Books, 2001.

Budd, M.L. *Low Blood Sugar (Hypoglycemia): The 20th Century Epidemic?* Wellingborough, U.K.: Thorsons, 1984.

Rivkah Roth DO DNM®

Carroll, D. *The Complete Book of Natural Medicine.* New York, N.Y.: Summit Books, 1980.

Case S. *Gluten-Free Diet: A Comprehensive Resource Guide.* Regina, SK: Case Nutrition Consulting, 2001.

Cheng, X., and Deng, L. *Chinese Acupuncture and Moxibustion.* Beijing, China: Foreign Language Press, 1999.

Coulter, H.L. *Homeopathic Science and Modern Medicine: The Physics of Healing with Microdoses.* Berkely, CA.: North Atlantic Books, 1987.

Cousins, B. *Cooking Without: Recipes Free from Added Gluten, Sugar, Dairy Products, Yeast, Salt, and Saturated Fat.* Toronto, Canada: Harper Collins Canada, 2000.

D'Adamo, P.J.D., and Whitney, C. *Diabetes: Fight it with the Blood Type Diet.* New York, N.Y.: G.P. Putnam's Sons, 2004.

Deadman, P., et al *A Manual of Acupuncture.* Seattle, WA: Eastland Press, 1998.

DePalma, A. *Your Complete Guide to Vitamins and Supplements: The Natural Pharmacist.* USA: Prima Publishing, 1999.

Elliott, W.H., and Elliott, D.C. *Biochemistry and Molecular Biology.* New York, N.Y.: Oxford University Press, 1997.

Erasmus, U. *Fats that Heal, Fats that Kill.* Vancouver, Canada: Alive Books, 1996.

Ezrin, C. and Kowalsi,R.E. *The Type II Diabetes Diet Book.* Toronto, Canada: McGraw-Hill, 1999.

Flaws, B. *The Tao of Healthy Eating: Dietary Wisdom According to Chinese Medicine.* Bolder, CO.: Blue Poppy Press, 1998.

Gittleman, A.L. *Get the Sugar Out: 501 Simple Ways to Cut the Sugar out of Any Diet.* New York, N.Y.: Three Rivers Press, 1996.

Grant, A., DeHoog, S. *Nutritional Assessment and Support.* Seattle, WA: Grant/deHoog, 1991.

Green, P.H.R. *Celiac Disease: A Hidden Epidemic.* New York, NY: Harper Collins, 2006.

Grieve, M. *A Modern Herbal.* New York, N.Y.: Random House, 1973.

Griffith, H.W. *Complete Guide to Prescription and Nonprescription Drugs.* New York, N.Y.: Penguin, 2007.

Hammer, L.I. *Chinese Pulse Diagnosis.* Seattle, WA: Eastland Press, 2001.

Hart, C. *Secrets of Serotonin: The Natural Hormone that Curbs Food and Alcohol Cravings, Elevates your Mood, Reduces Pain, and Boosts Energy.* New York, N.Y.: St. Martin's Paperbacks, 1996.

Hay, L. *You Can Heal Your Life.* Carlsbad, C.A.: Hay House, 1987.

Heel *Biotherapeutic Index*. Baden-Baden, Germany: Biologische Heilmittel, 2000.

Heine, H. *Homotoxicology and Ground Regulation System (GRS)*. Baden-Baden, Germany: Aurelia Publishers Ltd., 2000.

Heller, R.F., and Heller, R.F. *Healthy for Life*. New York, N.Y.: Plume, 1996.

Holt, G.A. *Food and Drug Interactions*. Chicago, IL.: Precept Press, 1998.

Jayasuriya, A. *Clinical Homoeopathy*. Kalubowila, Sri Lanka: Chandrakanthi Press.

Jensen, B., and Andersen, M. *Empty Harvest*. Garden City Park, N.Y.: Avery Publishing Group, 1990.

Karp, R. *Cell and Molecular Biology: Concepts and Experiments*. New York, N.Y.: John Wiley & Sons, 1999.

Kellman, R., and Colman, C. *Gut Reactions*. New York, N.Y.: Broadway Books, 2002.

Kent, J.T. *Lectures on Homeopathic Philosophy*. Wellingborough, U.K.: Thorsons Publishers, 1984.

Kersschot, J. *Biopuncture and Antihomotoxic Medicine*. Aartselaar, Belgium: Inspiration, 1998.

Khalsa, D.S. *Food as Medicine: How to use Diet, Vitamins, Juices, and Herbs for a Healthier, Happier, and Longer Life*. New York, N.Y.: Atria Books, 2004.

Kirkman, M.F., and Cedgard, L. *The Digestive Contract - Intestinal Microbiology & Probiotics*. Kent, U.K.: Bio Pathica Ltd., 2002.

Kleiner, S.M., and Greenwood-Robinson, M. *High-Performance Nutrition*. New York, N.Y.: John Wiley & Sons, 1996.

Koeppen, B.M., and Stanton, B.A. *Renal Physiology*. Toronto, Canada: Mosby Year Book, 1992.

Laron, Z. *Journal of Pediatric Endocrinology & Metabolism, Vol. 12 - Suppl. 1*. Petah Tikvah, Israel: Freund, 1999.

Lemmer, B. *Chronopharmakologie, Tagesrhythmen und Arzneiwirkung*. Stuttgart, Germany: Wissenschaftliche Verlagsgesellschaft, 1984.

Lieberman, S. *Is Gluten Making Me Ill?* London, U.K.: Rodale, 2007.

Lieberman, S. *The Gluten Connection: How Gluten Sensitivity May Be Sabotaging Your Weight*. London, U.K.: Rodale, 2006.

Lowell, J.P. *The Gluten-Free Bible*. New York, N.Y.: Henry Holt, 2005.

Lu, H.C. *Chinese Natural Cures*. New York, N.Y.: Black Dog & Leventhal, 1994.

Lu, H.C. *Chinese System of Foods for Health & Healing*. New York, N.Y.: Sterling, 2000.

Rivkah Roth DO DNM®

Lu, H.C. *Chinese System of Food Cures Prevention & Remedies*. New York, N.Y.: Sterling, 1986.

Maciocia, G. *The Foundations of Chinese Medicine*. Oxord, U.K.: Churchill Livingstone, 1980.

McKenna, J. *Natural Alternatives to Antibiotics*. Garden City, N.Y.: Avery Publishing Group, 1998.

Mein, C. *Different Bodies, Different Diets*. New York, N.Y.: HarperCollins, 2001.

Millstone, E., and Abraham, J. *Additives*. London, U.K.: Penguin, 1988.

Mindell, E. *Earl Mindell's New Herb Bible*. New York, N.Y.: Fireside Press, 2000.

Mindell, E. *Earl Mindell's Diet Bible: Cut the Carbs and Lose the Fat*. Beverly, MA: Rockport, 2002.

Mitchell, D.R. *The Dell Natural Medicine Library: Natural Medicine for Diabetes*. New York, N.Y.: Dell Publishing, 1997.

Mowrey, D. *Next Generation Herbal Medicine*. New Canaan, C.T.: Keats Publishing, 1988.

Murray, M.T. *The Healing Power of Herbs*. Rocklin, CA.: Prima Publishing, 1992.

Murray, M.T. *Natural Alternatives to Over-the-Counter and Prescription Drugs*. New York, N.Y.: Morrow, 1994.

Murray, M.T. *Diabetes and Hypoglycemia: How You Can Benefit From Diet, Vitamins, Minerals, Herbs, Exercise and Other Natural Methods*. Rocklin, CA.: Prima Publishing, 1994.

Murray M, and Lyon, M. *How to Prevent and Treat Diabetes with Natural Medicine*. New York, N.Y.: Riverhead Books, 2004.

Ni, M. *The Yellow Emperor's Classic of Medicine*. Boston, MA: Shambala Publications, 1995.

Pauling, L. *How to Live Longer and Feel Better*. New York, N.Y.: W.H. Freeman, 1986.

Peters, A. *Conquering Diabetes*. New York, N.Y.: Penguin 2005.

Pizzorno, J.E., and Murray, M.T. *A Textbook of Natural Medicine*. Rocklin, CA.: Prima Publishing, 1988.

Poole, M.C., et al. *Biology in Action*. Toronto, Canada: Harcourt Brace Jovanovich, 1992.

Reckeweg, H.-H. *Materia Medica Homeopathica Antihomotoxica*. Baden-Baden, Germany: Aurelia Publishers Ltd., 2002.

Rice-Evans, C., and Packer, L. *Flavenoids for Health and Disease*. New York, N.Y.: Marcel Dekker, 1997.

Rohracher, H. and Inanaga, K. *Die Mikrovibration - Ihre biologische Funktion und ihre klinisch-diagnostische Bedeutung.* Bern, Schweiz: Hans Huber, 1969.

Schmid, F. *Biological Medicine - Scientific Position, Medication and Therapeutic Techniques.* Baden-Baden, Germany: Aurelia Publishers Ltd., 1991.

Sears, B., and Lawren, B. *Enter the Zone: A Dietary Road Map to Lose Weight Permanently.* New York, N.Y.: Regan Books, 1995.

Selections from Article Abstracts on Acupuncture and Moxibustion. Beijing, China: China Association, 1987.

Selya, H. *Einfuehrung in die Lehre vom Adaptionssyndrom.* Stuttgart, Germany: G. Thieme, 1952.

Semelka, R.C., et al. *MRI of the Abdomen and Pelvis.* Toronto, Canada: Wiley-Liss, 1997.

Smith, M.D. *Going Against the Grain: How Reducing and Avoiding Grains Can Revitalize Your Health.* Toronto, Canada: McGraw-Hill, 2002.

Steward, H.L., et al. *Sugar Busters! Cut Sugar to Trim Fat.* New York, N.Y.: Ballantine Books, 1998.

Surwit, R.S. *The Mind Body Diabetes Revolution: A Proven New Program for Better Blood Sugar Control.* New York, N.Y.: Free Press, 2004.

Thibodeau, G.A., and Patton, K.T., *Anatomy & Physiology.* St. Louis, MI.: Mosby, 1999.

Tierra, L. *The Herbs of Life: Health and Healing Using Western and Chinese Techniques.* Freedom, CA.: The Crossing Press, 1992.

Tierra, M. *Planetary Herbology.* Twin Lakes, WI.: Lotus Press, 1988.

Valdes-Dapena, A.M., and Stein, G.N. *Morphologic Pathology of the Alimentary Canal.* Toronto, Canada: W.B. Saunders, 1970.

Van Brandt, B. *Inflammation Means Healing.* Aartselaar, Belgium: Inspiration, 2002.

Vegotsky, K., et al. *The All-In-One Guide to™ Natural Remedies and Supplements.* Niagara Falls, N.Y.: Ages Publications, 2000.

Webb, M.A., Craze, R. *The Herb & Spice Companion.* London, U.K.: Quantum 2000.

Weiss, R.F. *Lehrbuch der Phytotherapie.* Stuttgart, Germany: Hippocrates Verlag, 1980.

Williams, R.J. *Nutrition Against Disease.* London, U.K.: Pitman, 1971.

Williams, T. *The Complete Illustrated Guide to Chinese Medicine.* Boston, MA: Element 1999

Yin, H., et al. *Fundamentals of Traditional Chinese Medicine.* Beijing, China: Foreign Language Press, 1995.

Zhen, Z. *Advanced Textbook on Traditional Chinese Medicine and Pharmacology.* Beijing, China: New World Press 2002.

Research Articles

Agren, M.S., et al. "Selenium, zinc, iron and copper levels in serum of patients with arterial and venous leg ulcers." *Acta Derm Venereol.* 1986;66:237-40.

Alexandraki, K.I., et al. "Cardiovascular risk factors in adult patients with multisystem Langerhans-cell histiocytosis: evidence of glucose metabolism abnormalities." *OJM.* 2008;101(1):31-40.

Ali, A., et al. "Diabetic muscle infarction associated with multiple autoimmune disorders, IgA deficiency and a catastrophically poor glycaemic control: a case report." *Diab Nutr Metab.* 2003;16(2):134-37.

Al-Mahroos, F., and Al-Roomi, K. "Diabetic neuropathy, foot ulceration, peripheral vascular disease and potential risk factors among patients with diabetes in Bahrain: a nationwide primary care diabetes clinic-based study." *Ann Saudi Med.* 2007;27(1):25-31.

Andersen, C.A., and Roukis, T.S. "The diabetic foot." *Surg Clin North Am.* 2007;87(5):1149-77.

Anderson, R.A., et al. "Chromium supplementation of human subjects: effects on glucose, insulin and lipid parameters." *Metabol.* 1983;32:894-99.

Anderson, R.A., et al. "Elevated intakes of supplemental chromium improve glucose and insulin variables in individuals with type 2 diabetes." *Diab.* 1997;46:1786-91.

Anderson, R.A., et al. "Supplemental-chromium effects on glucose, insulin, glucagon, and urinary chromium losses in subjects consuming controlled low-chromium diets." *Am J Clin Nut.* 1991;54:909-16.

Atkinson, M.A., and Eisenbarth, G.S. "Type 1 diabetes: new perspectives on disease pathogenesis and treatment." *Lancet.* 2001;358(9277):221-29.

Avery, R.A., et al. "Severe vitamin K deficiency induced by occult celiac disease." *Am J Hematol.* 1996; 53(1): 55.

Bakris, G.L. "Current perspectives on hypertension and metabolic syndrome." *J Manag Care Pharm.* 2007;13(5 Suppl):S3-5.

Balci, K., and Utku, U. "Carpal tunnel syndrome and metabolic syndrome." *Acta Neurol Scand.* 2007;116(2):113-17.

Banks, J., et al., "Disease and Disadvantage in the United States and England." *JAMA.* 2006;295:2037-45.

Baumgartner, B.G., et al. "Identification of a novel modulator of thyroid hormone receptor-mediated action." *PLoS ONE.* 2007;2(11):e1183.

Beckett, G.J., and Arthur, J.R. "Selenium and endocrine systems." *J Endocrinol.* 2005;184(3):455-65.

Bellentani, S., et al. "Behavior therapy for nonalcoholic fatty liver disease; the need for a multidisciplinary approach." *Hepatol.* 2008;472):746-54.

Bhandankar, R., et al. "Diabetic amyotrophy masquerading as quadriceps tendon rupture: a word of caution." *J R Coll Surg Edinb.* 2001;46(6):375-76.

Biro, L., et al. ["Hungarian national dietary survey, 2003-2004. Micronutrients: mineral salts."] *Orv Hetil.* 2007;148(15):703-8.

Bitar, M.S., et al. "Oxidative stress-mediated alterations in glucose dynamics in a genetic animal model of type II diabetes." *Life Sci.* 2005;77(20):2552-73.

Blostein-Fujii, A., et al. "Short-term zinc supplementation in women with non-insulin-dependent diabetes mellitus: Effects on plasma 5'-nucleotidase activities, insulin-like growth factor I concentrations, and lipoprotein oxidation rates in vitro." *Am J Clin Nutr.* 1997;66:639-42.

Boden, G. "Fatty acid-induced inflammation and insulin resistance in skeletal muscle and liver." *Curr Diab Rep.* 2006;6(3):177-81.

Boden, G., et al. "Effects of vanadyl sulfate on carbohydrate and lipid metabolism in patients with non-insulin-dependent diabetes mellitus." *Metabol.* 1996;45:1130-35.

Bogusz, M.J., et al. "How natural are 'natural herbal remedies'?" *Adverse Drug React Toxicol Rev.* 2002;21(4):219-29.

Boyko, E.J., et al. "Prediction of diabetic foot ulcer occurrence using commonly available clinical information: the Seattle Diabetic Foot Study." *Diab Care.* 2006;29(6):1202-07.

Bresnick, W., et al. "The effect of acute emotional stress on gastric acid secretion in normal subjects and duodenal ulcer patients." *J Clin Gastro.* 1993;17:117-22.

Brichard, S.M., and Henquin, J.C. "The role of vanadium in the management of diabetes." *Trends Pharmacol Sci.* 1995;16:265-70.

Brindley, D.N., and Rolland, R. "Possible connections between stress, diabetes, obesity, hypertension and altered lipoprotein metabolism that may result in atherosclerosis." *Clin Sci.* 1989;77(5):453-61.

Broadhurst, C.L., and Domenico, P. "Clinical studies on chromium picolinate supplementation in diabetes mellitus—a review." *Diab Technol Ther.* 2006;8(6):677-87.

Broderick, T.L., et al. "Effect of a novel molybdenum ascorbate complex on ex vivo myocardial performance in chemical diabetes mellitus." *Drugs R D.* 2006;7(2):119-25.

Brosnan, J.T. "Glutamate, at the interface between amino acid and carbohydrate metabolism." *J. Nutr.* 2000;130:988

Buchanan, T.A. "Glucose metabolism during pregnancy: normal physiology and implications for diabetes mellitus." *Isr J Med Sci.* 1991;27(8-9):432-441.

Campbell, W.W., and Anderson, R.A. "Effects of aerobic exercise and training on the trace minerals chromium, zinc and copper." *Sports Med.* 1987;4(1):9-18.

Cerda, C., et al. "Nonalcoholic fatty liver disease in women with polycystic ovary syndrome." *J Hepatol.* 2007;47(3):412-17.

Chan, K. "Some aspects of toxic contaminants in herbal medicines." *Chemosphere.* 2003;52(9):1361-71.

Chandrasekharan, B., and Srinivasan, S. "Diabetes and the enteric nervous system." *Neurogastroenterol Motil.* 2007;19(12):951-60.

Chen, H.S., et al. "Subclinical hypothyroidism is a risk factor for nephropathy and cardiovascular diseases in type 2 diabetic patients." *Diab Med.* 2007;24(12):1336-44.

Ch'ng, C.L., et al. "Celiac disease and autoimmune thyroid disease." *Clin Med Res.* 2007;5(3):184-92.

Cho, L.W., and Atkin, S.L. "Risico cardiovascolare nelle donne con sindrome dell'ovario policistico." *Min Endocrinol.* 2007;32(4):263-73.

Ciglar, L., et al. "Influence of diet on dental caries in diabetics." *Coll Antropol.* 2002;26(1):311-17.

Civitarese, A.E., et al. "Diet, energy metabolism and mitochondrial biogenesis." *Curr Opin Clin Nutr Metabol Care.* 2007;10(6):679-87.

Collin, P., et al. "Autoimmune thyroid disorders and coeliac disease." *Eur J Endocrinol.* 1994;130(2):137-40.

Collin, P., et al. "Endocrinological disorders and celiac disease." *Endocr Rev.* 2002;23(4):464-83.

Conway, G.S., et al. "Hyperinsulinemia in the polycystic ovary syndrome confirmed with a specific immunoradiometric assay for insulin." *Clin Endocrinol.* 1992;37(2):119-25.

Coulston, A.M., et al. "Deleterious metabolic effects of high-carbohydrate, sucrose-containing diets in patients with non-insulin-dependent diabetes mellitus." *Am J Med.* 1987;82:213-20.

Coulston, A.M., et al. "Plasma glucose, insulin and lipid responses to high-carbohydrate low-fat diets in normal humans." *Metab.* 1983;32(1):52-56.

Cousen, P., et al. "Tear production and corneal sensitivity in diabetes." *J Diab Complic.* 2007;21(6):371-73.

Cuajungco, M.P., et al. "Zinc metabolism in the brain: relevance to human neurodegenerative disorders." *Neurobiol Dis.* 1997;4:137-69.

Cuoco, L., et al. "Celiac disease and autoimmune endocrine disorders." *Dig Dis Sci.* 2000;45(7):1470-71.

Dahele, A., and Gosh, S. "Vitamin B12 deficiency in untreated celiac disease." *Am J. Gastroenterol.* 2001;96(3):745-50.

Daly, P.A., and Landsberg, L. "Hypertension in obesity and NIDDM. The role of insulin and sympathetic nervous system." *Diab Care.* 1991;14(3):240-48.

Davis, B.R., et al. "Lack of effectiveness of a low-sodium/high-potassium diet in reducing antihypertensive medication requirements in overweight persons with mild hypertension." *Am J Hypertens.* 1994;7:926-32.

De Berardis, G., et al. "Are type 2 diabetic patients offered adequate foot care? The role of physician and patient characteristics." *J Diab Complic.* 2005;19(6):319-27.

DeFronzo, R.A., and Ferrannini, E. "Insulin resistance. A multifactered syndrome responsible for NIDDM, obesity, hypertension, dyslipidemia, and atherosclerotic cardiovascular disease." *Diab Care.* 1991;14(3):173-94.

Del Prato, S. "Hyperinsulinemia. Causes and mechanisms." *Presse Med.* 1992;21(28):1312-17.

Delany, H., et al. "The interrelationship of the liver and the gut." *Nutr.* 1998;54-55.

Di Pietro, S., and Suraci, C. "Metabolic abnormalities in first-degree relatives of type 2 diabetics." *Boll Soc Ital Biol.* 1990;66(7):631-38.

Dietz, A.-R. "Possibilities for a lymph therapy with diabetic polyneuropathy. Matrix therapy with type II diabetes. - A practice-based study in engl. translation. *Biolog Medizin.* 2000 29(1):4-9.

Docherty, J.P., et al. "A double-blind, placebo-controlled, exploratory trial of chromium picolinate in atypical depression: effect on carbohydrate craving." *J Psych Pract.* 2005;11(5):302-14.

Doig, C.J. "Intestinal permeability defects linked to multiple organ dysfunction." *Am J Respir Crit Care Med.* 1998;158(2):444-51.

Duseja, A., et al. "The clinicopathological profile of Indian patients with nonalcoholic fatty liver disease (NAFLD) is different from that in the West." *Dig Dis Sci.* 2007;52(9):2368-74.

Eaton, S.B., et al. "Stone agers in the fast lane: chronic degenerative diseases in evolutionary perspective." *New Engl J Med.* 1988;84(4):739-49.

Eckhard, M., et al. "Fungal foot infections in patients with diabetes mellitus— results of two independent investigations." *Mycoses.* 2007;50(Suppl2):14-19.

Elghblawl, R. "Polycystic ovary syndrome and female reproduction." *Br J Nurs.* 2007;16(18):1118-21.

El-Sakka, A.I., et al. "Type 2 diabetes-associated androgen alteration in patients with erectile dysfunction." *Int J Androl.* 2007;Sep 18 [Epub ahead of print].

Emmelot-Vonk, M.H., et al. "Effect of testosterone supplementation on functional mobility, cognition, and other parameters in older men. A randomized controlled trial." *JAMA.* 2008;299(1):39-52.

Eric C Westman, E.C., et al. "Low-carbohydrate nutrition and metabolism." *Am J Clin Nutr.* 2007;86:276-84.

Fine, K.D., et al. "High prevalence of celiac sprue-like HLA-DQ genes and enteropathy in patients with the microscopic colitis syndrome." *Am J Gastroenterol.* 2000;95(8):1974-82.

Finsterer, J. "Recurrent pancreatitis as a manifestation of multisystem mitochondrial disorder." *Minerva Gastroenterol Dietol.* 2007;53(3):285-89.

Flora, S.J. "Role of free radicals and antioxidants in health and disease." *Cell Mol Biol.* 2007;53(1):1-2.

Frankenburg, F.R., and Zanarini, M.C. "Obesity and obesity-related illnesses in borderline patients." *J Personal Disord.* 2006;20(1):71-80.

Fraser, A., et al. "The associations between height components (leg and trunk length) and adult levels of liver enzymes." *J Epidemiol Conn Health.* 2008;62(1):48-53.

Freeland-Graves, J.H., "Manganese: An essential nutrient for humans." *Nutr Today.* 1989;23:10-13.

Frommer, D.J. "The healing of gastric ulcers by zinc sulphate." *Med J Aust.* 1975;2:793-96.

Fukudome, S., and Yoshikawa, M. "Opioid peptides derived from wheat gluten: Their isolation and characterization. *Febs Letts.* 1992;296(1):107-11.

Fukudome, S., et al. "Effect of gluten exorphins A5 and B5 on the post prandial plasma insulin level in conscious rats." *Life Science.* 1995;57(7):729-34.

Fukudome, S., et al. "Release of opioid peptides, gluten exorphins by the action of pancreatic elastase." *Febs Letts.* 1997;412:475-79.

Fung, T.T., et al. "A prospective study of overall diet quality and risk of type 2 diabetes in women." *Diab Care.* 2007;30:1753-57.

Futterweit, W. "Polycystic ovary syndrome: a common reproductive and metabolic disorder necessitating early recognition and treatment." *Prim Care.* 2007;34(4):761-89.

Gambarin-Gelwan, M., et al. "Prevalence of nonalcoholic fatty liver disease in women with polycystic ovary syndrome." *Clin Gastroenterol Hepatol.* 2007;5(4):496-501.

Garcia-Borreguero, D., et al. "Epidemiology of restless legs syndrome: the current status." *Sleep Med Rev.* 2006;10(3):153-67.

Gemignani, F., et al. "Restless legs syndrome in diabetic neuropathy: a frequent manifestation of small fiber neuropathy." *J Peripher Nerv Syst.* 2007;12(1):50-53.

Gholam, P.M., et al. "Nonalcoholic fatty liver disease in severely obese subjects." *Am J Gastroenterol.* 2007;102(2):399-408.

Gigli, G.L., et al. "Restless legs syndrome in end-stage renal disease." *Sleep Med.* 2004;5(3):309-15.

Giugliano, D., et al. "The effects of diet on inflammation: emphasis on the metabolic syndrome." *J Am Coll Cardiol.* 2006;48:677-85.

Glauser, S.R., et al. "Diabetic muscle infarction: a rare complication of advanced diabetes mellitus." *Emerg Radiol.* 2008;15(1):61-65.

Godbout, J.P., and Glaser, R. "Stress-induced immune dysregulation: implication for wound healing, infectious disease and cancer." *J Neuroim Pharmacol.* 2006;1(4):421-27.

Grigoriadis, E., et al "Skeletal muscle infarction in diabetes mellitus." *J Rheumatol.* 2000;27(4):1063-68.

Grimaldi, A., et al. "Intolerance to carbohydrates: the seven questions." *Rev Med Interne.* 1990;11(4):297-307.

Grimm, A., et al. "Progression and distribution of plantar pressure in Type 2 diabetic patients." *Diab Nutr Metab.* 2004;17(2):108-13.

Gruengreiff, K., and Rheinhold, D. "Liver cirrhosis and 'liver' diabetes mellitus are linked by zinc deficiency." *Med Hypotheses.* 2005;64(2):316-17.

Grundy, S.M. "Metabolic Syndrome Pandemic. *Arterioscler Thromb Vasc Biol.* 2008;28(4):629-36.

Gulliford, M.C., et al. "Risk of diabetes associated with prescribed glucocorticoids in a large population." *Diab Care.* 2006;29(12):2728-29.

Gulliford, M.C., et al. "Increased incidence of carpal tunnel syndrome up to 10 years before diagnosis of diabetes." *Diab Care.* 2006;29(8):1929-30.

Guzelmeric, K., et al. "Chronic inflammation and elevated homocysteine levels are associated with increased body mass index in women with polycystic ovary syndrome." *Gynecol Endocrinol.* 2007;23(9):505-10.

Halberstam, M. "Oral vanadyl sulfate improves insulin sensitivity in NIDDM but not in obese diabetic subjects." *Diab.* 1996;45:659-66.

Hanzl, G. "Die Regulation des Koerpers." *Aeztezeitschr Naturheilverf.* 1997;38:465-76.

Harder, B. "Bright lights, big cancer: Melatonin-depleted blood spurs tumor growth." *Science News.* 2006;169(1):8-10.

Harris, P., and Ferguson, L. "Dietary fibers may protect or enhance carcinogenesis." *Mutat Res.* 1999;443(1-2):95-110.

Henderson, D.C., et al., "Clozapine, diabetes mellitus, hyperlipidemia, and cardiovascular risks and mortality: results of a 10-year naturalistic study." *J Clin Psychiatry.* 2005;66(9):1116-21.

Hendry, J. "Mediterranean-style eating staves off CVD in diabetes." *Am Diab Assoc DOC News.* 2008;5(1):5.

Hodgson, J.M., et al. "Increased lean red meat intake does not elevate markers of oxidative stress and inflammation in humans." *J Nutr.* 2007;137:363-67.

Hoffman, H.N., et al. "Zinc-induced copper deficiency." *Gastroenterol.* 1988;94:508-12.

Horasanli, K., et al. "Do lifestyle changes work for improving erectile dysfunction?" *Asian J Androl.* 2008;10(1):28-35.

Horvath, K., and Mehta, D.I. "Celiac disease—a worldwide problem." *Ind J Pediatr.* 2000;67(10):757-63.

Hsu, S.P., et al. "Chronic green tea extract supplementation reduces hemodialysis-enhanced production of hydrogen peroxide and hypochlorous acid, atherosclerotic factors, and proinflammatory cytokines." *Am J Clin Nutr.* 2007;86:1539-47.

Hunter, J.O. "Food allergy or enterometabolic disorder?" *Lancet.* 1991;338:495-96.

Idiculla, J., et al. "Diabetic amyotrophy: a brief review." *Natl Med J India.* 2004;17(4):200-02.

Imada, M., et al. "Median-radial sensory nerve comparative studies in the detection of median neuropathy at the wrist in diabetic patients." *Clin Neurophysiol.* 2007;118(6):1405-09.

Jacob, S., et al. "Enhancement of glucose disposal in patients with type 2 diabetes by alpha lipoic acid." *Arzneimittelforsch.* 1995;45:872-74.

Jaeken, J., and Carchon, H. "The carbohydrate-deficient glycoprotein syndromes: an overview." *J Inher Metab Dis* 1993;16:813-20.

Jameson, S. "Coeliac disease, insulin-like growth factor, bone mineral density, and zinc." *Scand. J Gastroenterol.* 2000;35(8):894-6.

Jones, A.A., et el. "Copper supplementation of adult men: effects on blood copper enzyme activities and indicators of cardiovascular disease risk." *Metabolism.* 1997;46:1380-83.

Jones, O.A.H., et al. "Environmental pollution and diabetes: a neglected association." *Lancet.* 2008;371(9609):287-288.

Judd, A.M., et al. "Zinc, acutely, selectively and reversibly inhibits pituitary prolactin secretion." *Brain Res.* 1984;294:190-92.

Kahler, W., et al. "Diabetes mellitus—a free radical-associated disease: Results of adjuvant antioxidant supplementation." *Ges. Innere Med.* 1993;48:223-32.

Kapoor, D., et al. "Erectile dysfunction is associated with low bioactive testosterone levels and visceral adiposity in men with type 2 diabetes." *Int J Androl.* 2007;30(6):500-7.

Katchinski, B.D., et al. "Duodenal ulcer and refined carbohydrate intake: A case control study assessing dietary fiber and refined sugar intake." *Gut.* 1990;31:993-96.

Kaukinen, K., et al. "Celiac disease and autoimmune endocrinologic disorders." *Dig Dis Sci.* 1999;44(7):1428-33.

Kawagashira, Y., et al. "Intravenous immunoglobulin therapy markedly ameliorates muscle weakness and severe pain in proximal diabetic neuropathy." *J Neurol Neurosurg Psych.* 2007;78(8):899-901.

Kershaw, E.E., and Flier, J.S. "Adipose tissue as an endocrine organ." *J Clin Endocrinol Metab.* 2004;89(6):2548-56.

Koshihara, M., et al. "Reduction in dietary calcium/phosphorus ratio reduces bone mass and strength in ovariectomized rats enhancing bone turnover." *Biosci Biotechnol Biochem.* 2005;69(10):1970-73.

Koshihara, M., et al. "Effect of dietary calcium/phosphorus ratio on bone mineralization and intestinal calcium absorption in ovariectomized rats." *Biofactors.* 2004;22(1-4):39-42.

Kotronen, A., and Yki-Jaervinen, H. "Fatty liver: a novel component of the metabolic syndrome." *Arterioscler Thromb Vasc Biol.* 2008;28(1):27-28.

Krasinski, S.D., et al. "The prevalence of vitamin K deficiency in chronic gastrointestinal disorders." *Am J Clin Nutr.* 1985;41(3):639-43.

Krebs, M., and Roden, M. "Molecular mechanisms of lipid-induced insulin resistance in muscle, liver and vasculature." *Diab Obes Metab.* 2005;7(6):621-32.

Kumar, A., et al. "Sweeteners, Flavourings and Dyes in Antibiotic Preparations." *Paediatrics.* 1991;87(3):352-59.

Kurlan, R., et al. "Medication tolerance and augmentation in restless legs syndrome: the need for drug class rotation." *J Gen Intern Med.* 2006;21(12):C1-4.

Kushida, C., et al. "Burden of restless legs syndrome on health-related quality of life." *Qual Life Res.* 2007;16(4):617-24.

Lars Berglund, L., et al. "Comparison of monounsaturated fat with carbohydrates as a replacement for saturated fat in subjects with a high metabolic risk profile: studies in the fasting and postprandial states." *Am J Clin Nutr.* 2007;86:1611-20.

Ledoux, W.R., et al. "Relationship between foot type, foot deformity, and ulcer occurrence in the high-risk diabetic foot." *J Rehabil Res Dev.* 2005;42(5):665-72.

Lee, S., et al. "Evaluation of hallux alignment and functional outcome after isolated tibial sesamoidectomy." *Foot Ankle Int.* 2005;26(10):803-09.

Leslie,C.A.,et al. "Psychological insulin resistance: a missed diagnosis?" *Diab Spectr* 1994;7:52-57.

Lewy, A., et al. "Antidepressant and circadian phase-shifting effects of light." *Science.* 1987;235(4786):352-54.

Lipsky, B.A., et al. "Diagnosis and treatment of diabetic foot infections." *Clin Infect Dis.* 2004;39(7):885-910.

Lodyga-Chruscinska, E., et al. "Copper (II) complexes and opiate-like food peptides." *J Agric Food Chem.* 1998;46:115-18.

Lomax, A.E.,et al. "Effects of gastrointestinal inflammation on enteroendocrine cells and enteric neural reflex circuits." *Auton Neurosci.* 2006;126-127:250-57.

Lopez, M.C., et al. "Splenocyte subsets in normal and protein malnourished mice after long-term exposure to cocaine or morphine." *Life Science.* 1991;49(17):1253-62.

Loukas, S., et al. "Opioid activities and structures of a-casein-derived exorphins." *Biochem.* 1983;22:4567-73.

Lovell, M.A., et al. "Copper, iron and zinc in Alzheimer's disease senile plaques." *J Neurol Sci.* 1998;158:47-52.

Lucove, J., et al. "Metabolic syndrome and the development of CKD in American Indians: the Strong Heart Study." *Am J Kidney Dis.* 2008;51(1):21-28.

Lund, B.C., et al. "Clozapine use in patients with schizophrenia and the risk of diabetes, hyperlipidemia, and hypertension: a claims-based approach." *Arch Gen Psychiatry.* 2001;58(12):1172-76.

Luzi, L., et al. "Metabolic effects of restoring partial beta-cell function after islet allotransplantation in type 1 diabetic patients." *Diab.* 2001;50(2):277-82.

Magnotti, M., and Fotterweit, W. "Obesity and the polycystic ovary syndrome." *Med Clin North Am.* 2007;91(6):1151-68, ix-x.

Makepeace, A., et al. "Incidence and determinants of carpal tunnel decompression surgery in type 2 diabetes: The Freemantle Diabetes Study." *Diab Care.* 2008;31(3):498-500.

Malabu, U.H., et al. "Diabetic foot osteomyelitis; usefulness of erythrocyte sedimentation rate in its diagnosis." *West Afr J Med.* 2007;26(2):113-16.

Mallette, P., et al. "Muscle atrophy at diagnosis of carpal and cubital tunnel syndrome." *J Hand Surg.* 2007;32(6):855-58.

Marchesini, G., et al. "NAFLD treatment: cognitive-behavioral therapy has entered the arena." *J Hepatol.* 2005;43(6):926-28.

Marsh, M.N. "Gluten sensitivity and latency: Can patterns of intestinal antibody secretion define the great 'silent majority'?" *Gastroenterol.* 1993;104(5):1550-53.

Marsh, M.N. "Gluten, major histocompatibility complex, and the small intestine." *Gastroenterol.* 1992;102(1):330-54.

Marshall, T.G. "Vitamin D discovery outpaces FDA decision making." *Bioessays.* 2008;30(2):173-82.

Martelossi, S., et al. "Dental enamel defects and screening for celiac disease." *Acta Paediatr.* 1996;412(Suppl):47-48.

Melo, F.M. ["Association between serum markers for celiac and thyroid autoimmune diseases."] *Arq Bras Endocrinol Metabol.* 2005;49(4):542-47.

Merlino, G., et al. "Association of restless legs syndrome in type 2 diabetes: a case-control study." *Sleep Med.* 2007;30(7):866-71.

Merlino, G., et al. "Restless legs syndrome: diagnosis, epidemiology, classification and consequences." *Neurol Sci.* 2007;28(Suppl1):S37-46.

Millichap, J.J., et al. "Spinal cord infarction with multiple etiologic factors." *J Gen Intern Med.* 2007;22(1):151-54.

Rivkah Roth DO DNM*

Mina, A., et al. "Hemostatic dysfunction associated with endocrine disorders as a major risk factor and cause of human morbidity and mortality: a comprehensive meta-review." *Semin Thromb Hemost.* 2007;33(8):798-809.

Mitrou, P.N., et al. "Mediterranean dietary pattern and prediction of all-cause mortality in a US population." *Arch Intern Med.* 2007;167(22):2461-68.

Mooradian, A.D., and Morley, J.E. "Micronutrient status in diabetes mellitus." *Am J Clin Nutr.* 1987;45:977-95.

Morley, J., et al. "Effect of exorphins on gastrointestinal function, hormonal release and appetite." *Gastroenterol.* 1983;84(6):1517-23.

Morse, C.G., and Kovacs, J.A., "Metabolic and skeletal complications of HIV infection: The price of success." *JAMA.* 2006;296(7):844-54.

Mozaffarian, D., et al. "Incidence of new-onset diabetes and impaired fasting glucose in patients with recent myocardial infarction and the effect of clinical and lifestyle risk factors." *Lancet.* 2007;370(9588):667-75.

Mukherjee, B., et al. "Vanadium—an element of atypical biological significance." *Toxicol Lett.* 2004;150(2):135-43.

Musselman, B.C., et al. "Potassium-depletion paralysis associated with gluten-induced enteropathy." *Am J Dis Child.* 1968;116:414-17.

Musso, G., et al. "Nitrosative stress predicts the presence of nonalcoholic fatty liver at different stages of the development of insulin resistance and metabolic syndrome: possible role of vitamin A intake." *Am J Clin Nutr.* 2007;86(3):661-71.

Musso, G., et al. "Adipokines in NASH: postprandial lipid metabolism as a link between adiponectin and liver disease." *Hepatol.* 2005;42(5):1175-83.

Nagamatso, M., et al. "Lipoic acid improves nerve blood flow, reduces oxidative stress and improves distal nerve conduction in experimental diabetic neuropathy." *Diab Care.* 1995;18:1160-67.

Nieuwenhuijsen, M.J., et al. "Uptake of chlorination disinfection by-products; a review and a discussion of its implications for exposure assessment in epidemiological studies." *J Expo Anal Environ Epidemiol.* 2000;10(6Pt1):586-99.

Nihalani, N.D., et al., "Diabetic ketoacidosis among patients receiving clozapine: a case series and review of socio-demographic risk factors." *Ann Clin Psych.* 2007;19(2):105-12.

Nöthlings, U. et al. "Dietary glycemic load, added sugars, and carbohydrates as risk factors for pancreatic cancer: the Multiethnic Cohort Study." *Am J Clin Nutr.* 2007:86:1495-1501.

Novak, M., et al. "Diagnosis and management of sleep apnea syndrome and restless legs syndrome in dialysis patients." *Semin Dial.* 2006;19(3):210-16.

Nube, V.L., et al. "Biomechanical risk factors associated with neuropathic ulceration of the hallux in people with diabetes mellitus." *J Am Podiatr Med Assoc.* 2006;96(3):189-97.

Odetti, P., et al. "Oxidative stress in subjects affected by celiac disease." *Free Radical Res.* 1998;29(1):17-24.

Oerdoeg, T. "Interstitial cells of Cajal in diabetic gastroenteropathy." *Neurogastroenterol Motil.* 2008;20(1):8-18.

Oka, Y., et al. "Sevelamer hydrochloride exacerbates metabolic acidosis in hemodialysis patients, depending on dosage." *Ther Apher Dial.* 2007;11(2):107-13.

Olivieri, O.D., et al. "Selenium, zinc, and thyroid hormones in healthy subjects. Low T3/T4 ratio in the elderly is related to impaired selenium status. *Biol Trace Elem Res.* 1996;51:31-41.

Overlack, A., et al. "Potassium citrate versus potassium chloride in essential hypertension. Effects on hemodynamic, hormonal and metabolic parameters." *Dtsch Med Wochenschr.* 1995;120:631-35.

Palmer, G.W., and Greco, T.P. "Diabetic thigh muscle infarction in association with antiphospholipid antibodies." *Semin Arthritis Rheum.* 2001;30(4):272-80.

Pastore, M.R., et al. "Six months of gluten-free diet do not influence autoantibody titers, but improve insulin secretion I subjects at high risk for type 1 diabetes." *J Clin Endocrinol Metab.* 2003;88(1):162-65.

Pataky, Z., and Vischer, U. "Diabetic foot disease in the elderly." *Diab Metabol.* 2007;33Suppl1:S56-65.

Paudel, B. "Metabolic syndrome: are we at risk?" *Nepal Med Coll J.* 2007;9(3):204-11.

Pecqueur, C., et al. "Uncoupling protein-2 controls proliferation by promoting fatty acid oxidation and limiting glycolysis-derived pyruvate utilization." *FASEB J.* 2008;22:9-18.

Pi, J., et al. "Activation of Nrf2-mediated oxidative stress response in macrophages by hypochlorous acid." *Toxicol Appl Pharmacol.* 2008;226(3):236-43.

Piarulli, F., et al. "Mild peripheral neuropathy prevents both leg muscular ischaemia and activation of exercise-induced coagulation in type 2 diabetic patients with peripheral artery disease." *Diabet Med.* 2007;24(10):1099-104.

Rivkah Roth DO DNM®

Pozzilli, P. et al. "Double or hybrid diabetes associated with an increase in type 1 and type 2 diabetes in children and youths." *Pediatr Diab.* 2007;8(Suppl9):88-95.

Prasad, A.S. "Role of zinc in human health." *Contemp Nut.* 1991;16(5).

Quilliot, D., et al. "Diabetes mellitus worsens antioxidant status in patients with chronic pancreatitis." *Am J Clin Nutr.* 2005;81(5):1117-25.

Rader, D.J. "Effect of insulin resistance, dyslipidemia, and intra-abdominal adiposity on the development of cardiovascular disease and diabetes mellitus." *Am J Med.* 2007;120(3 Suppl1):S12-S18.

Randell, E.W., et al. "Relationship between serum magnesium values, lipids and anthropometric risk factors." *Atherosclerosis.* 2008;196(1):413-09.

Randi, G., et al. "Glycemic index, glycemic load and thyroid cancer risk." *Ann Oncol.* 2008;19(2):380-03.

Rauscher, A.M., et al. "Zinc metabolism in non-insulin-dependent diabetes mellitus." *J Trace Elem Med Biol.* 1997;11:65-70.

Ravina, A., et al. "Chromium in the treatment of clinical diabetes mellitus." *HaRefuah.* 1993;125:142-45.

Razavi, R., et al. "TRPV1+ sensory neurons control beta-cell stress and islet inflammation in autoimmune diabetes." *Cell.* 2006;127:1123-35.

Reiter, R., et al. "Free radical-mediated molecular damage. Mechanisms for the protective actions of melatonin in the central nervous system." *Ann N Y Acad Sci.* 2001;939:200-15.

Relea, P. "Zinc, biochemical markers of nutrition, and type-I osteoporosis." *Age Ageing.* 1995;24:3003-07.

Remillard, R.B.J., and Bunce, N.J. "Linking dioxins to diabetes: epidemiology and biologic plausibility." *Environ Health Perspect.* 2002;110:853-58.

Richardson, S.D., et al. "Occurrence, genotoxicity, and carcinogenicity of regulated and emerging disinfection by-products in drinking water: A review and roadmap for research." *Mutat Res.* 2007;636(1-3):178-242.

Roberts, E.A. "Pediatric nonalcoholic fatty liver disease (NAFLD): a "growing" problem?" *J Hepatol.* 2007;46(6):1133-42.

Rodriguez-Rodriguez, E., et al. ["Dietary habits and their relationship with the knowledge on the concept of a balanced diet in a group of young women with overweight/obesity."] *Nutr Hosp.* 2007;22(6):654-60.

Roussel, A.M., et al. "Food chromium content, dietary chromium intake and related biological variables in French free-living elderly." *Br J Nutr.* 2007;98(2):326-31.

Rozlog, L.A., et al. "Stress and immunity: implications for viral disease and wound healing."

J Periodontol. 1999;70(7):786-92.

Salley, K.E., et al. "Glucose intolerance in polycystic ovary syndrome. A Position Statement of the Androgen Excess Society." *J Clin Endocrinol Metab.* 2007;92(12):4546-56.

Sam, S., et al. "Evidence for pancreatic beta-cell dysfunction in brothers of women with polycystic ovary syndrome." *Metabolism.* 2008;57(1):84-9.

Sanchez, A. et al. "Role of Sugar in human neutrophilic phagocytosis." *Am J Clin Nutr* 1973;26:180.

Sanders, M.H., and Givelber, R. "Sleep disordered breathing may not be an independent risk factor for diabetes, but diabetes may contribute to the occurrence of periodic breathing in sleep." *Sleep Med.* 2003;4(4):349-50.

Sandstead, H.H. "Requirements and toxicity of essential trace elements, illustrated by zinc and copper." *Am J Clin Nutr.* 1995; 61(Suppl.):621S-24S.

Sargin, M., et al. "Association of nonalcoholic fatty liver disease with insulin resistance: is OGTT indicated in nonalcoholic fatty liver disease?" *J Clin Gastroenterol.* 2003;37(5):399-402.

Schmidt, L.E., et al. "Evaluation of nutrient intake in subjects with non-insulin-dependent diabetes mellitus." *J Am Diet Assoc.* 1994;94:773-74.

Schulze, M.B., et al. "Dietary pattern, inflammation and incidence of type 2 diabetes in women." *Am J Clin Nutr.* 2005;82(3):675-84.

Schusdziarra, V., et al. "Effect of beta-casomorphins on somatostatin release in dogs." *Endocrinol.* 1983;112:1948-51.

Schusdziarra, V., et al. "Evidence for an effect of exorphins on plasma insulin and glucagon levels in dogs." *Diab.* 1981;Apr.362-4.

Schusdziarra, V., et al. "Modulation of post-prandial insulin release by ingested opiate-like substances in dogs." *Diabetol.* 1983;24:113-6.

Schwegler, B., et al. "Unsuspected osteomyelitis is frequent in persistent diabetic foot ulcer and better diagnosed by MRI than by 18F-FDG PET or 99mTc-MOAB." *J Intern Med.* 2008;263(1):99-106.

Scott, H., and Brandtzaeg, P. "Pathogenesis of food protein intolerance." *Acta Paed Scand Suppl.* 1989;351:48-52.

Scott, K.C., and Turnlund, J.R. "A compartmental model of zinc metabolism in adult men used to study effects of three levels of dietary copper." *Am J Physiol.* 1994;267(1Pt.1):E165-73.

Selby, P.L., et al. "Bone loss in celiac disease is related to secondary hyperparathyroidism." *J Bone Miner Res.* 1999;14(4):652-57.

Shamberger, R.J. "The insulin-like effects of vanadium." *J Adv Med.* 1996;9:121-31.

Shechter, Y. "Insulin-mimetic effects of vanadate. Possible implications for future treatment of diabetes." *Diab.* 1990;39(1):1-5.

Sigal, R.J., et al. "Effects of aerobic training, resistance training, or both on glycemic control in type 2 diabetes." *Ann Intern Med.* 2007;147(6):357-69.

Singh, R., et al. "Lifetime risk of symptomatic carpal tunnel syndrome in type 1 diabetes." *Diabet Med.* 2005;22(5):625-30.

Sjoegren, A., et al. "Evaluation of zinc status in subjects with Crohn's disease." *J Am Coll Nutr.* 1988;7:57-60.

Smajlovic, D., et al. "Stroke in patients with diabetes mellitus: a hospital based study." *Med Arh.* 2006;60(6 Suppl2):63-65.

Smith, S.C. Jr. "Multiple risk factors for cardiovascular disease and diabetes mellitus." *Am J Med.* 2007;120(3 Suppl1):S3-S11.

Smotkin-Tangorra, M., et al. "Prevalence of vitamin D insufficiency in obese children and adolescents." *J Pediatr Endocrinol Metab.* 2007;20(7);817-23.

Soysal, N., et al. "Differential diagnosis of Charcot arthropathy and osteomyelitis." *Neura Endocrinol Lett.* 2007;28(5):556-59.

Spencer, H., et al. "Effect of calcium and phosphorus on zinc metabolism in man." *Am J Clin Nutr.* 1984;40:1213-18.

Spencer, H., et al. "Inhibitory effects of zinc on magnesium balance and magnesium absorption in man." *J Am Coll Nutr.* 1994;13(5):479-84.

Spickett, C.M. "Chlorinated lipids and fatty acids: an emerging role in pathology." *Pharmacol Ther.* 2007;115(3):400-9.

Spinler, S.A. "Challenges associated with metabolic syndrome." *Pharmacother.* 2006;26(12 Pt2):209S-17S.

Stankiewicz, M., and Norman, R. "Diagnosis and management of polycystic ovary syndrome: a practical guide." *Drugs.* 2006;66(7):903-12.

Stener-Victorin, E., et al. "Acupuncture in polycystic ovary syndrome: current experimental and clinical evidence." *J Neuroendocrinol.* 2008;20(3):290-08.

Stochmal A., et al. ["The influence of physical training on metabolic indices in men with myocardial infarction and impaired glucose tolerance."] *Przegl Lek.* 2007;64(6):410-15.

Stump, C.S., et al. "The metabolic syndrome: role of skeletal muscle metabolism." *Ann Med.* 2006;38(6):389-402.

Stupar, J., et al. "Longitudinal hair chromium profiles of elderly subjects with normal glucose tolerance and type 2 diabetes mellitus." *Metab.* 2007;56(1):94-104.

Stur, M., et al. "Oral zinc and the second eye in age-related macular degeneration." *Invest Ophthalmol Vis Sci.* 1993;37:1225-35.

Su, C.C., et al. "Association of nonalcoholic fatty liver disease with abnormal aminotransferase and postprandial hyperglycemia." *J Clin Gastroenterol.* 2006;40(6):551-54.

Suba, Z., and Ujpal, M. "Disorders of glucose metabolism and risk of oral cancer." *Fogorv Sz.* 2007;100(5):250-57/243-49.

Sun, P., et al. "Erectile Dysfunction—An observable marker of diabetes mellitus? A large national epidemiological study." *J Urol.* 2006;176:1081-85.

Szybinski, Z., and Szurkowska, M. ["Insulinemia—a marker of early diagnosis and control of efficacy of treatment of type II diabetes."] *Pol Arch Med Wewn.* 2001;106(3):793-800.

Tang Y.J., et al. "Serum testosterone levels and related metabolic factors in men over 70 years old." *J Endocrinol Invest.* 2007;30(6):451-58.

Thompson, A.M., et al. "Cardiorespiratory fitness as a predictor of cancer mortality among men with pre-diabetes and diabetes." *Diab Care.* 2008;31(4):764-09.

Tortosa, A., et al. "Mediterranean diet inversely associated with the incidence of metabolic syndrome: the SUN prospective cohort." *Diab Care.* 2007;30(11):2957-59.

Tosevski, D.L., Milovancevic, M.P. "Stressful life events and physical health." *Curr Opin Psychiatry.* 2006;19(2):184-89.

Trirogoff, M.L., et al. "Body mass index and fat mass are the primary correlates of insulin resistance in nondiabetic stage 3–4 chronic kidney disease patients." *Am J Clin Nutr.* 2007;86:1642-48.

Troncone, R., et al. "Gluten sensitivity in a subset of children with insulin dependent diabetes mellitus." *Am J Gastroenterol.* 2003;98(3):590-95.

Tronlone, R., at al. "Increased intestinal sugar permeability after challenge in children with cow's milk allergy or intolerance." *Allergy.* 1994;49:142-44.

Trujillo-Santos, A.J. "Diabetic muscle infarction an underdiagnosed complication of long-standing diabetes." *Diab Care.* 2003;26(1):211-15.

Rivkah Roth DO DNM®

Tsang, C.S., et al. "Phospholipase, proteinase and haemolytic activities of Candida albicans isolated from oral cavities of patients with type 2 diabetes mellitus." *J Med Microbiol.* 2007;56(Pt10):1393-98.

Tseng, C.H., et al. "Epidemiological evidence of diabetogenic effect of arsenic." *Toxicol Lett.* 2002;133:69-76.

Tuomi, T., "Type 1 and type 2 Diabetes: what do they have in common?" *Diab.* 54:S40-S45.

Uusitupa, M.I. "Chromium supplementation in impaired glucose tolerance of elderly: effects on blood glucose, plasma insulin, c-peptide and lipid levels." *Br J Nutr.* 1992;68(1):209-16.

Valko, M., et al. "Metals, toxicity and oxidative stress." *Curr Med Chem.* 2005;12(10):1161-208.

Valko, M., et al. "Free radicals, metals and antioxidants in oxidative stress-induced cancer." *Chem Biol Interact.* 2006;160(1):1-40.

Valko, M., et al. "Free radicals and antioxidants in normal physiological functions and human disease." *Int J Biochem Cell Biol.* 2007;39(1):44-84.

Van de Wal, Y., et al. "Effect of zinc therapy on natural killer cell activity in inflammatory bowel disease." *Aliment Pharmacol Ther.* 1993;7:281-86.

Varthakavi, P.K., et al. "A study of insulin resistance in subjects with acanthosis nigricans." *J Assoc Phys Ind.* 2001;49:705-12.

Varthakavi, P.K., et al. "Acanthosis nigricans: a dermatologic marker of metabolic disease." *Ind J Dermatol Venereol Leprol.* 2002;68(2):67-72.

Vinciguerra, G., et al. "Cramps and muscular pain: prevention with pycnogenol in normal subjects, venous patients, athletes, claudicants and in diabetic microangiopathy." *Angiol.* 2006;57(3):331-39.

Wada, Y., et al. "A case of diabetic amyotrophy with severe atrophy and weakness of shoulder girdle muscles showing good response to intravenous immune globulin." *Diab Res Clin Pract.* 2007;75(1):107-10.

Waltenberger, J. "Stress testing at the cellular and molecular level to unravel cellular dysfunction and growth factor signal transduction defects: what molecular cell biology can learn from cardiology." *Thromb Haemost.* 2007;98(5):975-79.

Waring, W.S., et al. "Glycolysis inhibitors negatively bias blood glucose measurements: potential impact on the reported prevalence of diabetes mellitus." *J Clin Pathol.* 2007;60(7):820-23.

Wei, M., et al. "The association between cardiorespiratory fitness and impaired fasting glucose and type 2 diabetes mellitus in men." *Ann Intern Med.* 1999;130(2):89-96.

Wei, Y., et al. "Skeletal muscle insulin resistance: role of inflammatory cytokines and reactive oxygen species." *Am J Physiol Regul Integr Comp Physiol.* 2008;294(3):R673-80.

Weiner, H.L., and Meyer, L.F. (eds.) "Oral tolerance: mechanisms and applications. *Acad Sci* 1996;778:1-451.

Whiteman, M., et al. "Do mitochondriotropic antioxiants prevent chlorinative stress-induced mitochondrial and cellular injury?" *Antioxid Redox Signal.* 2008;10(3):641-50.

Whiteman, M., et al. "The pro-inflammatory oxidant hypochlorous acid induces Bax-dependent mitochondrial permeabilisation and cell death through AIF-/EndoG-dependent pathways." *Cell Signal.* 2007;19(4):705-14.

Will, J.C., et al. "Does diabetes mellitus increase the requirement for vitamin C?" *Nutr Rev.* 1996;54:193-202.

Williams, M.J.A., et al. "Impaired endothelial function following a meal rich in used cooking fat." *J Am Coll Cardiol.* 1999;33(4):1050.

Wilson, B.E., et al. "Effects of chromium supplementation on fasting insulin levels and lipid parameters in healthy non-obese young subjects." *Diab Res Clin Pract.* 1995;28:179-84.

Winkelman, J.Q., et al. "Association of restless legs syndrome and cardiovascular disease in the Sleep Heart Health Study." *Neurol.* 2008;70(1):35-42.

Wood, W.A., et al. "Testing for loss of protective sensation in patients with foot ulceration: a cross-sectional study." *J Am Podiatr Med Assoc.* 2005;95(5):469-74.

Wright, D.C. "Mechanisms of calcium-induced mitochondrial biogenesis and GLUT4 synthesis." *Appl Physiol Nutr Metab.* 2007;32(5):840-45.

Yadrick,M.K., et al. "Iron, copper, and zinc status: response to supplementation with zinc or zinc and iron in adult females." *Am J Clin Nutr.* 1989;49:145-50.

Yaghmaie, F., et al. "Age-dependent loss of insulin-like growth factor-1 receptor immunoreactive cells in the supraoptic hypothalamus is reduced in calorically restricted mice." *Int J Dev Neurosci.* 2006;24(7):431-36.

Yamada, A., et al. "Assessment of the risk factors for colonic diverticular hemorrhage." *Dis Colon Rectum.* 2008;51(1):116-20.

Rivkah Roth DO DNM®

Yehuda, S., et al. "Fatty acid mixture counters stress changes in cortisol, cholesterol, and impaired learning." *Inter J Neurosci.* 2000;108:73-87.

Zalber-Sagi, S., et al. "NAFLD and hyperinsulinemia are major determinants of serum ferritin levels." *J Hepatol.* 2007;46(4):700-07.

Ziegler, D., et al. "Alpha-lipoic acid in the treatment of diabetic peripheral and cardiac autonomic neuropathy." *Diab.* 1997;46(Suppl2);62-66.

Index

A

absorption, 19, 249, 275, 320, 338
   lack of, 75, 104, 290, 298
   supplements, 268
acanthosis nigricans, 92, 94
   polycystic ovary syndrome and, 92
acid-base balance, 200, 208, 211, 254,
   264, 308, 312, 316
acidity, 21, 69, 104, 110, 153, 176, 206,
   262, 264, 267, 286, 301, 310, 349
   exercise and, 252
   from heated oils, 281
   gluten-sensitivity and. See gluten-
      sensitivity
   heart disease and, 223
   hydrochloric acid, 73, 75, 76, 327, 328
   hypertension and, 176
   mineral deficiencies. See mineral
      deficiencies
   oxidative stress. See oxidative stress
   proteins and, 283
   smoking and, 170
   warning signs, 207
acne, 92
   intestinal inflammation and, 121
addiction
   carbohydrates, 50, 99, 104, 252, 291,
      297
   food, 292
additives, 259, 261, 262, 264, 268, 274,
   283, 305, 328
   effect on zinc, 320
adrenal deficiency, 135, 137, 170, 183,
   184, 347
adrenals, 65, 313, 336

depression and, 141
hormones, 37, 85, 90, 197
nickel deficiency and, 327
obesity and, 99, 100
sodium balance and, 316
stress, 65, 105
tin and, 327
type 1 diabetes and, 37
alcohol, 170
   calories and carbs of, 276
   intestinal inflammation and, 121
   mineral absorption, 311, 320
   vitamin deficiencies, 76
allergies
   food, 261, 299
   molybdenum deficiency and, 325
amputations, 32, 155, 234
anemia, 326, 327
   fatigue, 137
   gluten-sensitivity and, 215
autoimmune deficiencies, 21, 36, 264

B

beer-belly, 40, 57, 58, 90, 98, 110, 174,
   223
bloating, 174, 217, 252, 267, 276, 281,
   296, 300, 307
   grain proteins and, 281
   gynecological issues, 90
   inflammation, 106
   mineral deficiencies, 328
   vagus nerve and, 232
blood sugar, 20, 35, 37, 276, 292, 313,
   324
   control, 20, 254, 321
   dawn phenomenon, 129

375

C

F

I

K

L

M

T

U

foaming, 82
frequent, 19, 81
increased amounts, 35, 81
urine tests. See laboratory tests

V

vegetables
nutrient deficiencies, 50
vision, 198, 236
blurred, 176, 237
changes, 167
retinopathy, 32, 236
vitamins, 38, 69, 146, 186, 249, 258, 259,
268, 269, 270, 272, 301, 338, 340, 342
calcium and, 269
combining, 271
deficiencies, 76, 145, 216, 218, 257
fats and, 286
food and, 299
for detox, 323
kidneys and, 226
minerals and, 23
one-a-day, 321
processing and, 280, 304
restless legs syndrome, 145
sodium and, 317
vitamin A, 188, 218, 286, 319, 321
vitamin B, 69, 145, 151, 201, 218,
308, 311, 317, 318, 321, 327
vitamin C, 23, 218, 321, 323, 327
vitamin D, 148, 218, 226, 257, 269,
286, 307, 308, 312, 318, 329

vitamin E, 190, 218, 286, 317
vitamin K, 218, 286, 307

W

water, 64, 186, 272, 300, 323, 329
chlorination, 61, 191, 304
chlorine, 263
contamination, 191, 258, 263, 270,
304
cramps and insufficient hydration, 148
hormones and medication residues in,
192
minerals in, 323
retention, 21, 90, 124, 129, 311, 316,
326, 328
water metabolism, 200
wheat
animal food and, 283
consequences of export, 27, 259, 298
consumption statistics, 219
destructive role of gluten, 103
wound
infections, 57
wound healing, 144, 151, 234
infections, 157
periodontal disease, 75
threat of amputation and, 234

Z

zinc. See minerals, zinc

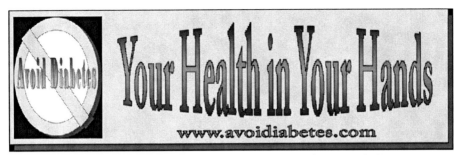

About the Author

Rivkah Roth DO DNM®

More people than ever go through life without recognizing that they are at risk of developing diabetes. In her passionate campaign for early diabetes risk recognition, her multidisciplinary training ideally benefits this author; and so do her multilingual background and the fact that over the years she has lived on several continents and amidst different cultures. Author, Rivkah Roth, is a natural medicine professional and lecturer with doctorates in osteopathy, natural medicine, acupuncture and traditional Chinese medicine.

She shows a keen interest in seeking connections between cause and effect. Asking new questions and questioning old answers is how she has been able to help many of her patients and students overcome their issues. Her out-of-the-box questioning mind gives her a fresh perspective on prevention. She fosters true cooperation between patient and doctor and puts an increased onus on the patient. Patients who recognize the connection between different symptoms and conditions are more aware of their own body and their own responsibility in their healing process—a necessary first step towards proactively avoiding diabetes.

Practicing transdisciplinary medicine offers the most viable and promising approach towards stemming the epidemics of chronic and metabolic diseases. Diabetes, along with other gastrointestinal conditions (such as irritable bowel disease, ulcerative colitis, Crohn's disease, celiac disease) and many painful conditions (among them fibromyalgia, rheumatoid arthritis, or chronic fatigue) all show a link to our food intake. Recognizing our body for the marvelous biochemical plant that it is, Rivkah Roth has spent years studying the biochemical and physiological processes that lead from food to health or from food to disease.

During her university years in Europe she actively participated in dozens of cooking competitions. Several big wins in national competitions and three years of placing among the top finalists at the Swiss Amateur Cooking Championships culminated in a 4th place in 1973 and a 3rd place finish from among over 2000 entries the following year. Shortly after that bronze medal win in 1974 an enterprising German publisher asked her to write two cook books in German language for Hoelker Publishing. Both books have become coveted gift items and, several editions later, may still be found in online stores. These books deal with the historical and local cuisine of two of her favorite areas of her native Switzerland—the culinary traditions of the city of Zurich and those of the rural areas surrounding Bern, the Swiss capital.

Over the years, Rivkah Roth has taught and practiced natural medicine in Canada, Europe, and the Middle East. She has won accolades for her dedication and contribution to the field of natural medicine including the title of "Doctor of the Year" awarded to her by a professional association in 2005. Apart from several further book projects that she has in the works she makes it her major objective to spread public awareness of how to avoid diabetes and many of its complications.

Aside from her recent book, *At Risk?—Avoid DIABETES by Recognizing Early Risk,* Rivkah Roth DO DNM® has published the *DIABETES-Series Little Books*, a series of 1-topic, point-form, easy to read titles. She also designed a quick *Early Diabetes Risk Recognition Questionnaire.* Her teaching includes web-based education and support programs for the general public. For licensed and accredited health professionals she offers specialized training programs for *Early Diabetes Risk Recognition Counselors, Natural Diabetes Avoidance Coaches,* and *Natural Medicine Diabetes Avoidance and Reversal Counselors.*

Rivkah Roth lives, writes, and practices on a quiet country property in Ontario, Canada, where she enjoys long walks with her dogs and dedicates much of her energy and focus on advocating for *Early Diabetes Risk Recognition and Avoidance.* For more information and to find out about the diabetes avoidance programs visit her online at www.avoidiabetes.com.

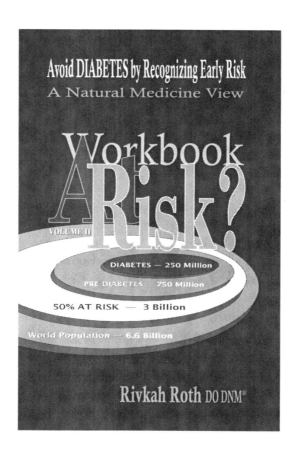

INFO

At Risk? Expanded Workbook
Avoid DIABETES by Recognizing Early Risk – A Natural Medicine View
(Separate, expanded Workbook and "FACT" Summary)
Softcover ISBN 978-1-981-2297-9-9

NATURAL MEDICINE CENTRE – PUBLISHING
Toronto

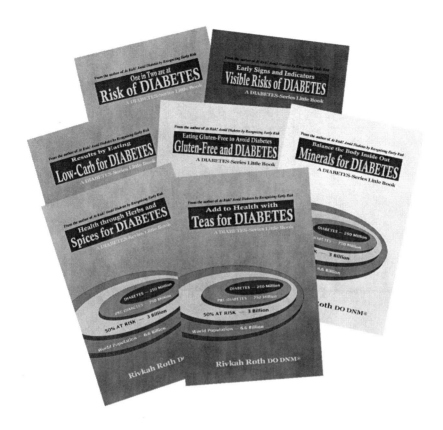

INFO DIABETES-Series Little Books

1-topic, point-form, easy to read, 48-page titles

By the author of "At Risk? Avoid Diabetes by Recognizing Early Risk -
A Natural Medicine View" and the DIABETES-Series Little Books

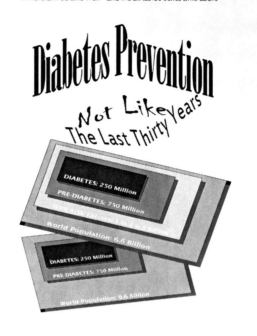

Rivkah Roth DO DNM®

INFO

Diabetes Prevention—Not Like The Last Thirty Years
Softcover ISBN 978-0-9812297-1-3
(also available as downloadable e-book)

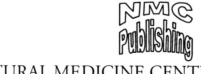

NATURAL MEDICINE CENTRE – PUBLISHING
Toronto

Ready to Check Your Risk?

Mini Risk Questionnaire

SECTION 1:

Do you have PARENTS or SIBLINGS diagnosed with

- ❑ Diabetes
- ❑ Heart Disease
- ❑ Celiac Disease
- ❑ Kidney Disease

SECTION 2:

Do YOU experience or have YOU been diagnosed with

- ❑ High Blood Pressure / Hypertension
- ❑ High Cholesterol / Triglycerides
- ❑ Overweight / Obese
- ❑ Intestinal bloating / Gas
- ❑ Irregular stools (diarrhea / loose stools / explosive stools / constipation)
- ❑ Frequent urination (every 1 or 2 hours)
- ❑ Ample and clear urine
- ❑ Burning tongue
- ❑ Frequent thirst
- ❑ Craving for ice / cold drinks
- ❑ Hunger / cravings
- ❑ Sleep disturbance
- ❑ Snoring / sleep apnea
- ❑ Men: ED—erectile dysfunction
- ❑ Women: polycystic ovary syndrome
- ❑ Women: heavy menses
- ❑ Fatigue / tiredness
- ❑ Carpal Tunnel Syndrome on both wrists
- ❑ Restless Legs Syndrome

Evaluation: If you have 3 checks in "Section 2," or 2 checks in "Section 2" plus 1 or more in "Section 1" you want to schedule an in-depth diabetes risk assessment.

Printed in the United States
150794LV00001B/18/P